The Student's Pocket Medical Lexicon

Giving the Correct

Pronunciation and Definition

of All Words and Terms in General Use in Medicine and the Collateral Sciences, the Pronunciation Being Plainly Represented in the American Phonetic Alphabet

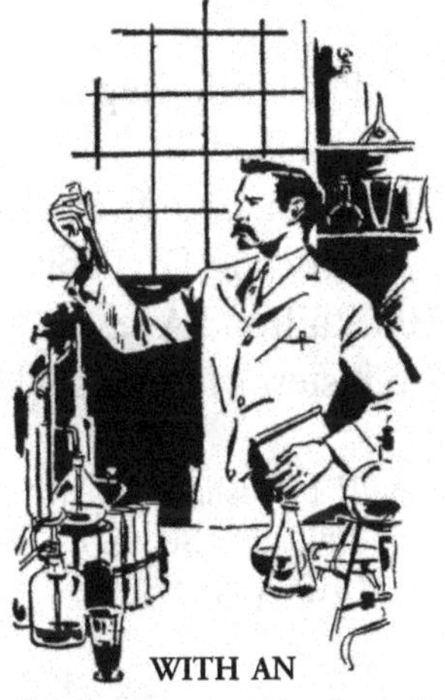

with an

Appendix, Containing a List of All Poisons and Their Antidotes, Abbreviations Used in Prescriptions, and a Metric Scale of Doses

by

Elias Longley

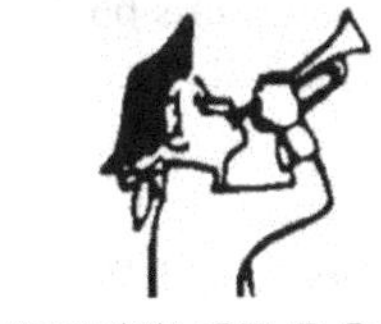

HERITAGE BOOKS
2011

HERITAGE BOOKS
AN IMPRINT OF HERITAGE BOOKS, INC.

Books, CDs, and more—Worldwide

For our listing of thousands of titles see our website
at
www.HeritageBooks.com

A Facsimile Reprint
Published 2011 by
HERITAGE BOOKS, INC.
Publishing Division
100 Railroad Ave. #104
Westminster, Maryland 21157

Originally published Philadelphia:
P. Blakiston, Son & Co.
1012 Walnut Street
1889

Entered according to Act of Congress, in the year 1879, by
Lindsay & Blakiston
In the office of the Librarian of Congress, at Washington, D.C.

— Publisher's Notice —
In reprints such as this, it is often not possible to remove blemishes from the original. We feel the contents of this book warrant its reissue despite these blemishes and hope you will agree and read it with pleasure.

International Standard Book Numbers
Paperbound: 978-0-7884-1545-6
Clothbound: 978-0-7884-8829-0

STUDENT'S

POCKET MEDICAL LEXICON;

GIVING THE CORRECT

PRONUNCIATION AND DEFINITION

OF ALL WORDS AND TERMS IN GENERAL USE IN MEDICINE AND THE COLLATERAL SCIENCES, THE PRONUNCIATION BEING PLAINLY REPRESENTED IN THE AMERICAN PHONETIC ALPHABET.

WITH AN APPENDIX,

CONTAINING A LIST OF POISONS AND THEIR ANTIDOTES, ABBREVIATIONS USED IN PRESCRIPTIONS, AND A METRIC SCALE OF DOSES.

BY

ELIAS LONGLEY,

Author of a "Pronouncing Vocabulary of Geographical and Personal Names," "Eclectic Manual of Phonography," and a Series of Phonetic School Books.

A NEW EDITION.

PHILADELPHIA:

P. BLAKISTON, SON & CO.,

1012 WALNUT STREET.

1889.

Entered according to Act of Congress, in the year 1879,
BY LINDSAY & BLAKISTON,
In the office of the Librarian of Congress, at
Washington, D. C.

PREFACE.

It has been nearly a quarter of a century since the author of this little volume assisted in the compilation of a similar work, that has had a more extensive sale than any other book of its kind. Since that time many and remarkable changes have taken place, in the sciences and arts as well as in the more transient affairs of men. And medical science, though generally in the keeping of conservative minds, has not been exempt from the mutations of time.

A well known medical author writes: "There exists a fashion in medicine, as in other affairs of life, regulated by the caprice and supported by the authority of a few leading practitioners, which has been frequently the occasion of dismissing from practice valuable medicines and of substituting others less certain in their effects and more questionable in their nature."

Even where there has been no change in the materia medica of the profession, there have been very many changes in its terminology. Botanical names have, within twenty-five years, been greatly modified and rendered more uniform in orthography and pronunciation; while the incessant experiments of the chemist in his laboratory have been constantly multiplying new articles, and taxing the ingenuity of lexicographers to give them names.

Thus it has come to pass that a new lexicon is needed, to enable students, and even old practitioners, to understand all they hear and read on professional subjects.

It is an unfortunate fact that a large proportio: those who study medicine have not been favored wi liberal education, and hence know very little in re; to the structure and pronunciation of the terms of m cal science. To enable such to overcome this defec their early studies, a special effort is made in the fol ing pages to supply the simplest and most effectual m for mastering the correct pronunciation of all the Gr Latin, and French words they may find it necessar use in their profession. By giving this feature of book the attention its importance demands, they save themselves the frequent mortification of being pected of ignorance, not only of the technicalities bu the essential facts of medical science. A little ca study of the Phonetic Alphabet, on page eight, in diately, or before beginning the use of the book, make it not only easy but a satisfaction to consul pages. There are but twenty new letters to be lear and as the old letters have the sounds they usually re sent in common print, the task is a light one. This m od of indicating pronunciation is much simpler, more easily remembered than the use of marked let as employed in the dictionaries.

This is the only medical lexicon in existence in w the pronunciation of words is fully and distinctly ma Two or three others mark the accent, and indicate tha of two or three vowel sounds may be used in those ac ed syllables, but this is a very uncertain guide to student. It is believed that the phonetic method, much as it notes distinctly every vowel and conso sound in a word, as well as accent, will be highly s factory, and make better readers and speakers on pr sional topics than have heretofore been known.

In regard to pronunciation, Dr. Thomas, in his preface, after referring to the fact that there are three systems of pronouncing the Latin and Latinized Greek terms used in the sciences, says: "Under the existing state of things, the editor has not felt justified in attempting to lay down *any positive rules* for the pronunciation of the vowels occurring in Latin terms. He has .... confined his labors ....to marking the accent and syllabication, and to indicating such vowel sounds ....as are essentially the same, whether they are pronounced according to the continental or the English mode."

The author of the present work, believing that to be a guide at all he should point in one direction or another, has adopted the English mode of pronunciation, that used at the University of Oxford in England and at Harvard in this country. It gives to the vowels, when accented, their long English sounds, thus; *mammalia*—mamália, (a as in fate, not as in far;) *foramen*—forámen, (not forámen;) *alveolar*—alvéolar, (e as in me not as in they;) *bronchitis*—bronkítis, (i as in find, not as in field.) The phonetic orthography thus secured more nearly resembles the common spelling, and the pronunciation thus indicated is more in harmony with the usage of the best speakers in this country, than if we were to adopt the continental usage.

If any one prefers the continental pronunciation, he has only to give to "a" the sound of "a" (ah), to "ē" the long sound of "a", and to *u* its long sound as in *true*. In regard to the other letters there is no difference in the two systems.

In the matter of definitions the author has sought as great brevity as accuracy and clearness of meaning would permit. The limited space in these pages, no less than the time of the student who consults them, rendered this advisable. No one would think of learning all he wants to know on any subject by simply turning to his dictionary. He refers to it, generally in haste, to satisfy his mind as to the general meaning or the pronunciation of a word; and when he wants to post himself fully on a subject he reads his text books at length and thoughtfully.

The larger works of Thomas and Dunglison are, of course, necessary in the physician's library, for the elaborate investigation of a topic — and the writer here cheerfully acknowledges his indebtedness to the former especially, for his clear and terse elucidation of the meaning of words, by explaining their etymology — but on account of their very copiousness they are unsuited for hasty and frequent reference.

The author takes great satisfaction in acknowledging his obligations to Prof. J. U. Lloyd, for his complete and critical revision of the chemical and pharmaceutical portion of the work in these pages; and also to his brother, Mr. Curtis G. Lloyd, for the exact orthography and careful descriptions of the botanical plants named herein. They are patient and critical students in the lines they have chosen, and will no doubt reach eminence and disdinguished usefulness in the not distant future.

Let the following fact be borne in mind, in the use of this Lexicon: In looking for the definition of a word, the description of a plant, mineral or part of the body, it will sometimes be necessary to turn to one or another of the synonyms given. Thus: "Deadly Nightshade, the common name for *Atropa Belladonna*," is desirable information; but, by turning to *Atropa Belladonna*, its use as a medicine will be found.

Explanation of the Phonetic Alphabet.

All who have thought of the matter are aware that there is very little analogy between the spelling of words and their pronunciation, especially in the English language; the result of which is, that no one can tell the spelling of an unfamiliar word from hearing it pronounced, nor pronounce such a word from seeing its spelling; hence the necessity for Pronouncing Dictionaries, and the almost ceaseless drilling of children in the difficult task of reading and spelling correctly.

This want of consistency between orthography and pronunciation is the result of using an imperfect alphabet, containing but twenty-six letters for the representation of forty-three elementary sounds. By the rejection of three redundant letters, (c, q, x,) and the addition of twenty new ones, and restricting the use of each of the forty-three to the representation of a single sound, a simple and philosophical orthography is established which makes spelling and pronunciation synonymous, and the art of reading very simple and easily acquired. (For information in regard to the use of this improved alphabet in teaching children and foreigners to read the common orthography, address the author, Cincinnati, O.)

The Alphabet thus perfected affords, of course, the simplest means of representing pronunciation, and it is now employed for that purpose by various publishers. The use of figures, or diacritical marks, to indicate the ever-varying sounds of the vowels, has always proved perplexing, and driven students from the critical study of pronunciation. By a little observation of the alphabet on the following page, learning the sounds of the letters from the key-words, the pronunciation of the most strange and difficult terms in the Lexicon is made as manifest and easy as the most simple.

American Phonetic Alphabet.

Each letter has the sound of the *italicised* letter or letters in the illustrative words.

VOWELS.

Letter.	*Sound.*		*Name.*
Ꭿ	ɋ	as in *a*rm	ɋ
Ɑ	ɑ	. . *a*sk	ɑ
Ą	ą	. . . *ai*r	ą
A	a	. . . *a*t	a
Ɐ	ɐ	. . . *a*le	ɐ
Ɛ	ɛ	. . *ear*n	ɛ
E	e	. . . *e*ll	e
Ɩ	ɩ̄	. . fi*e*ld	ɩ̄
I	i	. . . f*i*ll	i
Θ	ɵ	. . . . *o*r	ɵ
O	o	. . . *o*dd	o
Ꮻ	ω	. . *oa*k	ω
U	u	. . . *u*p	u
Ɯ	ɯ	. . tr*ue*	ɯ
Ɯ	ɰ	. . f*u*ll	ɰ

DIPHTHONGS.

Letter.	*Sound.*		*Name.*
Ɨ	ị	. . . *i*ce	ị
Ơ	ơ	. . . *oi*l	ơ
Ɣ	ɣ	. . . *ow*l	ɣ
Ɥ	ɥ	. . m*u*le	ɥ

SEMI-VOWELS.

Letter.	*Sound.*		*Name.*
Y	y	. . . *y*ea	yɐ
W	w	. . *w*ay	wɐ

BREATHING.

Letter.	*Sound.*		*Name.*
H	h	. . . *h*ay	hɐ

EXPLODENTS.

Letter.	*Sound.*		*Name.*
P	p	. . *p*ole	pɩ̄
B	b	. . *b*owl	bɩ̄
T	t	. . . *t*oe	tɩ̄
D	d	. . . *d*oe	dɩ̄
Ꞓ	ç	. . *ch*eer	çɐ
J	j	. . *j*eer	jɐ
K	k	. . *k*ing	kɐ
G	g	. . *g*ame	gɐ

CONTINUANTS.

Letter.	*Sound.*		*Name.*
F	f	. . . *f*ear	ef
V	v	. . *v*eer	vɩ̄
Ħ	ŧ	. . *th*igh	iŧ
Ƌ	đ	. . . *th*y	đɐ
S	s	. . *s*eal	es
Z	z	. . *z*eal	zɩ̄
Σ	ʃ	. . *sh*all	iʃ
Ʒ	ʒ	. vi*s*ion	ʒɐ

LIQUIDS.

Letter.	*Sound.*		*Name.*
R	r	. . *r*are	ur
L	l	. . . *l*ull	el

NASALS.

Letter.	*Sound.*		*Name.*
M	m	. . *m*aim	em
N	n	. . *n*one	en
Ŋ	ŋ	. . si*ng*	iŋ
	ṅ	(*Fr.*) nearly	ŋ

STUDENT'S

POCKET MEDICAL LEXICON.

A or An, a prefix, signifying *without;* as "acephalous," without a head;" achymosis," deficient in chyme.

Abactus Venter, Ab-ák-tus Vén-ter; abortion by art.

Abalienation, Ab-el-yen-á-ʃon; corporeal or mental decay.

Abarticulation, Ab-qr-tik-ɥ-lá-ʃon; (see *Diarthrosis;*) a joint admitting extensive motion.

Abbreviation, A-brī-vi-á-ʃon; part of a word written, or printed to represent the whole word. For medical abbreviations, see page 288.

Abdomen, Ab-dṓ-men: the larger cavity of the body; [the belly.

Abdominal Aorta, Ab-dóm-i-nal Ɐ-ór-tɑ; that part of the aorta below the diaphragm.

Abdominal Cavity, — Káv-i-ti; the cavity within the peritoneum, excluding th pelvic viscera.

Abdominal Ganglia, — Gáŋ-gli-ɑ; the semi-lunar ganglia of the abdomen.

Abdominal Pregnancy, — Prég-nan-si; pregnancy when the fœtus is above the uterus in the ovaduct.

Abdominal Regions, — Rí-jonz; divisions of the abdomen, as the epigastric, umbilical, hypogastric, hypochondriac, lumbar, and inguinal regions.

Abdominal Ring, — Riŋ; also called inguinal ring; the ring-like opening on each side of the abdomen, through which in males passes the spermatic cord.

Abdominoscopy, Ab-dom-in-ós-kɷ-pi; examination of the abdomen, by percussion, etc.

Abducent, Ab-dɥ́-sent; drawing from, as of muscles that draw limbs from the axis of the body.

Abductor, Ab-dúk-tor: applied to a muscle that draws from a part.

Abductor Oculi, — Ok'ɥ-lị; the muscle that draws the eyeball from the nose.

Abductor Labiorum, Ab-dúk-tor Lab-i-ó-rum; lifter of the angles of the mouth.
Abductor Indicis Manus, — In-dị-sis Má-nus; the muscle of the first finger.
Aberration, Ab-er-á-ʃon; disordered state of the mind, or other departure from nature. [evacuation.
Abevacuation, Ab-ē-vak-ɥ-á-ʃon; partial, or unnatural
Abies, Ab'i-ēz; a genus of evergreen trees, the source of the different turpentines. [tree.
Abietis Rezina, Ab-ị-e-tis Re-zị-nɑ; resin of the fir-
Abirritation, Ab-ir-i-tá-ʃon; lessened irritation.
Ablactation, Ab-lak-tá-ʃon; drying up of milk; weaning of a child.
Ablation, Ab-lá-ʃon; process of removing by excision.
Abnormal, Ab-nór-mɑl; not natural: irregular.
Aborticide, Ab-ór-ti-sịd; killing the unborn fœtus.
Abortion, Ab-ór-ʃon; premature birth; miscarriage.
Abortives, Ab-ór-tivz; medicines used to cause miscarriage. [of the blood vessels.
Abouchement, A-bɯʃ-mɑṅ; union of the extremities
Abrasion, Ab-rá-ʒon; rubbing or tearing off of skin or other membranous surface.
Abscess, Ab'ses; a cavity or tumor containing pus.
Absinthate, Ab-sín-ŧat; absinthic acid, combined with a base. [thium.
Absinthin, Ab-sín-ŧin; the bitter element of absin-
Abscission, Ab-sí-ʒon; the cutting away of a part.
Absinthium, Ab-sín-ŧi-um; wormwood. See *Artemisia Absinthium*.
Absorbents, Ab-sórb-ents; the lacteal and lymphatic vessels; in medicines, the calcareous earths.
Absorption, Ab-sórp-ʃon; the sucking up of substances, or taking in of liquids or vapors.
Abstergent, Ab-stér-jent; cleansing; purifying.
Abstraction, Ab-strák-ʃon; separating, as of a fluid from a salt. [ginous plant.
Abutilon, A-bɥ́-til-on; the yellow marrow, a mucila-
Acacia Catechu, A-ká-ʃi-ɑ Kát-ē-kɥ; an East Indian plant, the source of the astringent Gum Catechu.
Acacia Vera, — Vē-rɑ; a tree of Egypt which yields gum arabic.

Acajou, A-kä-ʃü; the cashew nut, containing a caustic liquor.

Acalypha Indica, Ak-a-lif-a In'di-ka; a plant of India, used in pulmonary diseases.

Acampsia, A-kámp-si-a; an inflexible state of a joint.

Acanthoid, A-kán-θoid; formed like a thorn, or spine.

Acanthulus, A-kán-θu-lus; an instrument for removing thorns, etc., from wounds.

Acarus, Ak'a-rus; an insect infesting the skin.

Acarus Scabiei, — Ska-bi-é-i; the itch insect;

Acatalepsy, A-kat-a-lép-si; uncertainty in the diagnosis of disease.

Accelerator Urinæ, Ak-sel-er-a-tor Yu-rí-nē; a muscle of the penis that propels the urine.

Acclimated, A-klí met-ed; accustomed to a climate.

Accouchement, A-kuʃ-mäṅ; delivery; child-birth.

Accoucheur, A-ku-ʃér; a male practitioner of midwifery; an obstetrician.

Accretion, A-kré-ʃon; increase; addition by growth.

Acephalobrachus, A-sef-a-lo-brák-us; a monster fœtus, without head or arms.

Acephalochirus, A-sef-a-lo-kí-rus; the same without head or hands.

Acephalus, A-séf-a-lus; without a head.

Acephalocyst, A-séf-a-lo-sist; the headless hydatid.

Acerate, As'er-at; aceric acid, combined with a base.

Acerbity, A-sér-bi-ti; sourness, with bitterness and astringency.

Acervulus, A-sér-vu-lus; sand-like particles found in the pineal gland.

Aceric Acid, A-sér-ik As'id; acid found in the maple.

Acetabulum, As-ē-táb-u-lum; the cavity receiving the head of the thigh bone, at the hip joint.

Acetates, As'ē-tats; salts and ethers of acetic acid.

Acetic Acid, A-sét-ic As'id; a volatile liquid of a punjent odor, obtained by fermentation or the destructive distillation of wood.

Acetica, A-sét-i-ka; preparations of vinegar.

Acetone, As'ē-ton; acetic acid diluted: pyro-acetic ether.

Acetum, A-sé-tum; vinegar; impure dilute acetic acid, prepared by fermentation. U. S. P.

Achillea, A-kil-ē-a; a native plant, used as a bitter tonic.

Achillis Tendo, A-kil-is Tén-dō; the strong tendon of the heel.

Achne, Ak'nē; a mucous-like flake on the cornea.

Acholous, Ak'ō-lus; deficient in bile.

Achromatopsia, Ak-rō-ma-tóp-si-a; deranged vision, with inability to distinguish colors.

Achylosis, Ak-i-lṓ-sis; defective formation of chyle.

Achymosis, Ak-i-mṓ-sis; defective formation of chyme.

Acicular, A-sík-ų-lar; needle-shaped.

Acids, As'idz; formerly defined as compounds which unite with alkalies to form salts; now called *salts of hydrogen*, in which the hydrogen may be replaced by a metal. When acted upon by metallic hydrates, water is always formed. Acids unite bodily with alkaloids, (organic bases,) without formation of water.

Acidifiable, A-sid-i-fį-a-bl; capable of being converted into acids.

Acidimeter, As-id-im-ē-ter; an instrument for measuring the acidity of liquids.

Acidulous, A-sid-ų-lus; slightly acid.

Acinesia, A-si-nē-si-a; rest, or loss of motion.

Acinus, As'i-nus; small granulations of the liver, etc.

Acme, Ak'mē; the height of a disease; the crisis.

Acne, Ak'nē; pimples, chiefly appearing on the face.

Acne Rosacea, — Rō-zá-ʃē-a; a carbuncled face.

Acology, A-kól-ō-ji; the science of remedies.

Aconitia, Ak-ō-niʃ-i-a; an alkaloid obtained from aco-

Aconitum Napellus, Ak-ō-nį-tum Na-pél-us; wolfsbane; monkshood; a poisonous plant of Europe, extensively used as a nervous sedative.

Acor, Ē'kor; acidity in the stomach.

Acoria, A-kṓ-ri-a; insatiable hunger.

Acorus Calamus, Ak'ō-rus Kál-a-mus; sweet-flag.

Acoumeter, A-kú-mē-ter; an instrument for measuring the degree of hearing.

Acouophonia, Ak-u-ō-fṓ-ni-a; the testing of the condition of the lungs and heart by percussion.

Acoustics, A-kōs-tiks; pertaining to sounds.

Acrania, A-krá-ni-a; without a cranium.

Acrimony Ak'ri-mō-ni; a pungent, corrosive quality.

Acrinia, A-krin-i-ɑ; suppression of the secretions.
Acrodynia, Ak-rɷ-din-i-ɑ; a painful rheumatic affection of the wrists and ankles.
Acromania, Ak-rɷ-mǽ-ni-ɑ; incurable madness.
Acromial, A-krɷ́-mi-al; belonging to the acromion.
Acromion, A-krɷ́-mi-on; the top of the shoulder-blade.
Acro-Narcotic, Ak'rɷ-Nɑr-kót-ik; a poison that is not only excessively stupefying, but that irritates the brain and spinal marrow.
Acrotism, Ak'rɷ-tizm; defective pulse. [plant.
Actæa Alba, Ak-tĭ-ɑ Al'bɑ; white cohosh, a native
Actual Cautery, Ak'tų-al Kó-ter-i; the application of red hot iron in the treatment of disease.
Acupression, Ak ų-pré-ʃon; preventing hemorrhage of wounds, by inserting a needle through the skin so as to press against the blood-vessel.
Acupuncture, A-kų-púŋk-tųr; an oriental method of bleeding, by plunging needles into the soft parts, now practiced in certain diseases.
Acus, Ɛ'kus; a surgeon's needle.
Adacria, A-dák-ri-ɑ; insufficiency of the lachrymal secretion. [the larynx.
Adam's Apple, Ad'am'z Ap'l; the thyroid cartilage of
Adansonia Digitata, Ad-an-sɷ́-ni-ɑ Dij-i-tǽ-tɑ; the baobab, an African tree, the bark of which is reputed antiperiodic.
Adder's Tongue, Ad'er'z Tuŋ; *Erythronium Americanum*, having emetic properties, but little used.
Additamentum, A-dit-a-mén-tum; superadded, as the prolongation of certain sutures of the skull.
Adductor, A-dúk-tor; the name of muscles which draw parts toward the axis of the body. [muscle of the eye.
Adducens Oculi, A-dų́-sens Ok'ų-lį; a straight internal
Aden, Ɛ'den; a gland; a bubo.
Adenalgia, Ad-en-ál-ji-ɑ; a pain in a gland.
Adenitis, Ad-en-į-tis; inflammation of a gland.
Adenology, Ad-en-ól-ɷ-ji; a description of the glands.
Adenomeningeal, A-dén-ɷ-men-in-jĭ-al; affecting the glands and mucous membrane.
Adenotomy, Ad-en-ót-ɷ-mi; dissection of the glands.
Adeps, Ad'eps; hog's lard, the prepared fat of the hog.

Adiantum Pedatum, Ad-i-án-tum Pē-dā́-tum; maiden-hair fern; a native fern, used as a pectoral.

Adiaphorous, Ad-i-áf-ω-rus; ineffective; neutral, as of salts.

Adiaphoresis, Ad-i-a-fω-rḗ-sis; deficient perspiration.

Adipose, Ad'i-pωs; fatty.

" **Arteries**; branches of arteries that supply the fat about the kidneys.

Adipsous, A-díp-sus; a medicine which relieves thirst.

Adjuvant, Ad'jų-vant; assisting other remedies.

Ad Lib.; Ad Líb-i-tum; at pleasure.

Admov.; (*admoveatur*) "let there be applied."

Adnata Tunica, Ad-nā́-ta Tų́-ni-ka; the external covering of the eye.

Adnate, Ad'nat; grown together.

Adolescence, Ad-ω-lés-ens; youth verging on maturity.

Adonis Vernalis, A-dώ-nis Ver-nā́-lis; a plant containing medicinal drastic properties.

Adonsonia Digitata, Ad-on-sώ-ni-a Dij-i-tā́-ta; the baobab tree.

Adragant, Ad'ra-gant; tragacanth; juice of the Ástragalus, that imparts a gummy substance to water.

Adventitious, Ad-ven-tí-ʃus: accidental.

Ædœitis, Ē-dē-ī-tis; inflammation of the genital parts.

Ægle Marmelos, Ē'gl Mą́r-mē-los; an East Indian tree, source of bael fruit.

Adynamic, A-din-ám-ik; relating to vital debility.

Aerate, Ē'er-at; to impregnate with air by mechanical pressure, as in the manufacture of mineral waters.

Aeriform, Ē'er-i-fərm; having the form of the air; gas.

Aerometer, Ē-er-óm-ē-ter; an instrument for measuring the bulk of gasses.

Æruginous, Ē-rū́-jin-us; resembling verdigris.

Ærugo, Ē-rū́-gω; copper; the rust of copper.

Æsculapius, Es-kų-lā́-pi-us; the god of medicine; name of an ancient physician.

Æsculin, Es'kų-lin; an alkaloid from the bark of the horse-chestnut.

Æsculus Glabra, Es'kų-lus Glā́-bra; the buckeye.

Æsculus Hippocastanum. Es'kų-lus Hip-ω-kás-ta-num; the horse-chestnut.

Æsthetica, Es-thét-i-ka; diseases or agents affecting the sensation.

Æstuarium, Es-tų-á-ri-um; a stove for applying dry heat to all parts of the body at once; a vapor bath.

Æther, Ĺ'ter; oxide of ethyl. (See *Ether*.)

Ætherea, Ĺ-tĥ-rĕ-a; a general term for preparations of ether.

Æthiops Martis, Ĺ'thi-ops Mąr-tis; black scales, struck from red hot iron, by the blacksmith's hammer.

Æthiops Mineral, sulphide of mercury.

Æthusa Cynapium, Ĺ-thų-sa Sin-á-pi-um; garden hemlock, or "fool's parsley."

Ætiology, Ĺ-ti-ól-ω-ji; science of the causes of disease.

Afferens, Af'er-ens; name of lymphatics that convey lymph to the glands.

Afflatus, A-flá-tus; applied to erysipelas that looks as if it had been blown upon by a destructive blast.

Affinity Chemical; the power or force which unites different kinds of matter, and forms a new substance or substances.

Affluxus, A-flúk-sus; the act of flowing to.

Affluxion, A-flúk-ʃon; accumulation of fluids.

After-Birth; the placenta, cord, and membranes following delivery.

After-Pains; pains occurring after delivery.

Affusion, A-fų-ʒon; the pouring of water upon patients, as a bath, in fevers.

Agaric; A-gár-ik; a fungus; the *Boletus laricis* is the purging agaric of medical writers.

Agaricus Quercus, A-gár-i-kus Kwér-kus; a fungus of the oak, used for arresting external hemorrhage.

Agave Americana; A-gá-vĕ; American aloe.

Agave Virginiana; false aloe, used in colic.

Agenesia, A-jen-ĕ-si-a; impotence; sterility.

Agenesis, A-jen-ĕ-sis; imperfect development of any part of the body.

Agglutinate, A-glų-tin-at; to unite; to stick together.

Aglutition, Ag-lų-tí-ʃon; impossibility of swallowing.

Agnus Castus; the chaste tree, formerly noted as an antiphrodisiac.

Agonia, A-gó-ni-a; sterility; barrenness.

Agonida Lancifolia, A-gω-nį-da Lan-si-fó-li-a; a tree containing agoniadin: anti-intermittent.

Agria, Ag'ri-ɑ; an intractible pustular eruption.
Agrimony, Ag'ri-mɷ-ni; a native plant an astringent.
Agriothymia, Ag-ri-ɷ-ŧím-i-ɑ; wild or furious insanity.
Agrippa, A-gríp-ɑ; birth of a child with the feet foremost.
Ague, Ē'gų; the cold stage of an intermittent fever.
Ague-Cake; enlarged spleen, after intermittents.
Ague-Drops, Ē'gų-Drops; Fowler's Solution; arsenite of potassium.
Ailanthus Glandulosa, Ī-lán-ŧus Glan-dų-lɷ́-sɑ; tree of heaven, native of China and Japan, the bark of which is an anthelmintic.
Ajuga Chamæpitys; A-jų́-gɑ Kam-ḗ-pi-tis; ground pine, a low creeping plant.
Ala, Ē'lɑ, (*pl.* Alæ, Ē'lē); a wing, in anatomy applied to parts having some resemblance to wings.
Alantol, A-lán-tɷl; an aromatic liquid, with odor of peppermint, obtained from Inula camphor.
Alares Venæ, A-lá-rēz Vén-ē; superficial veins where the arm bends.
Alaris, A-lá-ris; wing-shaped.
Albino, Al-bį-nɷ; a person whose skin, hair, and iris are white, the pigmentum nigrum being absent.
Albuginea Oculi, Al-bų-jín-ē-ɑ Ok'ų-lį; tunic of the eye, under the conjunctiva.
Albuginea Testis, —Tés-tis; internal coat of the testicle.
Albugineous, Al-bų-jín-ē-us; a term applied to textures humors, &c., which are perfectly white.
Albuginitis, Al-bų-jin-į-tis; inflammation of the albugineous tissues.
Albugo, Al-bų́-gɷ; the white of the eye; the white of an egg.
Albumen, Al-bų́-men; a substance found in animals and vegetables, and which constitutes the chief part of the white of eggs.
Albuminous principles; the albuminoid group, the varieties of which are albumen, fibrin and casein.
Albuminuria, Al-bų-mi-nų́-ri-ɑ; urine containing albumen.
Alcarnoque, Al'kɑr-nók; bark of a West Indies plant, bitter and tonic, used in phthisic.

Alchemy, Al'kem-i; a supposed science, cultivated by the ancients, for the purpose of finding out how to turn all the baser metals into gold, and to find a remedy for all diseases.

Alcohol, Al'kω-hol; the product of vinous fermentation of saccharine matter.

Alcoholates, Al'kω-hol-ats; medicated alcohol.

Alcohometer, Al-kω-hóm-ē-ter; an instrument to determine the proportion of spirit in any vinous liquid.

Aldehyde, Al'dē-hīd; alcohol deprived of one or more molecules of hydrogen,

Alder, Al'der; *Alnus serrulata*; tag alder.

Alembic; a chemical utensil used in distillation.

Alembroth, A-lém-broth; a compound of bichloride of mercury and sal ammoniac.

Aletrin, Al'e-trin; a precipitated alcoholic extract of *Aletris Farinosa*.

Aletris Farinosa, Al'e-tris Far-i-nó-sa; star grass, an intensely bitter tonic.

Alexipharmic, A-leks-i-fár-mik; an antidote to poison.

Alexipyretic, A-leks-i-pi-rét-ik; warding off fevers; a febrifuge. [madder.

Algarin; Al'ga-rin; the principal coloring matter of

Algæ, Al'gē; sea weeds. [der.

Algaroth, Al'ga-roth; oxide of antimony, in white pow-

Algedo, Al-jē-dω; violent pain in the urethra, bladder, testes, &c., caused by the too sudden suppression of gonorrhea. [small-pox.

Alices, Al'i-sēz; spots that precede the eruption in

Aliform, Al'i-form; wing-like.

Aliment; any kind of food; nourishment.

Alimentary Canal; the entire passage through which the food passes from the mouth to the anus.

Alisma Plantago, A-lís-ma Plan-tá-gω; water plantain.

Alisphenoid, Al-i-sfē-noid; middle or great wing of the sphenoid bone.

Alkalescent, Al-ka-lés-ent; slightly alkaline.

Alkali, Al'ka-lī; a substance which neutralizes acids, as potassa, soda, etc.; and change vegetable blues to green.

Alkalimeter, Al-ka-lím-ē-ter; an instrument for ascertaining the proportion of alkali in any substance.

Alkaline, Al'ka-lin; having the properties of alkalies.
Alkaloids; organic substances possessing alkaline properties, capable of combining with acids to form salts.
Alkanet, Al'ka-net; the root of *Anchusa tinctora*.
Alkekenge, Al'kē-kenj; the winter cherry, used in nephritis, dysuria, etc.
Allantois, A-lán-tō-is; the name applied to a certain membrane in the fœtus.
Alliaceous, Al-i-á-ʃus; similar to garlic.
Allium Sativum, Al'i-um Sa-tį-vum; the plant garlic.
Allium Cepa, Al'i-um Sé-pa; the onion.
Alloys, Al'oz; compounds obtained by fusing metals together.
Allopathy, A-lóp-a-ti; the system of curing by opposites, "*contraria contrariis curantur.*"
Allotropism, A-lót-rō-pizm; the existence of an element in two conditions.
Alloxan, A-lóks-an; the product of the oxidation of uric acid by nitric acid.
Alloxantin, Al-oks-án-tin; substance resulting from the evaporation of a solution of alloxan.
Allspice; berries of the *Eugenia pimenta*.
Almond, fruit of the *Amygdalus communis*.
Alnus Glutinosa, Al'nus Glų-tin-ó-sa; a European tree, the leaves and bark of which are bitter and astringent.
Alnus Serrulata, — Ser-ų-lá-ta; the tag alder, having the same qualities as the last mamed.
Aloes, Al'ōz; the inspissated juice of the aloe.
Aloe Socotrina, A-ló-e Sok-ō-trį-na; the aloe of Socotra, furnishing Socotrine aloes.
Aloe Spicata, — Spi-ká-ta; spiked aloe, furnishing Cape aloes.
Aloe Vulgaris, — Vul-gá-ris; the aloe yielding Barbadoes aloe.
Aloin, Al'ō-in; the crystaline principle of aloes, said to be its cathartic constituent.
Alpinia Cardamomum, Al-pín-i-a Kąr-da-mó-mum; a plant producing cardamon seed.
Alphonsin, Al-fón-sin; an instrument for taking balls out of wounds.
Alteratives; medicines intended to change the morbid action, by restoring the healthy functions of the system gradually.

Alternis Horis, Al-tẽr-nis Hṓ-ris; every alternate hour.

Althæa Officinalis, Al-thē-a Of-is-i-nā́-lis; the marsh mallow.

Althæa Rosea,— Rō-sḗ-a; the hollyhock.

Althein, Al-thḗ-in; the alkaline substance in the marsh mallow.

Alum, Al'um; a double sulphate of aluminum and am- [monium.

Alumen, A-lū́-men; a salt composed of sulphuric acid and alumina, with potassa or ammonia, or both.

Alumina, A-lū́-min-a; oxide of aluminum.

Aluminates, A-lū́-min-ats; compounds formed by the combination of aluminic hydrates and basic radicals.

Aluminum, A-lū́-min-um; the metallic base of alumina.

Alum Root; *Heuchera Americana.*

Alusia, A-lū́-si-a; illusion; low spirits.

Alvearium, Al-vē-ā́-ri-um; the external opening of the [ear.

Alveolar, Al-vḗ-o-lar; belonging to the alveoli, or bony sockets of the teeth.

Alveolar Structure, small superficial cavities in the mucous membrane of the stomach and minor intestines.

Alveolus, Al-vḗ-o-lus; the bony socket of a tooth.

Alveus, Al'vē-us; a hollow; enlarged part of a canal or channel.

Alvine, Al'vin; relating to the intestines.

Amadou, A-mā́-dū; a substance used to support varicose veins, protect injured surfaces, etc.

Amalgam, A-mál-gam; mercury alloyed with another metal.

Amara, A-mā́-ra; bitter; sometimes used as a specific name for plants.

Amarin, Am'a-rin; the bitter quality of vegetables.

Amarus, A-mā́-rus; bitter; medicine with bitter flavor.

Amaurosis, Am-e-rṓ-sis; paralysis of the optic nerve; loss of vision.

Amber, Am'ber; a fosil resin from an extinct plant.

Amblosis, Am-blṓ-sis; abortion; miscarriage.

Amblyopia, Am-bli-ṓ-pi-a; impaired eye-sight, from loss of sensibility of the retina.

Ambrein Am-brḗ-in; a fatty matter constituting the base of ambergris.

Ambrosia, Am-brṓ-zi-a; "food of the gods;" applied to certain alexipharmic medicines.

Ambrosia Artemisiæfolia, Am-brō-ʒi-a Ar-te-mís-i-ē-fō-li-a; rag-weed.
Ambrosia Trifida, — Tri-fį-da; horse-weed.
Amenorrhœa, A-men-ō-rē-a; absence of the menses by delay or suppression.
Amentia, A-mén-ʃi-a; without mind; imbecility.
American Columbo; *Frasera Carolinensis;* root of the plant that affords a mild tonic for the digestive organs.
American Ipecac; root of the *Euphorbia Ipecacuanhæ.*
Amides, A-mį-dēz; compounds formed when the hydrogen of ammonia is replaced by oxidized, or other negative principles.
Amines, A-mį-nēz; compounds formed when the hydrogen of ammonia is replaced by positive radicals.
Ammonia, A-mō-ni-a; a compound formed by the combination of nitrogen and hydrogen, possessing alkaline qualities.
Ammoniacum, Am-ō-nį-a-kum; a gum resin, obtained from the *Dorema ammoniacum.*
Ammonii Carbonates, A-mō-ni-į Kąr-bon-ets; volatile salts, smelling salts.
Ammonii Chloride, — Klō-rįd; muriate of ammonium; sal ammoniac.
Ammonium, A-mō-ni-um; a presumed metallic substance, supposed to be similar in character to potassium.
Amnesia, Am-nē-ʒi-a; loss, or want of memory. [*utero.*
Amnion, Am'ni-on; the inner envelope of the *Fœtus in*
Amniotic Acid; an acid found in the liquor contained in the amnion.
Amorphous, A-mór-fus; destitute of regular structure.
Ampelopsis Quinquefolia, Am-pē-lóp-sis Kwin-kwē-fō-li-a; American ivy.
Amphi, Am'fi; both, on all sides.
Amphiarthrosis, Am-fi-ar-ŧrō-sis; a two-sided articulation, allowing of slight motion.
Amphidiarthrosis, Am'fi-dį-ar-ŧrō-sis; a two-sided articulation, as of the lower jaws.
Amphoric, Am-fór-ik; a sound resembling that made by blowing into a decanter, heard in auscultating the chest. [als of the ear.
Ampulla Am-púl-la; the bottle-like mouths of the can-
Amputation, the act of cutting off.

Amygdalæ, A-míg-da-lĕ; the tonsils; the exterior glands of the neck.

Amygdala Amara, A-míg-da-la A-má-ra; the bitter almond.

Amygdala Dulcis, — Dúl-sis; sweet almond.

Amygdalin, A-míg-da-lin; a crystalline substance existing in bitter almond.

Amygdalitis, A-mig-da-lį-tis; inflammation of the tonsils.

Amygdalus Persica, A-míg-da-lus Pér-si-ka; the peach tree.

Amyl, Am'il; the radical of amylic alcohol, C^5H^{11}.

Amyl Alcohol, derived from fusel oil.

Amyl Nitrite, — Nį-trįt; an etherial liquid used in medicine, highly recommended for sea-sickness.

Amylaceous, Am-i-lá-ʃus; starch-like.

Amylum, Am'i-lum; medical term for starch.

Amylum Marantæ; — Mar-án-tĕ; arrow root.

Amyous, Am'i-us; weak in muscles.

Anacatharsis, An-a-ka-tą́r-sis; cough with expectoration.

Anacathartic, An-a-ka-tą́r-tik; promoting expectoration.

Anacardium, An-a-ką́r-di-um; the Malacca Bean, containing a very caustic liquor.

Anæsthesia, An-es-té-ʒi-a; suspended sensibility.

Anæsthetics, An-es-tét-iks; chloroform, ether, etc., which render the patient insensible to pain.

Anagallis Arvensis, An-a-gál-is Ar-vén-sis; pimpernel, poor man's weather glass; used mostly in the form of poultices for old ulcers.

Anaplosis, An-a-pló-sis; restoration of decayed parts.

Anasarca, An-a-są́r-ka; dropsy of the cellular tissue.

Anastomosis, An-as-to-mó-sis; communications of vessels with each other.

Anatomy, An-át-o-mi; to cut; dissection of organized bodies with a view to displaying the structure, relations and uses of parts.

Anazoturia, An-a-zo-tų́-ri-a; chronic diuresis, where there is a deficiency of urea.

Anchusa Tinctoria, An-kų́-sa Tiŋk-tó-ri-a; a plant, the root of which contains a red coloring matter.

Anchylosis, An-ki-ló-sis; stiff or useless joint.

Ancon, An'kon; the elbow joint.

Anconæus, An-ko-né-us; the small muscle on the elbow.

Anconoid, An'kω-nəd; a process of the ulna.

Andromeda Arborea, An-dróm-ĕ-da Ar-bω-rĕ-a; the sorrel tree. (See *Oxydendrum*. [pecially of the male.

Andranatomy, An-dra-nát-ω-mi; human anatomy, es-

Andria Mulier, An'dri-a Mú-li-er; an hermaphrodite, the female organs being predominant.

Andromania, An-drω-má-ni-a; nymphomania, morbid sexual excitement of females.

Androgynus; An-drój-i-nus; partaking of each sex.

Anemone Nemorosa, A-ném-ω-nĕ Nem-ω-rώ-sa; the wind flower.

Anemone Pulsatilla, — Pul-sa-tíl-a; a flowering plant of Europe, used in nervous diseases; synonym for *Pulsatilla nigricans*. [out brains.

Anencephalus, An-en-séf-a-lus; a monster, born with-

Anesis, An'ĕ-sis; remission, as of symptoms.

Anethi Fructus, An-ĕ-thị Frúk-tus; fruit of the dill, from which oil of the dill is obtained. [sweet fennel.

Anethum Graveolens, An-ĕ-thum Grav-ĕ-ώ-lenz; dill;

Anetus, An'ĕ-tus; intermittent fever.

Aneurism, An'ų-rizm; a morbid dilatation of an artery, with rupture of one or more of its coats.

Aneurism Cordis; a dilatation of the heart.

Aneurism Spurium, — Spų́-ri-um; a rupture of all the coats of the artery, with blood retained in the surrounding tissues.

Aneurism by Anastomosis, a vascular tumor by the enlargement and inosculation of numerous arteries.

Anfractuosity; a groove or furrow, as in the brain.

Angelica, An-jél-i-ka; the plant masterwort, mostly used for diseases of the urinary organs. [the body.

Angiology, An-ji-ól-ω-ji; science of the blood vessels of

Angiitis, An-ji-ị-tis; inflammation of vessels, especially of the capillaries.

Angina, An-jị́-na; morbid affections of the throat.

Angina Maligna, — Ma-líg-na; putrid sore throat, as in scarlatina.

Angina Parotydea, — Par-ω-tíd-ĕ-a; the mumps.

Angina Tonsillaris, — Ton-sil-á-ris; the quinsy.

Angina Trachealis, — Trak-ĕ-á-lis; the croup.

Angina Pectoris, — Pék-tω-ris; spasms of the nerves of the chest.

Anginosa, An-ji-nώ-sa; accompanied with angina.

Angone, An'gō-nē; nervous quinsy; strangulation.
Angular Artery; terminations of veins near the inner angle of the eye.
Angustura, An-gus-tū-ra; a tree of South America, *Galipea Officinalis*.
Anhelation, An-hē-lá-ʃon; rapid breathing.
Anhydrotics, An-hi-drót-iks; agents which check profuse perspiration.
Anhydrous, An-hí-drus; destitute of water.
Animalcula, An-i-mál-kų-la; an insect only visible by the microscope.
Animal Heat; caloric formed by respiration.
Animalization; assimilation; vital conversion of food into organized matter.
Animus, An'i-mus; the mind or principle of life.
Anise, An'is; a plant originally from Egypt, *Pimpinella Anisum*.
Aniseed; fruit of the Anise plant, used as a carminative.
Ankylosis, An-ki-lō-sis, (*Anchylosis*); a stiff joint.
Annular, An'ų-lar; like a ring, when applied to ligaments.
Annular Cartilage, — Kár-ti-laj; one of the cartilages of the larynx.
Annular Ligament; a strong ligament of the wrist; also of the ankle.
Annular Vein; the vein between the little finger and the one adjoining, or "ring finger."
Anodic, An-ód-ik; ascending; styptic or astringent.
Anodyne, An'ō-dīn; a drug that eases pain by benumbing the sensibility and inclining to sleep.
Anodynia, An-ō-dín-i-a; absence of pain.
Anomalous, An-óm-a-lus; unnatural; applied to irregular symptoms.
Anomesia, An-ō-mē-si-a; dementia; loss of mind.
Anophthalmia; An-of-tál-mi-a; being without eyes.
Anopsia, An-óp-si-a; defective eye-sight.
Anorchous, An-ór-kus; without testicles.
Anorexia, An-ō-rék-si-a; want of appetite.
Anosmia, An-ós-mi-a; loss of the sense of smell.
Antacid, Ant-ás-id; an agent that neutralizes acidity.
Antaphrodisiac, An-ta-frō-dís-i-ak; medicines which reduce the venereal passion.

Antarthritic, Ant-qr-ŧrít-ik; tending to relieve from the gout.
Antasmatic, Ant-as-mát-ik relieving the asthma.
Anteflexio Uteri, An-tē-flék-ſi-ω Yú-ter-i; bending forward of the womb.
Antemetica, An-tē-mét-ik-a; remedies for vomiting.
Antesternum, An-tē-stér-num; anterior, or first division of the sternum.
Anteversio Uteri, An-tē-vér-ſi-ω Yú-ter-i; reversion of the mouth of the womb.
Anthelix, Ant'hē-liks; the inner ridge of the external [ear.
Anthelmintic, An-ŧel-mín-tik, antagonistic to worms.
Anthemis Nobilis, An'ŧē-mis Nó-bil-is; the garden chamomile.
Anthiarin, Au-ŧí-a-rin; the active principle of a gum obtained from the Upas tree.
Anthorisma, An-tor-ís-ma; a tumor with no definite [boundary.
Anthracene, An'ŧra-sēn; a hydro-carbon.
Anthracoid, An'ŧra-kəd, having the nature of a car- [búncle.
Anthracokali, An-ŧra-kók-a-li; preparation of coal dust and potassa, for herpetic ailments.
Anthracosis, An-ŧra-kó-sis; carbuncle of the eye-lids.
Anthrax, An'ŧraks; a carbuncle, or little tumor.
Anthropography, An-ŧrω-póg-ra-fi; history of the structure of man.
Anthypnotic, Ant-hip-nót-ik; preventing sleep.
Antiades, An-tí-a-dēz; the tonsils.
Antiaditis, An-ti-a-dí-tis; inflammation of the tonsils.
Antiarthritic, An-ti-qr-ŧrít-ik; medicines for the cure of diseases of the joints.
Antibrachial, An-ti-brák-i-al; relating to the fore- [arm.
Antibromic, An-ti-bróm-ik; destructive of offensive odors.
Anticardium, An-ti-kár-di-um; the pit of the stomach.
Antidinic, An-ti-dín-ik; remedy for giddiness or vertigo.
Antidote, An'ti-dωt; medicine given to destroy a morbid cause, or to counteract a poison.
Antidynous, An-tíd-i-nus; like an anodyne.
Antidysenteric, a remedy for dysentery.
Antifebril, An-ti-féb-ril; mitigating fever.

Antigalactic, An-ti-ga-lák-tik; reducing the secretion of milk.

Antihectic, An-ti-hék-tik; opposed to hectic fever. [ear.

Anthelix, Ant-hĕ-liks; the small circular ridge of the

Antihelminticus, An-tĭ-hel-mín-tik-us; opposed to worms. [flow of blood.

Antihemorrhagic, An-ti-hem-or-áj-ik; stopping the

Antihydropic, An-ti-hį-dróp-ik; remedy for dropsy.

Antihydropin, An-ti-hį-drǿ-pin; a crystalline principle obtained from cockroaches, medicinal for dropsy.

Anti-Icteric, An-ti-Ik-tér-ik; remedy for jaundice.

Antilethargic, An-ti-leŧ-ár-jik; opposed to sleep.

Antilithic, An-ti-líŧ-ik; preventive of the formation of stone in the bladder.

Antilyssic, An-ti-lís-ik; curative of hydrophobia.

Antimephitic, An-ti-mĕ-fít-ik; preventive against impure air or gas. [and a base.

Antimonates, An-ti-mǿ-nets; salts of antimonic acid

Antimonial Powder; substitute for James's Powder.

Antimonii et Potassæ Tartras; tartar emetic.

Antimonii Vinum; wine of antimony.

Antimony, An′ti-mo-ni; a brilliant blueish metal, very brittle.

Antinephritic, An-ti-nĕ-frít-ik; remedial for inflammation of the kidneys.

Antipathic, An-ti-páŧ-ik; contrary to. [diseases.

Antiperiodic, An-ti-pĕ-ri-ód-ik; remedial for periodic

Antiperistaltic, An-ti-per-i-stál-tik; inverted action of the bowels. [inflammation.

Antiphlogistic, An-ti-flo-jís-tik; that which subdues

Antiphthisic An-ti-tíz-ik; remedy for phthisic, or consumption.

Antipleuritic, An-ti-plų-rít-ik; remedy for pleurisy.

Antipsoric, An-tip-sór-ik; remedy for the itch. [pus.

Antipyic, An-ti-pį́-ik; preventive to the formation of

Antipyretic, An-ti-pi-rét-ik; a febrifuge, to allay fever.

Antipyrotic, An-ti-pi-rót-ik; remedy for burns.

Antiseptic, An-ti-sép-tik; preventive of putrefaction.

Antispasmodic, An-ti-spaz-mód-ik; that which allays spasms or pains. [vation.

Antisialagogue, An-ti-sį-ál-a-gog; a remedy for sali-

Antisyphilitic, An-ti-sif-i-lít-ik; cure for syphilis.
Antithenar, An-tít-ē-nar; relating to muscles of the hand and great toe. [helix.
Antitragus, An-tít-ra-gus; the thick part of the anti-
Antivenereal, An-ti-ven-ē-rē-al; remedy for the venereal disease.
Antizymic, An-ti-zím-ik; preventing fermentation.
Antodontalgic, An-tō-don-tál-jik; remedy for the tooth-ache.
Antonii, Ignis Sancti; St. Anthony's Fire; erysipelas.
Antritis, An-trī-tis; inflammation of any cavity in the animal organization.
Antrum, An'trum; a cave; the cavity of a bone, especially that in the upper maxillary bone, termed *Antrum Highmorianum*. [of the ear.
Antrum Buccinosum, — Buk-si-nó-sum; the cavity
Antrum Pylori, — Pi-ló-rī; the small part of the stomach near the pylorus.
Anuria, A-nú-ri-a; suppression of the urine.
Anus, Ē'nus; a circle; the lower extremity of the rectum or bowel.
Aorta, Ē-ór-ta; the great artery of the body, that arises from the left ventricle of the heart. [of the aorta.
Aorturisma, Ē-or-tu-ríz-ma; aneurism, or enlargement
Aortic, Ē-ór-tik; belonging to the aorta.
Aortitis, Ē-or-tī-tis; inflammation of the aorta.
Aortra, Ē-ór-tra; a lobe of the lungs.
Apathy, Ap'a-thi; absence of feeling or emotion.
Apepsia, A-pép-si-a; imperfect digestion; dyspepsia.
Aperient, A-pē-ri-ent; a laxitive, or gentle purgative.
Apex, Ē'peks; the summit, or extremity, as the pointed end of the heart. [surgery.
Aphæresis, A-fér-ē-sis; the removal of a part, as in
Aphelxia, A-félk-si-a; mental abstraction.
Aphonia, A-fó-ni-a; without voice.
Aphoria, A-fó-ri-a; barrenness; sterrility. [ment.
Aphrodisia, Af-rō-díz-i-a; immoderate venereal excite-
Aphrodisiac, Af-rō-díz-i-ak; descriptive of drugs or food supposed to excite venery.
Aphtha, (*pl.* Aphthæ) Af'tha; ulcers in the mouth; characteristic symptoms of the thrush.

Aphthous, Af'ŧus; affected with or resembling aphthæ.
Apiol, Ap'ī-ꞷl; a principle obtained from parsley seed.
Apis Mellifica, Ꞓ'pis Me-lif-i-kɑ; the honey bee; a tincture obtained chiefly from the poison of the sting of the bee, used by the homeopathists and others.
Apium Petroselinum, Ꞓ'pi-um Pē-trꞷ-sē-lį-num; former name for *Petroselinum Sativum*, the common parsley.
Apleuria, A-plų́-ri-ɑ; absence of ribs.
Apnœa, Ap-nḗ-ɑ; suspension of breath. [evacuation.
Apocenosis, A-pos-ē-nꞷ́-sis; increased discharge, or
Apocynum Androsæmifolium, A-pós-i-num An-drꞷ-sem-i-fꞷ́-li-um; bitter root; dog's bane; an indigenous plant, used in a variety of diseases.
Apocynum Cannabinum, — Kan-a-bį́-num; white Indian hemp, used in dropsy.
Apomorphia, Ap-ꞷ-mér-fi-ɑ; a powerful emetic, obtained by heating morphia with hydrochloric acid.
Aponeurosis, Ap'on-ų-rꞷ́-sis; expansion of muscles.
Apophysis, A-póf-i-sis; a projection or protuberance of bone.
Apoplexia, Ap-ꞷ-plék-si-ɑ; apoplexy; congestion, or rupture of the vessels of the brain.
Apoplexy Cutaneous, rapid flow of blood to the skin and cellular membrane. [tion of blood in the lungs.
Apoplexia Pulmonaris, — Pul-mꞷ-ná-ris; extravasa-
Apostema, Ap-os-tḗ-mɑ; aposteme, an abscess.
Apothecary; one who prepares and sells drugs.
Appendices Epiploicæ, A-pén-di-sēz Ep-i-plꞷ́-i-sē; prolongations of the peritoneum, filled with a fatty substance.
Appendicula Vermiformis, A-pen-dík-ų-lɑ Vɛr-mi fér-mis; a worm-like excrescence from the *cæcum*, or first part of the large intestine.
Appetence, Ap'ē-tens; appetency; strong desire; disposition to appropriate what is essential to animal existence.
Apyretic, (*Apyrexia*), Ap-i-rét-ik; absence of fever.
Aq., or Aqua, Ꞓ'kwɑ; water, hydrogen and oxygen combined as represented by H^2 O.
Aqua Fortis, — Fér-tis; an old name for nitric acid.

Aqua Regia, — Rē-ji-a; a mixture of nitric and hydrochloric acids, having the properties of dissolving gold and platinum.

Aqua Vitæ, Ȧ'kwa Vī-tē; spirits of the first distillation.

Aquæ Minerales, — Min-er-á-lēz; mineral waters, impregnated with acid, iron, salt, sulphur, etc.

Aqueduct of the Cochlea; an opening in the temporal bone, for the passage of the vessels of the ear. [ear.

Aqueduct of Fallopius, bony canals of the internal

Aqueduct of Sylvius; a canal between the third and fourth ventricles of the brain.

Aqueduct of the Vestibulum; a canal that opens on the posterior surface of the temporal bone of the cranium. [of water.

Aqueous, Ȧ'kwē-us; containing water, formed by means

Aqueous Humor, — Yú-mor; a watery fluid of the anterior and posterior chambers of the eye.

Arabin, Ar'a-bin; the gummy principle of acacia, isomeric with cane sugar.

Arachnoid, A-rák-nœd; applied to the middle membrane of the brain. [arachnoid membrane.

Arachnoiditis, A-rak-nœ-dī-tis; inflammation of the

Aræometer, Ar-ē-óm-ē-ter; an instrument for measuring the gravity of liquids.

Aralia, A-rá-li-a; a genus of indigenous plants, most species of which are medicinal.

Aralia Hispida, — His-pi-da; dwarf elder, used in pulmonary diseases.

Aralia Nudicaulis, — Nų-di-ké-lis; American sarsaparilla, an alterative, and also used for pulmonary affections.

Aralia Quinquefolia, — Kwin-kwē-fṓ-li-a; ginseng, formerly and commonly described as *Panax quinquefolium*; used in certain forms of dyspepsia.

Aralia Racemosa, — Ra-sē-mṓ-sa; spikenard, used in pulmonary affections.

Aralia Spinosa, — Spi-nṓ-sa: prickly elder, the Angelica tree; used in syphilitic and rheumatic affections, and certain skin diseases.

Arbor Vitæ, Ȧr'bor Vī-tē; white cedar, an American evergreen, a domestic remedy for intermittent fever.

Arbutin, Ar-bú-tin; a glucoside found in *Uva Ursi* leaves.

Arbutus, Trailing, Ar-bú-tus; a pretty spring flower. See *Epigæa repens.*

Arbutus Uva Ursi, former name for *Arctostaphylos Uva Ursi.*

Arcanum, (*pl.* Arcana), Ar-ká-num; a secret; medicines the composition of which is concealed.

Arch, femoral; the arch over the border of the pelvis.

Arch of the Aorta; the turn made in the thorax by that artery.

Arch of the Colon; transverse portion of that intestine.

Archorrhagia, Ar-kor-á-ji-a; hemorrhage of the anus.

Archostenosis, Ar-kos-tē-nó-sis; structure of the rectum.

Arctatio, Ark-tá-ʃi-o; constipation; also an unnatural contraction of the vagina.

Arctium Lappa, Ark'ti-um Láp-a; former name for *Lappa Officinalis.*

Arctostaphylos Uva Ursi, Ark-to-stáf-i-los Yú-va Ur-si; bearberry, a very small evergreen shrub, the leaves of which are used in diseases of urinary organs.

Arcus Senilis, Ar'kus Sen-í-lis; a circular opaque appearance in the eyes of old men.

Ardor Febrilis, Ar'dor Feb rí-lis; feverish heat.

Ardor Urinæ, — Yu-rí-nē; inflammation of the urethræ, causing the sensation of heat in passing urine.

Ardor Ventriculi, — Ven-trík-u-lí; the heart-burn.

Areca Catechu, A-ré-ka Kát-ē-ku; a palm of India, which yields betel nuts.

Areca Nuts; (See Betel nuts.)

Arenosa Urina, Ar-ē-nó-sa Yu-rí-na; urine with gravel.

Areola, Ar-ē-ó-la; a colored ring, as around the nipple.

Areolæ, Ar-ē-ó-lē; interstices between the fibres of an organ.

Argema, Ar'jē-ma; a small white ulcer in the eye.

Argenti Nitras, Ar-jén-tí Ní-tras; nitrate of silver; when fused called lunar caustic.

Argentum, Ar-jén-tum; silver, a white metal.

Argillaceous, Ar-ji-lá-ʃus; of the nature of clay.

Argol, Ar'gol; an impure acid tartrate of potassium, deposited from wine; crude cream of tartar.

Aricina, Ar-i-sį-na; an alkaloid found in cusco bark, similar to that in cinchona.

Arisæma Triphyllum, Ar-i-sē-ma Trį-fil-um; Indian turnip, (Dragon root), the fresh corm of which is intensely acrid. Formerly *Arum Triphyllum*.

Aristolochia Serpentaria, Ar-is-tœ-lœ́-ki-a Ser-pen-tá-ri-a; Virginia snake root; serpentaria root; used as an adjuct in intermittent fevers, as a diaphoretic.

Armillæ, Ar-míl-ē; a membranous ligament that confines the tendons of the wrist.

Arnica Montana, Ar'ni-ka Mon-tá-na; a plant of central Europe, the flowers of which afford a stimulant of the nervous system, the tincture of which is used externally for sprains, etc.

Arnotto, See *Bixa*, the seeds of which yield a pigment.

Aromatic, Ar-œ-mát-ik; possessing a fragrant odor, and usually a warm, pungent taste.

Arrack, Ar'ak; an intoxicating beverage of India, made chiefly by the distillation of the sweet sap of the palm.

Arrow Root, a pure kind of starch, obtained from the tubers of Maranta arundinacea.

Arsenic, Ar'sen-ik; a metallic substance of a steel gray color, which with all its compounds is poisonous; generally applied to arsenious acid.

Arsenicum, Ar-sén-i-kum; See Arsenic.

Artanthe Elongata, Ar-tán-thē E-loŋ-gá-ta; a shrub, native of Peru, which yields Matico.

Artemisia, Ar-tē-míʃ-i-a; an extensive genus of intensely bitter herbs.

Artemisia Abrotanum, — A-brót-a-num; southern wood, a fragrant bitter herb of the south.

Artemisia Absinthium, —Ab-sín-thi-um: wormwood, native of Europe; anthelmintic.

Artemisia Contra, — Kón-tra; a plant of the Levant, which yields Santonica.

Artemisia Santonica, — San-tón-i-ka; a plant formerly supposed to yield Levant; wormseed.

Artemisia Vulgaris, — Vul-gá-ris; mugwort, a common weed, sometimes used as a vermifuge.

Arteria Aspera, Ar-tĕ-ri-a As'per-a; the "rough artery;" the trachea or windpipe.
Arteria Innominata, —In-nom-i-ná-ta; the "unnamed artery," the first branch of the aorta.
Arteria Magna, — Mág-na; the aorta.
Arterial, Ar-tĕ-ri-al; belonging to arteries.
Arterial Blood; the red blood flowing in the arteries of the body and the pulmonary veins.
Arterial Duct; the duct leading from the pulmonary artery to the aorta in the fœtus.
Arterial Ligament; the arterial duct when obliterated.
Arterialization, Ar-tē-ri-al-i-zá-ʃon; change of the blood by respiration.
Arteriotomy, Ar-tē-ri-ót-ọ-mi; opening, or dividing an artery; blood letting.
Arteritis, Ar-tē-rį-tis; inflammation of an artery.
Artery, Ar'ter-i; one of the vessels, or ducts, which carries blood from the heart.
Arthralgia, Ar-trál-ji-a; chronic pain in the joints; rheumatism, gout.
Arthritic,, Ar-trít-ik; relating to gout.
Arthritis, Ar-trį-tis; same as *Arthralgia*.
Arthrocace, Ar-trók-a-sē; ulceration of a cavity of a bone.
Arthrodia, Ar-tró-di-a; a joint admitting of motion on all sides.
Arthrodynia, Ar-trọ-dín-i-a; same as *Arthralgia*.
Arthrography, Ar-tróg-ra-fi; a written description of the joints.
Arthrology, Ar-tról-ọ-ji; the science of joints.
Arthroncus, Ar-trón-kus; a cartilaginous substance that sometimes forms in the knee joint.
Arthropathia, Ar-trọ-pá-ti-a; a disease of the shoulder joint.
Arthrosia, Ar-tró-si-a; general term for inflammation of the joints.
Arthrosis, Ar-tró-sis; connection by joints.
Artiads, Ar'ti-adz; elements whose quantivalence is even.
Articular, Ar-tík-ų-lar; relating to joints.
Articularis, Ar-tik-ų-lá-ris; relating to arteries, muscles, etc, connected with joints.
Articulation · a joint; the fastening together of the various bones of the animal skeleton.

Arum Maculatum, Ȩ'rum Mak-ụ-lá-tum; the Wake-robin, having an acrid root, stimulant internally.

Arum Triphyllum, Ȩ'rum Trị-fíl-um; synonym for *Arisœma Triphylla.*

Arytænoid, A-rít-ē-nɵd; applied to the third and fourth cartilages of the larynx.

Asagræa Officinalis, As-a-grē-ɑ Of-is-i-ná-lis; a Mexican plant, supposed to yield Cevadilla seed.

Asaphatum, A-sáf-a-tum; matter found in the sebaceous follicles of the skin, which appear like small worms.

Asarum Çanadense, As'a-rum Kan-a-dén-sē; wild ginger; Canada snakeroot; used in colic, and as a stimulating agent.

Ascaris, As'ka-ris, (*pl Ascarides;*) a kind of worm infesting the rectum.

Ascaris Vermicularis, — Vɛr-mik-ụ-lá-ris; the thread worm.

Ascensus Morbi, A-sén-sus Mɵ́r-bị; increase of a disease.

Ascites, A-sị-tēz; dropsy in the abdomen.

Asclepias, As-klē-pi-as; a genus of plants with milky juice.

Asclepias Cornuti, — Kɵr-nụ́-tị; the common silkweed.

Asclepias Incarnata, — In-kɑr-ná-tɑ; flesh-colored asclepias, found in damp soil, and used as a vermifuge.

Asclepias Tuberosa, — Tụ-ber-ṓ-sɑ; pleurisy-root; an indigenous plant, the root of which is used in inflammation of the lungs, pleurisy, etc., as an expectorant.

Asepta, A-sép-tɑ; matter free from putrefaction.

Ash, Aʃ; common name for trees of the genus *Fraxinus.*

Ashes, Aʃ'ez; the substance remaining after burning any thing.

Asitia, A-sị-ʃi-ɑ; loss of appetite; abstinence from food.

Asparagus Officinalis, As-pár-a-gus —; the garden asparagus, a diuretic.

Asphyxia; As-fík-si-ɑ; suspension of the action of the heart, as by suffocation.

Asphyxia Idiopathica, — Id-i-ɷ-páth-i-kɑ; sudden death without apparent cause.

Asphyxia Neonatorum, — Nē-ɷ-na-tṓ-rum; want of respiration in a new born child.

Asphyxia Suffocationis, — Suf-ɷ-ka-ʃi-ṓ-nis; death by hanging or drowning.

Aspidium Felix Mas, As-píd-i-um Fē-liks Mas; the male fern, used for tape worm.

Assafœtida; As-a-fét-i-da; a fetid gum resin, obtained from a plant of Persia, *Narthex Assafœtida*.

Assodes, A-sṓ-dēz; continued fever, with loathing of [food.

Aster, As'ter; a large genus of plants, a few of which are medicinal.

Asternia, A-stẽr-ni-a; absence of the sternum in a fœtus.

Asthenia, As-thē-ni-a; debility; want of strength.

Asthma, Ast'ma; a disease the prominent symptoms of which are difficulty of breathing, wheezing, aud expectoration.

Astragalus Verus, As-trág-a-lus Vē-rus; a little spiny shrub, from which gum tragacanth exudes.

Astriction, As-trík-ʃon; condition produced by astringent medicines.

Astringent, As-trín-jent; causing contraction in the muscles, and thereby checking discharges.

Ataxia, A-ták-si-a; irregularity; want of uniform manifestation.

Athermanous, A-thẽr-ma-nus; not conducting heat.

Atheroma, Ath-er-ṓ-ma; a pulpy, encysted tumor.

Atlas, At'las; the first cervical vertebra.

Atocia *or* **Atokia**, A-tṓ-ki-a; sterility.

Atonic, A-tón-ik; with diminished tone or power.

Atrabiliary, At-ra-bíl-ya-ri; melancholy; gloomy.

Atrabilious, At-ra-bíl-yus; despondent; melancholy.

Atrabilis, At-ra-bị-lis; black bile, an imaginary fluid, the excess of which has been supposed to cause melancholy.

Atresia, A-trē-ʃi-a; adhesive perforation, as of the [anus, vulva, etc.

Atropa Belladonna, At'rọ-pa Bel-a-dón-a; the deadly night shade, a poisonous herbaceous plant of Europe; a narcotic poison, that acts upon the cerebro-spinal system.

Atrophy, At'rọ-fi; imperfect nutrition, resulting in emaciation and loss of strength.

Atropia, A-trṓ-pi-a; a very poisonous alkaloid of *Atropa Belladonna*, used mainly for eye diseases.

Atropism, At'rọ-pizm; diseased condition produced by excessive use of Belladonna.

2

Attenuant, A-tén-ụ-ant; a medicine for increasing the fluidity of the blood, etc.

Attollens, A-tól-ēnz; lifting; applied to muscles whose office is to raise up.

Attrahens Auris, At'ra-hens Θ'ris; muscles of the ear.

Attrition, A-tri-ʃon; an abrasion of the skin; the crushing of a part.

Auditory Nerve, Θ'di-tω-ri Nεrv; the acoustic nerve, *Portio Mollis.*

Aura, Θ'ra; a steam, or subtle vapor.

Aura Epileptica, — Ep-i-lép-ti-ka; premonitory sensation of epileptic patients, like a cold fluid rising to the brain.

Aura Seminalis — Se-mi-ná-lis; supposed fecundating principle of the seminal fluid, believed to pass through the Fallopian tubes to the ovum.

Aura Vitalis, — Vị-tá-lis; the principle of life.

Aurantium Amarus, Θ-rán-ʃi-um A-má-rus; bitter orange, the fruit of *Citrus Vulgaris,* the rind of which is used in medicine.

Aurantium Dulcis, — Dúl-sis; sweet orange, the fruit of *Citrus Aurantium.*

Auricula, Θ-rík-ụ-la; the external portion of the ear.

Auriculæ Cordis, Θ-rík-ụ-lē Kór-dis; cavities of the heart that lead to the ventricles.

Auricularis, Θ-rik-ụ-lá-ris; belonging to the ear.

Auris, Θ'ris: the ear, external and internal.

Auriscope, Θ'ri-skωp; an instrument for examining the tube of the ear.

Aurum, Θ'rum; gold, the chloride of which, and chloride of gold and sodium, are much used in medicine.

Auscultation, Θs-kul-tá-ʃon; diagnosis by sounding the lungs and heart.

Auscultation Immediate; auscultation without the aid of an instrument, by merely listening to the functional movements of lungs and heart.

Autoplasty, Θ'tω-plas-ti; same as Anaplasty.

Autopsoria, Θ-top-só-ri-a; administering a patient's own virus.

Autopsy, Θ'top-si; personal inspection.

Ava, Ɛ'va; a narcotic drink.

Avenæ Farina, A-vē-nē Fa-rī-na; oat meal.
Avenæ Sativa, — Sa-tī-va; the common oat.
Avulsion, A-vúl-ʃon; the forcible separation of parts.
Avens, Ā'venz; name for several species of *Geum*.
Axilla, Aks-il-a; the cavity under the shoulder.
Axillary Plexus, Aks'il-a-ri Plék-sus; the last three cervical and the first dorsal nerves of the arm.
Axis, Aks'is; in anatomy, a right line passing through the center of the body.
Azedarach, A-zéd-a-rak; the "pride of India;" *Melia Azederach*, cathartic and emetic.
Azoturia, Az-o-tū-ri-a; disease characterized by great increase of urea in the urine.
Azygous Muscle, Az'i-gus Mus'l; a muscle of the uvula.
Azygous Process; a process of the sphenoid bone.
Azygous Vein; a vein rising from the union of the lower intercostal veins of the left side.

B

B., symbol for the element *Boron*, used in medical preparations.
Baccæ, Bák-sē; berries, fruit, as *Baccæ Juniperi*.
Bacchia, Ba-kī-a; pimpled condition of the face, caused by hard drinking.
Baculus, Bák-u-lus; a lozenge in the form of a little roll.
Bael Fruit; the dried unripe fruit of the *Ægle Marmelos*, an astringent.
Baker's Itch, caused by the poisonous, or irritating nature of the yeast used.
Balanism, Bál-an-izm; the use of a pessary.
Balanitis, Bal-an-ī-tis; inflammation of the *glans penis*.
Balanus, Bál-a-nus; the *glans penis* and *glans clitoridis*.
Balbuties, Bal-bū-ʃi-ēz; stammering, or hesitation in speech.
Ballottement, Ba-lót-mon; movement of the fœtus after being elevated in the liquor amnii, in falling back to its place; a diagnosis of pregnancy.

Balm, Bqm; a soothing or tranquilizing medicine.
Balm; *Melissa Officinalis*; lemon balm.
Balm of Gilead; the resinous juice of the *Balsamodendron Gileadense.*
Balm of Gilead, (American); the resinous buds of a species of poplar, *Populus Balsamifera var candicans.*
Balmony, Bál-mω-ni; *Chelone Glabra*, called, also, snake-root, turtle-head, etc.
Balneum, Bál-nĭ-um; a bath; a washing place.
Balneum Animale, — An-i-má-lĭ; part of a lately killed animal, applied to a body or a limb.
Balneum Medicatum, — Med-i-ká-tum; a medicated bath.
Balneum Siccum, — Sík-um; immersion in dry ashes, salt, etc.
Bals., an abbreviation for *Balsamum.*
Balsam, Bǿl-sam; *Balsamum*; a mixture of resins with volatile oils, some containing benzoic acid.
Balsamatio, Bol-sam-á-ʃi-ω; the process of embalming a corps.
Balsamodendron Myrrha, Bol-sam-ω-dén-dron Mír-a; a small tree of Arabia, that yields gum myrrh.
Baneberry, Bán-ber-i; common name for *Actæa alba*, white cohosh.
Baobab, Bq́-ω-bq́b; a tree of western Africa, the bark of which is sometimes used instead of *Cinchona.*
Baptisia Tinctoria, Bap-tiʃ-i-a Tiŋk-tώ-ri-a; the wild indigo, a small indigenous shrub, used externally in the form of a decoction.
Barbadoes Leg, Bqr-bá-dωz Leg; a disease of hot climates, resulting in great swelling.
Barbadoes Aloes, — Al'ωz; the variety yielded by the *Aloe vulgaris.*
Barium, Bár-ri-um; an elementary body, a metal of the alkaline earths, the salts from which are poisonous.
Barosma Crenata, Ba-rós-ma Krĭ-ná-ta; the buchu shrub, native of South Africa, used in diseases of the urino-genital organs.
Barosma Serratifolia, — Ser-a-ti-fώ-li-a; the shrub that yields what is known as *long* buchu.
Bark, Bqrk; in the plural, a popular term for Peruvian bark, or any of the cinchona species.
Baryecoia, Bar-i-ĭ-kώ-ya, difficulty in hearing, deafness.

Baryphony, Ba-ríf-ω-ni; hesitancy in speech.

Baryta, Ba-rį-ta; oxide of barium, the soluble salts of which are highly corrosive poisons.

Basculation, Bas-kų-lé-ʃon, examination of the uterus in retroversion.

Base, Bás; The hydroxyl compounds of those elements which have a markedly metallic character."—*Remsen.* "The idea implied by the word 'base' belongs to the obsolete dualistic theory of salts."—*Tilden.*

Base, Organic; organic bodies capable of uniting with acids and forming neutral compounds, resembling salts.

Basiator Oris, Bas-i-á-tor Ω'ris; a muscle that contracts the mouth.

Basilic Vein, Bas-íl-ik Van; the large vein inside the elbow, opened in blood-letting.

Basilicon Ointment; (*Basilicum*); made of five parts resin, eight of lard, and two of yellow wax, used for burns, ulcers, etc.

Basio Glossus; Bá-si-ω Glós-us; a muscle connecting the *os hyoides* and the tongue.

Basioccipital, Bas-i-ok-síp-i-tal; relating to the base of the occipital bone.

Basis Cordis, Bá-sis Kér-dis; the base of the heart, as distinguished from the apex.

Basisphenoid, Bas-i-sfé-nød; the posterior part of the body of the sphenoid bone.

Bassorin, Bás-ω-rin; a kind of gum found in gum tragacanth, insoluble in water but swells when moistened, forming a gelatinous mass, used as an excipient in making pill-mass.

Basylus Radicals, Bás-i-lus Rád-i-kalz; those elements which have a metallic character and form oxides or hydrates capable of saturating acids.

Bath, Sea-water; made by a solution of one part of common salt to thirty parts of soft water. **Cold Bath**; at 50° Fahren. **Hot Bath**; at 98° to 112°. **Tepid Bath**; at 85° to 92°. **Sand Bath**; made by heating sand and applying to any part of the body.

Batrachus, Bát-ra-kus; ranula, or a semi-transparent tumor under the tongue.

Bauhin, Bó-an̍, (**Valvule of**); a valve in the cæcum, that prevents the return of excrementitious, matter into the intestines.

Baume De Vie, Bωm Dε Vē, *Balm of Life;* a decoction of aloes.

Bayberry Bark, the bark of the roots of the *Myrica Cerifera.*

Bayberry Wax, a light green wax obtained from the berries of *Myrica Cerifera.*

Bearberry, Bą̈r-ber-i; a common name for the *Uva Ursi* plant.

Bear's Foot, a common name in Europe for *Helleborus fœtidus;* lately applied in this country to *Polymnia Uvedalia.*

Bebeerin, Bē-bē-rín; known as *beberin, bebirin, bibirina,* an alkaloid obtained from *Bebeeru* bark. The sulphate of bebeerin is a febrifuge and antimittant.

Bebeeru Bark, the bark of *Nectandra Rodiei*, containing bebeerin.

Bechica, Bék-i-ka; medicines that relieve coughs.

Beech Drops, (*Epiphegus Virginiana*); a parasite on the roots of the beech tree.

Belladonna, Bel-a-dón-a; the leaves and roots of *Atropa Belladonna*, a powerful narcotic.

Belonoid, Bél-ω-nœd; like a bodkin, describing the process of a bone.

Benjamin Bush; the spice bush, *Lindera Benzoin.*

Benne, Bén-ē; *Sesamum Indicum;* a medicinal plant of India.

Benzoic Acid, Ben-zó-ik As'id; an acid formerly obtained exclusively from gum benzoin, but an acid of the same composition is now obtained from naphthalin, also from urine.

Benzoin, Ben-zó-in; a balsamic resin, exuded from the *Styrax Benzoin.*

Benzoin Odoriferum, — Ω-dor-íf-er-um; see *Lindera Benzoin.*

Berberin, Bér-ber-in; a yellow bitter alkaloid, first discovered in *Berberis vulgaris*, afterward found in *Hydrastis Canadensis*, and improperly termed "hydrastin;" used as a bitter tonic.

Berberis Aquifolium, Bér-ber-is A-kwi-fó-li-um; an evergreen shrub found in the western states, used in scrofulous diseases.

Berberis Vulgaris, — Vul-gá-ris; barberry; a shrub of Europe; tonic in small doses, laxative in large.

Bergamot Oil, Bér-ga-mot Ōl; a fragrant oil expressed from the fruit rind of the *Citrus Limetta.*

Bertin, (bones of,) Ber-tañ; two small bones often found under the opening of the sphenoidal bone.

Betel Nut, Bé-tel Nut; the Areca nut; the kernel from the fruit of the *Areca Catechu.*

Bezoar, Bē-zó-ar; a calculous substance, sometimes found in the stomach and intestines of the ox, horse, and other animals, supposed to antidote poisons, pestilence, etc.

Beth Root, Béth Ruut; (*Birth root*); the root of *Trillium erectum.*

Betula, Bét-u-la; the generic name for birch trees.

Bi.; symbol for the element bismuth, preparations of which are used in medicine.

Bi-; (the prefix) two; thus, bicarbonate of potassium indicates that this salt contains twice as much of the carbonic radical as the simple carbonate of potassium.

Bibasic, Bi-bá-sik; acids which contain two atoms of hydrogen, metals will displace either half or all to form normal and double salts.

Bib, (*bibe,* "drink"); used in prescriptions.

Bicapsular, Bi-káp-su-lar; having two capsules.

Bicarbonate, Bi-kár-bon-at; two parts of carbonic acid with one of base.

Bicaudal, Bi-kó-dal; two-tailed; applied to a muscle.

Bicephalous, Bi-séf-a-lus; possessing two heads.

Biceps, Bí-seps; two-headed; as *biceps brachii,* a muscle of the arm; *biceps femoris,* a muscle of the thigh.

Bichat, Bē-shá; (canal of); a small hole above the pineal gland, leading into the third ventricle of the brain.

Bichloride of Mercury; corrosive sublimate.

Bicipital, Bi-síp-i-tal; relating to the biceps muscle.

Bicuspid, Bi-kús-pid; having two points, as the bicuspid teeth.

Bidens Bipinnata, Bí-denz Bi-pín-a-ta; Spanish needles, a common weed, having expectorant properties.

Biferous, Bíf-er-us; bearing twice a year.

Bilabe, Bį-lab; an instrument for extracting, through the urethra, bodies from the bladder.
Bile, Bįl; the alkaline secretion of the liver, a viscid and exceedingly bitter fluid.
Bilin, *or* **Biline,** Bį-lin; a yellowish gummy mass, the chief constituent of bile.
Bilious, Bil-yus; relating to, or full of bile. [bile.
Biliphein, Bil-i-fē-in; the principal coloring matter of
Bilifulvin, Bil-i-fúl-vin; yellow coloring matter of the bile.
Bilirubin, Bil-i-rú-bin; red coloring matter of the bile.
Biliverdin, Bil-i-vér-din; green coloring matter of the bile.
Bilobate, Bį-ló-bat; possessed of two lobes.
Bilocular, Bį-lók-ų-lar; having two cells.
Bimanous, Bím-an-us; possessing two hands.
Binary, Bį- na-ri; composed of two elements, or measures.
Binate, Bį-nat; coming, or growing, in pairs.
Binocular, Bį-nók-ų-lar; using both eyes.
Biology, Bį-ól-ọ-ji; the science which treats of the nature of all living things.
Biolysis, Bį-ól-i-sis; the destruction of life.
Biolytic, Bį-ọ-lít-ik; destructive of life.
Birdlime, Bérd-lįm; a glutinous matter obtained from the bark of the holly.
Birth Root. See Beth Root. [individual.
Bisexual, Bį-séks-ų-al; both sexes conjoined in the same
Bismuth, Bíz-muth; (*Bismuthum,*); a hard, brittle metal, that crystalizes from the melted state in the form of rhombohedrons; used in medicine, and often found impure, from the presence of arsenic, with which it is usually contaminated. [Europe.
Bistort, Bís-tort; *Polygonum Bistorta;* a plant of
Bistouri; Bis-tur-i; a knife or scalpel, for surgical purposes. [one of the base.
Bisulphate, Bį-súl-fat; two parts of sulphuric acid with
Bisulphite, Bį-súl-fįt; two parts of sulphurous acid with one of the base.
Bitartrate, Bį-tár-trat; an acid having double as much tartaric acid as the neutral salt. [*Colocynthis.*
Bitter Apple; the dried pulp of the fruit of *Citrullus*

Bitter Root; *Apocynum androsæmifolium:* a native plant.
Bittersweet; *Solanum Dulcamara*, a climbing indigenous shrub.
Bittersweet, false; *Celastrus Scandens.*
Bivalence, (*Bivalent*), Bív-a-lens; atoms capable of taking the place of two atoms of hydrogen. See *Dyads.*
Bixa Orellana, Bíks-a Or-el-á-na; a West Indian tree, from the fruit of which annotto, or arnotto, a reddish dye-stuff is obtained; it is medicinal as an astringent.
Black Alder; a deciduous indigenous shrub, *Ilex verticillata.*
Blackberry; the common bramble, *Rubus villosus.*
Black Cohosh; a common native plant, *Cimicifuga racemosa.*
Black Haw; an indigenous small tree, *Viburnum prunifolium.*
Black Hellebore, — Hél-ĕ-bor; the poisonous root of the *Helleborus niger*, a European plant.
Black Mustard; *Sinapis nigra*, or *Brassica nigra*, (Gray); the seeds are pungent, and used as counter irritant.
Black Pepper; the dried unripe berries of the *Piper nigrum.*
Black Root; the common name for the root of *Veronica Virginica.*
Black Snakeroot. See Black Cohosh.
Black Spruce; *Abies nigra*, a native evergreen.
Bladder; in the animal organization, the receptacle of urine.
Bladder-Wrack, —Rack; a sea-weed, the *Fucus vesiculosus.*
Blastema, Blas-tí-ma; the rudimental tissue of the embryo.
Blazing Star; *Liatris squarrosa*, an indigenous plant.
Blastide, Blás-tjd; the small, clear space in the segments of the ovum, the precursor of the nucleus.
Blastoderm, Blás-to-derm; the germinal membrane from which the embryo is developed.
Blastodermic Vesicle, — Vés-i-kl; the envelope surrounding the yelk; which is covered by the vital membrane, and becomes the umbilical cord.
Blastomere, Blás-to-mīr; divisions of the ovum.
Blear-Eye; inflammation of the eye-lids, catarrhal and chronic.

Blennadenitis, Blen-ad-en-ị-tis; an inflamed condition of the mucous glands.

Blennelytria, Blen-ĕ-lít-ri-a. See *Leucorrhœa.*

Blennenteria, Blen-en-tḗ-ri-a; the flow of mucus from the intestines.

Blennogenic, Blen-ō-jén-ik; generating the flow of [mucus.

Blennophthalmia, Blen-of-thál-mi-a. See *Ophthalmia.*

Blennorrhagia, Blen-or-á-ji-a; a bursting forth, or excessive discharge of mucus.

Blennorrhœa, Blen-or-ḗ-a; a flow of mucus; generally applied to gleet; *Gonorrhœa.*

Blennymen, Blen-ị-men; a mucous membrane.

Blennymenitis, Blen-i-men-ị-tis; the inflammation of a mucous membrane.

Blepharitis, Blef-ar-ị-tis; inflammation of the eye-lids.

Blepharoplasty, Bléf-ar-ō-plas-ti; the reparing of an eye-lid, by substituting skin from a contiguous part.

Blepharoplegia, Blef-ar-ō-plḗ-ji-a; paralysis of the upper eye-lid, causing it to hang partially over the ball.

Blessed Thistle; *Cnicus benedictus,* a European plant, slightly naturalized in the United States.

Blister; serous fluid collected under the skin; a plaster to be applied to raise a blister.

Blood; the fluid that circulates in the heart, arteries, and veins; it is composed of albumen, fibrin, and saline matter suspended in water.

Blood-Shot; unusual fullness in the veins of the eye, caused by inflammation, etc.

Blood-Root; *Sanguinaria Canadensis;* red pucoon, an early flowering indigenous herb.

Blue Cohosh; an indigenous plant; *Caulophyllum thalictroides.*

Blue Flag; *Iris versicolor;* an ornamental plant, common in wet places.

Blue Mass; a mild preparation of mercury, from which blue pills are made.

Bog-Bean, *or* **Buck-Bean;** a little plant that grows in damp places; *Menyanthes trifoliata.*

Boletus Laricis, Bō-lḗ-tus Lár-i-sis; the agaric, a fungus found on the larch; a purgative, and in large doses, emetic.

Bombus, Bóm-bus; a buzzing sound in the ears; the sound of wind in the intestines.

Bone Ash; impure phosphate of calcium, prepared by calcining bones to whiteness in a current of air.

Bone Black; animal charcoal, prepared by heating bones to redness in a closed vessel. [*perfoliatum.*

Boneset, Bώn-set; a common native plant; *Eupatorium*

Bonplandia Trifoliata, Bań-plán-di-ɑ Trị-fω-lí-á-tɑ; a synonym for *Galipea officinalis.*

Boracic Acid, Bω-rás-ik As'id; used as an antiseptic, now called Boric Acid.

Borago Officinalis, Bω-rá-gω —; borage, a common European plant, used as a demulcent.

Boron, Bώ-ron; a non-metallic element.

Boswellia, Bos-wél-i-ɑ; a genus of trees, the source of olibanum.

Botany; Bót-a-ni; the branch of biology which treats of vegetable life; knowledge of the properties of vegetables used medicinally.

Botts; a species of small worms that infest the intestines of horses, supposed to come from the egg of the gad-fly, that are deposited on the hair of horses, and thence licked off and swallowed.

Bougie, Bu-ʒá; a flexible instrument for entering the urethra, rectum, vagina, etc., sometimes medicated.

Bowman's Root; *Gillenia, stipulacea;* an indigenous remedy.

Box-Wood; a local name for *Cornus Florida.*

B. P.; British Pharmacopœia.

Br.; symbol for the element Bromine.

Brachial, Brák-i-al; relating to muscles, nerves, and vessels of the arm.

Brachialgia, Brak-i-ál-ji-ɑ: pain in the arm.

Brachiate, Brák-i-at; spread out in pairs, to match those above and below. [lating to the arm.

Brachio-, Brák-i-ω; a prefix in compounding words re-

Brachium, Brák-i-um; the arm, strictly from shoulder to elbow, but often including the lower part to the wrist.

Brain, the nervous mass in the skull, including two divisions, the *cerebrum* and *cerebellum.*

Brake; a fern, the *Pteris aquilina.*

Brandy; an alcoholic liquid obtained by the distillation of wine.

Brassica Nigra, Brás-i-ka Nị-gra; (Gray); a synonym for *Sinapis nigra.*

Brayera Anthelmintica; Bre-ē-ra An-thel-mín-ti-ka; a tree of Africa that yields kooso flowers.

Brazil Wood; a reddish dye-wood, obtained from *Cæsalpina crista.*

Brimstone; roll sulphur.

British Gum. See Dextrin.

Bredouillement, Bra-dúl-móṅ; a kind of imperfect utterance of words, caused by too rapid articulation.

Bregma, Brég-ma; the sinciput, or crown of the head.

Brevissimus Oculi, Brē-vís-i-mus Ok'ụ-lị; the shortest muscle of the eye.

Bricklayer's Itch; a kind of inflammation of bricklayer's hands, caused by contact with lime.

Bright's Disease; a complicated disease of the kidneys.

Brise-pierre, Brēs-pē-ạr; an instrument for entering and crushing stones in the bladder.

British Oil; a popular liniment.

Brodium, Brṓ-di-um; the broth, or liquid in which a thing is boiled.

Bromides, Brṓ-midz; compounds in which bromine takes the part of an acidulous radical.

Bromine, Brṓ-min; a non-metallic element, consumed mostly in the preparation of medicinal bromides.

Bronchia, Bróŋ-ki-a; two branches of the wind pipe, that convey air into the lungs.

Bronchial Bróŋ-ki-al; relating to the bronchia, or air passages.

Bronchial Tubes; small vessels terminating in the air-cells of the lungs.

Bronchitis, Bron-kị-tis; inflammation of the bronchia.

Bronchocele, Bróŋ-kō-sēl; enlargement of the thyroid gland; goitre.

Bronchophonism, Broŋ-kóf-ō-nizm; sound of the voice heard by means of the stethoscope.

Bronchorrhœa; Broŋ-kō-rē-a; discharge of mucus from the bronchia.

Bronchotomy, Broŋ-kót-ō-mi; the process of cutting into the wind pipe.

Broom, Brɯm; *Sarothamœ scoparius;* a plant, native of Europe. [*Epiphegus.*

Broom Rape; European name for plants of the genus

Brucia, Brɯ́-ʃi-ɑ; (*Brucin, Brucine, Brucina;*) an alkaloid resembling strychnia, obtained from Nux vomica and St. Ignatius bean. [scope.

Bruit, Brwē; the sound heard by the use of the stetho-

Bruit de Soufflet, — dɛ Sɯ-flé; the sound heard in auscultating the chest.

Bruit de Placentaire, — Plɑ-sen-tɑ̧r; the utero-placental murmur heard in auscultation.

Bruit Tympanique, — Tań-pɑ-nēk; the sound heard in auscultating the stomach and intestines.

Brunner's Glands; Brún-erz Glandz; mucous follicles in the small intestines.

Brunonian Theory; Brɯ-nɷ́-ni-an —; the theory of John Brown, that all diseases are the consequences of excess or deficiency of excitability in the animal functions.

Brygmus, Bríg-mus; grinding or gnashing of the teeth.

Bryonia Alba, Brį-ɷ́-ni-ɑ Al'bɑ; a climbing plant of Europe, the active bitter principle of the roots being a drastic cathartic.

Bryony, Brį-ɷ-ni; purgative roots obtained from *Bryonia alba* and *B. dioica.* [groin or axilla.

Bubo, Bɥ́-bɷ; an inflamed gland, generally in the

Bubonalgia, Bɥ-bɷ-nál-ji-ɑ; pain in the groin.

Bubonocele, Bɥ-bón-ɷ-sēl; rupture in the groin, in which a portion of the bowels protrudes at the abdominal ring.

Buccal, Búk-al; relating to the cheek.

Buccal Glands; numerous follicles under the mucous membrane of the cheek, which secrete a viscid humor that mixes with the saliva. [maxillary.

Buccal Nerve; a nerve that springs from the inferior

Buccinator; Buk-sin-á-tor; a flat muscle, forming a large part of the cheek, much used in blowing wind instruments.

Buccula, Búk-ɥ-lɑ; the fleshy growth under some chins.

Buchu, Bɯ́-kɯ; the leaves of the *Barosma crenata;* a valuable diuretic.

Buck-Bean, Buk-Bēn. See Bog-bean.
Buckeye, Búk-ī; the fruit of *Æsculus glabra*, a common American tree.
Buckhorn Brake; *Osmunda regalis*, a native fern.
Buckthorn; *Rhamnus catharticus*, a spiny shrub, native of Europe, and naturalized in the United States.
Bucnemia; Buk-nē-mi-a; elephantiasis; an inflamed swelling of the leg.
Buena, Bu-ē-na. See *Yerba Buena.* [root.
Bug-Bane, Búg-Ban; *Cimicifuga racemosa*, black snake
Bugle-Weed, Bú-gl-Wēd; *Lycopus Virginicus*, a common indigenous herb of wet places. [bulb.
Bulb; portions of the body raised and rounded like a
Bulb of the Urethra; the enlarged part of the tube near the root of the penis.
Bulbo-Cavernosus, Búl-bō Kav-er-nṓ-sus; a muscle of the urethra; the *Accelerator urinæ.*
Bulbus Artereosus, Búl-bus; Ar-tē-ri-ṓ-sus; one of the three principal cavities of the heart.
Bulbus Olfactorius, — Ol-fak-tṓ-ri-us; the bulblike portion of the olfactory nerve.
Bulimia, Bu-lím-i-a; a morbid appetite.
Bull, (*Bulliate;*) in prescriptions, "let it boil."
Bulla, Búl-a; a bubble, a blister, or vesicle, caused by burns or scalds. [great toe.
Bunion, Bún-yon; an inflammation upon the ball of the
Burdock, Búr-dok; *Lappa officinalis*, formerly *Arctium Lappa*, a well known weed.
Burgloss, Búr-glos; the European name for two demulcent plants, *Anchusa officinalis* and *Borago officinalis.*
Burgundy Pitch, a resin which exudes from a European evergreen, *Abies excelsa.* [*pureus.*
Burning Bush; a local name for *Euonymus atropur-*
Bursa, Búr-sa; a membranous sac, containing fluid, lying between parts, to reduce friction.
Butter-Cup; a common name for several species of *Ranunculus.* [milk-weed.
Butterfly-Weed; *Asclepias tuberosa*, an indigenous
Butternut; *Juglans cinerea*, an American tree.
Butter of Antimony; a name applied to antimonious chloride.

Button-Bush; *Cephalanthus Occidentalis;* an indigenous shrub.

Button-Snakeroot; *Liatris spicata;* also sometimes applied to *Eryngium yuccæfolium.*

Butyric Acid, Bu̧-tír-ik —; an acid found in rancid [butter.

C

C., an abbreviation for "compound," or "composite;" also, a symbol for the element Carbon.

Ca., symbol for the element Calcium.

Cabbage-tree Bark; the bark of *Andira inermis;* a tree of West Indies; cathartic and anthelmintic.

Cacao Butter; Ka-ká-ω —; a concrete oil expressed from the seed of the *Theobroma Cacao;* chiefly used in making suppositories.

Cachelcoma, Kak-el-kώ-ma; a malignant ulcer.

Cachexia, Ka-kéks-i-a; bad condition of body.

Cachectic, Ka-kék-tik; relating to cachexia.

Cacocolpia, Kak-ω-kól-pi-a; vitiated condition of the vulva and vaginal orifice.

Cacoethes, Kak-ω-é-thēz; a bad or vitiated breath.

Cactus Grandiflora, Kák-tus Gran-di-flώ-ra; Night-blooming Cereus; synonym for Cereus grandiflora.

Cadaver, Ka-dáv-er; a dead body.

Cadmium; Kád-mi-um; an elemental metal, resembling [tin.

Caduca, Ka-dū̧-ka; a deciduous membrane of the uterus.

Cæcal, Sé-kal; belonging to the cæcum, or blind gut.

Cæcitis, Sē-kį-tis, inflammation of the cæcum.

Cæcum, Sé-kum; the blind gut, or head of the colon.

Cæsarean Operation, Ses-a-ré-an — the making of an incision through the abdomen into the uterus for the removal of a fœtus.

Cæsalpina Crista, Ses-al-pį-na Krís-ta; a tree of South America, that yields Brazil wood.

Caffea Arabica, Kaf-é-a Ar-áb-i-ka; a small tree that yields coffee.

Caffein, Ka-fē-in; a feeble organic base, obtained from tea and coffee.

Cajeput Oil, Káj-ŭ-put —; a greenish, volatile oil, distilled from the fermented leaves of *Melaleuca cajupui*, a stimulant.

Calabar Bean, Kál-a-bɑr —; the poisonous seed of an African vine, *Physostigma venenosum;* in small doses a sedative, but chiefly used to contract the pupils of the eye.

Calamine, Kál-a-min; *Lapis Calaminaris;* the native carbonate of zinc mineral.

Calamus, Kál-a-mus; the roots of the *Acorus Calamus.* or sweet flag, an aromatic tonic.

Calamus Draco, — Drá-kō; a small palm of the East Indies, the source of Dragon's Blood.

Calcaneum, Kal-ká-nĕ-um; the large tarsal bone.

Calcarea Carbonica, Kal-ká-rĕ-a Kɑr-bón-i-ka; carbonate of lime.

Calcarea Caustica, — Kós-ti-ka; oxide of lime.

Calcarea Phosphorica, — Fos-fór-i-ka; phosphate of lime.

Calcination, Kal-sin-á-ʃon; intense heat applied to mineral substances. [lime.

Calcium, Kál-ʃi-um; a metalic element, the base of

Calculus, Kál-kų-lus; (*pl. Calculi;*) stone or gravel; a concretion found in the bladder, gall duct, kidneys and the joints. [warmth.

Calefacient, Kal-ĕ-fá-ʃi-ent; applications that excite

Calendula Officinalis, Ka-lén-dų-la —; the garden Marigold, a tincture from which is recommended for dressing wounds.

Caligo, Ka-lį-gō; blindness, dimness of vision.

Caligo Lentis, — Lén-tis; cataract of the eye.

Calisaya, Kal-i-sá-ya; yellow Cinchona; the bark of *Cinchona calisaya.*

Callosity, Ka-lós-i-ti; hardness; callous condition of the skin in places usually soft.

Callus, Kál-us; bony matter found between the ends of fractured bones.

Calomel, Kál-ō-mel; mercurious chloride; mild chloride of mercury.

Caloric, Ka-lór-ik; the agent to which the phenomena of heat and combustion are ascribed.—(*Ure.*)

Calorific, Kal-or-íf-ik; heat-producing.

Calumba, Ka-lúm-ba; the root of an African vine, *Cocculus palmatus;* Columbo root.

Calvaria, Kal-vá-ri-a; the part of the cranium above the temples and ears.

Calvities, Kal-ví-ʃi-ēz; absence of hair; baldness.

Calx, Kalks; lime prepared by calcination.

Calx Viva, — Vī-va; quick lime.

Calyces, Kál-i-ēz; small membranous sacs that denote the papillæ of the kidneys.

Camera, Kám-ē-ra; a chamber; used in the plural to denote the anterior and posterior chambers of the eye.

Camphor, Kám-for; a concrete substance obtained by sublimation from the wood of the *Camphora officinarum,* an evergreen tree of China.

Camphorated Soap Liniment; an officinal preparation; Opodeldoc.

Canada Balsam; a semi-fluid turpentine, obtained from *Abies balsamea;* also called *balsam of fir.*

Canada Fleabane, — Flē-ban; *Erigeron Canadense;* a common weed.

Canada Snakeroot; wild ginger, the root of *Asarum* [*Canadense.*

Canal; Kan-ál; any tube, duct, or channel of the body.

Canal of Fontana; a small canal within the ciliary ligament.

Canal of Petit, — Pe-tē; a triangular vessel around the crystalline lens.

Canaliculated; grooved into channels.

Canalis Arteriosus, Ka-ná-lis Ar-tē-ri-ó-sus; the vessel that connects the aorta and pulmonary artery in the fœtus.

Canalis Venosus, — Vē-nó-sus; the vessel that unites the *vena porta* with the *vena cava,* in the fœtus.

Cancellated; formed of *cancelli,* lattices, or small appartments.

Canarium Commune, Kan-á-ri-um Kom-ūn; a tree of South America, supposed to yield *Elemi.*

Cancer, Kán-ser; a scirrhous tumor, terminating in a malignant ulcer.

Cancer-Root; *Epiphegus Virginiana*. See Beech Drops.
Cancroid, Kán-krød; resembling cancer.
Cancrum Oris, Kán-krum Ꞷ'ris; a deep and fetid ulcer of the gums and cheek.
Canella Alba, Ca-nél-ɑ Al'bɑ; a tree of the West Indies, the bark of which is an aromatic tonic.
Cane Sugar; a sweet substance found in the sap of many grasses and trees and the root of beets.
Canine Madness. See Hydrophobia.
Canine Teeth; the eye-teeth, or the four which are next to the incisors.
Caninus Spasmus; Ka-nį-nus Spáz-mus; spasms of patients having the hydrophobia.
Canities, Ka-ní-ʃi-ēz; grayness of the hair.
Canna Starch, Kán-ɑ Stɋrç; a peculiar fecula obtained from the roots of several species of Canna.
Cannabis Indica, Kán-a-bis In'di-kɑ; considered a variety of *Cannabis Sativa*,
Cannabis Sativa, Kán-a-bis Sa-tį-vɑ; the common cultivated hemp.
Cannabis Sativa var. Indica; the hemp plant of India commonly known as *Cannabis Indica*, an extract from which is a powerful narcotic, the Hashish of the Arabs.
Cannula, Kán-ɥ-lɑ; a hollow surgical instrument for drawing fluid from a tumor or cavity.
Cantharidal Collodion, Kan-ŧár-i-dal Ko-lꞶ́-di-on; a vesicating solution, made of cantharides, sulphuric ether, and gun cotton.
Cantharides, Kan-ŧár-i-dēz; green beetles, found in the temperate portions of Europe; also known as Spanish flies.
Cantharis Vesicatoria, Kán-ŧar-is Ves-i-ka-tꞶ́-ri-ɑ; the cantharides beetle; externally used to form blisters; internally a stimulant to the urinary organs.
Canthitis, Kan-ŧį-tis; inflammation of the *canthi*.
Canthoplasty, Kán-ŧꞶ-plas-ti; the transplanting of a part of the *conjunctiva* of the eye-ball to the external *canthus* of the eye-lids.
Canthus, (*pl. Canthi;*) the angle of the eye-lids.
Caoutchouc; Kɋ-ứ-ɋuk; India rubber; the thickened juice of several species of tropical trees.

Cape Aloes, Káp Al'ωz; the variety of aloes yielded by the *Aloe spicata.*

Capillary, Káp-i-la-ri; hair-like; in the plural, minute vessels on the surface of the body, which communicate with the arteries and veins.

Capilliculus, Kap-i-lík-ų-lus; arterial and venous radicals more minute than capillaries, that pervade the elements of every organ.

Capital, Káp-i-tal; belonging to the head; in surgery the more important operations.

Capitiluvium, Kap-i-ti-lų́-vi-um; a wash for the head.

Capitulum, Ka-pít-ų-lum; a rounded projection of bone.

Capsicum, Káp-si-kum; a plant of South America, the fruit of which is Cayenne, or red pepper; it is a powerful stimulant.

Capsula, Káp-sų-la; a membranous sac or case, for containing some part, organ, or joint.

Capsular Ligament; a fibrous sac surrounding every movable joint, and containing the synovial fluid.

Capsule of Glisson; the envelope enclosing the liver.

Capsules Renal; two triangular bodies that lie over the kidneys, in the fœtus, becoming, in the adult, lobes.

Capsulitis, Kap-sų-lį-tis; inflammation of the eye.

Caput, Ká-put; the head, comprising the head and face; also, any prominent object like a head.

Caput Coli, — Kώ-lį; the cæcum, or head of the colon.

Caramel, Kár-a-mel; burned sugar, used in coloring liquors.

Caraway, Kár-a-wa; the fruit of *Carum Carui;* aromatic and carminative.

Carbazotates, Kąr-ba-zώ-tats; salts of carbazotic or picric acid; the ammonium salt is used as an anti-periodic.

Carbo Animalis, Kár-bω An-i-má-lis; animal charcoal; bone-black.

Carbolic Acid; Phenol; the chief constituent of the acid portion of coal-tar oil.

Carbo Ligni, Kár-bω Líg-nį; wood charcoal.

Carbon, Kár-bon; an element which forms a large portion of all organic structures.

Carbonic Acid; a compound of oxygen and carbon, which is largely given off by all animals; carbon dioxide.

Carbo Vegetabilis, — Vej-ĕ-táb-i-lis; wood charcoal, a name used mainly by Homœopathists.

Carbuncle, Kq́r-buŋ-kl; a painful inflammation, of a gangrenous nature. [in an ulcer.

Carcinoma, Kqr-si-nó-mq; a scirrhous tumor, ending

Cardamom Seed, Kq́r-da-mom —; the fruit *Elettaria Cardamomum;* aromatic and stimulant. [the stomach.

Cardia, Kq́r-di-q; the heart; the superior opening of

Cardiac Plexus, — Plék-sus; the junction of the nerves situated behind the arch of the aorta.

Cardiagra, Kqr-dị-a-grq; gout of the heart. [stomach.

Cardialgia, Kqr-di-ál-ji-q; heart-burn, or pain in the

Cardiectasis, Kqr-di-ék-ta-sis; dilatation of the heart.

Cardinal Flower; *Lobelia cardinalis;* an indigenous, showy plant.

Cardiocele, Kq́r-di-ω-sĕl; the protrusion of the heart through an opening in the diaphragm.

Cardiopalmus, Kqr-di-ω-pál-mus; palpitation, or fluttering of the heart.

Cardiorhexis, Kqr-di-ω-rék-sis; rupture of the heart.

Cardiotromus. Same as *Cardiopalmus.*

Carduus Benedictus; synonym for *Cnicus benedictus.*

Carditis, Kqr-dị-tis; inflammation of the heart.

Cardo, Kq́r-dω; a hinge, or articulation.

Caries, Ká-rí-ĕz; ulceration of a bone.

Carious, Ká-ri-us; affected with caries.

Carminative, Kqr-mín-a-tiv; a medicine that relieves pain or flatulence. [from cochineal.

Carmine, Kq́r-mịn; a red coloring matter, obtained

Carneous, Kq́r-nĕ-us; fleshy; relati, g to flesh

Carnification, Kqr-ni-fi-ká-ʃon; turning into flesh.

Caroticus, Ka-rót-i-kus; the quality of stupefying.

Carotid, Ka-rót-id; applied to the artery on each side of the neck that conveys blood to the head.

Carpalia, Kqr-pá-li-q; the bones of the carpus.

Carphology, Kqr-fól-ω-ji; the motions of delirious patients, in picking at the bed clothes, etc., which are considered unfavorble symptoms.

Carpus, Kɑ́r-pus; the wrist, composed of eight bones uniting the hand with the fore-arm.

Carrot Seed; seed of *Daucus Carota.*

Carthamus Tinctorius, Kɑ́r-tħa-mus Tiŋk-tṓ-ri-us; the safflower, a cultivated plant, that yields American saffron.

|bones.

Cartilage, Kɑ́r-ti-lej; gristle attached to the joints of

Cartilaginous, Kɑr-ti-láj-in-us; having the nature of cartilage.

Carum Carui, Ká-rum Kár-ų-ị; an umbelliferous plant of Europe, which produces caraway.

Caruncula, Kar-úŋ-kų-lɑ; a small flesby excrescence; a carbuncle.

Caryophyllus Aromaticus, Car-i-óf-i-lus Ar-ɷ-mát-i-kus; a small tree of tropical islands, which yields cloves.

Cascarilla, Kas-ka-ríl-ɑ; an aromatic bark from *Croton Eleuteria.*

[from milk.

Casein, Ká-sī-in; an albuminous substance obtained

Cashew Nut, Ka-ʃų́-nut; a kidney-shaped nut obtained from the West Indies.

Cassia, Káʃ-i-ɑ; an extensive genus of plants possessing cathartic principles; also a name applied to the coarser varieties of cinnamon bark.

Cassia Acutifolia, and **C. Elongata;** plants of Africa and India which yield senna.

Cassia Fistula, — Fís-tų-lɑ; a tree of the tropics, which yields the purging cassia pods.

Cassia Marilandica, — Me-ri-lán-di-kɑ; an indigenous plant; American senna.

Castanea Vesca, Kas-tá-nī-ɑ Vés-kɑ; the chestnut tree, the leaves of which are recommended for whooping cough.

Castile Soap, a mild soap, made of olive oil and soda.

Castor, Kás-tor; the dried preputial follicles of the beaver, (*Castor fiber.*)

Castor Leaves, the leaves of *Ricinus communis,* used to increase the flow of milk.

Castor Oil; a fixed oil, expressed from the seed of *Ricinus communis,* a powerful cathartic.

Castration; the removal of the testicles.

Catalepsy, (*Catalepsia, Catalepsis;*) trance, suspension of sensibility and motion.

Cataleptic; relating to catalepsy.

Catalytic, Kat-a-lít-ik; having the quality of destroying or decomposing.

Catamenia, Kat-a-mḗ-ni-a; the menses, or monthly discharge from the uterus.

Cataphora, Ka-táf-ω-ra; a kind of lethargy in which there are intervals of partial consciousness.

Cataplasm, Kát-a-plazm; a poultice of any kind, sometimes medicated.

Cataract, Kát-a-rakt; opacity of the crystalline lens of the eye, or its capsule, obstructing vision.

Catarrh, Ka-tár; cold in the head or chest; also, a discharge of mucous fluid from the bladder, from disease of that organ.

Catastaltic, Kat-as-tál-tik; the quality of restraining or checking, as astringent medicines.

Catechu, Kát-ē-çu; an astringent extract obtained from the wood of *Acacia Catechu.*

Cathæretic, Kaŧ-ē-rét-ik; slightly caustic.

Catharsis; Ka-ŧár-sis; purging, removing the excrement, naturally or medicinally.

Cathartic; having the quality of purging.

Catheter, Káŧ-ē-ter; a tube for artificially emptying the bladder, in cases of retention.

Catholicon, Ka-ŧól-i-kon; universal; applied to medicines that it is claimed cure many diseases.

Catling, Kát-liŋ; a double-edged knife, used in amputations.

Catnep, Kát-nep; *Nepeta Cataria;* a common weed.

Cat's Purr; a peculiar sound of the chest, heard by means of the stethoscope.

Cauda, Ké-da; the tail; *cauda equina;* termination of the spinal cord.

Caul, Kel; omentum; a portion of the amnion that sometimes covers the head of the child at birth.

Cauliflower Excrescence; encephalosis; a disease of the *os uteri.*

Caulophyllum Thalictroides, Ke-lω-fíl-um Ŧa-lik-trω-í-dēz; blue cohosh; an emenagogue and parturient; formerly *Leontice thalictroides.*

Cauma, Ké-ma; the excessive heat of fever.

Caustic, Kés-tik; Lunar caustic, fused nitrate of silver, moulded in the form of sticks.

Caustic Lime, or **Quick Lime;** oxide of calcium, common lime.

Caustic Potash, or **Potassa;** potassium hydrate, a powerful caustic.

Caustic Soda, Sodium hydrate, similar in properties to potassium hydrate.

Causus, Ké-sus; a malignant remittent fever.

Cauterization, Ke-ter-i-zá-ʃon; the act of applying caustic, or of hot iron.

Cau'tery, Ké-ter-i; the application of caustic, or of hot iron; also employed as the name of the substance applied.

Cautery, Actual; the actual burning by fire, or heated iron, for the cure of a diseased part.

Cautery, Potential; the use of caustic substances, as above noted.

Cavernus Sinus, Káv-er-nus Sį-nus; a depression or cavity at the base of the brain.

Cayenne Pepper. See *Capsicum.*

Cd.; symbol for the element Cadmium.

Ce.; symbol for the element Cerium.

Ceanothus Americanus, Sē-án-ω-ŧus A-mer-i-ká-nus; Jersey tea; an astringent.

Cecal, Sé-kal; relating to the cæcum.

Cedron, Sé-dron; the seed *Simaba Cedron,* recommended as a tonic and antiperiodic.

Celandine, Sél-an-din; a common naturalized plant, with a yellow juice, *Chelidonium majus.*

Celastrus Scandens; Sē-lás-trus Skán-denz; a climbing shrub, the false bittersweet; used chiefly in scrofulous affections.

Cell, Sel; any hollow space; the beginning of every animal and vegetable organization.

Cellular Tissue; (or membrane;) the network of tissue which connects the most minute portions of the body.

Cellule, or **Cellula;** a small cell.

Cellulose, Sél-ų-lωs; the woody fiber of plants.

Celotomy, Sē-lót-ō-mi; the operation for the cure of hernia.

Centaurea Benedicta, Sen-té-rē-ɑ Ben-ē-dík-tɑ; a synonym for *Cnicus benedictus*.

Centaury, American, Sén-te-ri —; *Sabbatia angularis*; a native bitter herb.

Centigrade Thermometer, a thermometer in which the freezing point of water is made zero (0°), and the boiling point 100°.

Cephaelis Ipecacuanha, Sef-a-ē-lis Íp-ē-kak-ṳ-án-ɑ; a little shrubby plant of Brazil that produces ipecac root.

Cephalanthus Occidentalis; Sef-a-lán-thus Ok-si-den-tá-lis; button-bush, the bark of which is tonic and febrifuge.

Centrum Commune, Sén-trum Kóm-ṳn; the solar [plexus.

Cephalæa; Sef-a-lē-ɑ; diseases of the head.

Cephalæmia, Sef-a-lē-mi-ɑ; conjestion of the brain.

Cephalagra, Sē-fál-a-grɑ; gouty, or rheumatic affection of the head.

Cephalic, Sē-fál-ik; relating to the head.

Cephalic Vein; the anterior vein at the elbow.

Cephalitis; Sef-a-lī-tis; inflammation of the brain.

Cephalodinia, Sef-a-lō-dín-i-ɑ; headache of any nature.

Cephaloma, Sef-a-lṓ-mɑ; a species of tumor, the substance of which resembles brain.

Cephalometer, Sef-a-lóm-ē-ter; an instrument for measuring the head of a fœtus during parturition.

Cephalotomy, Sef-a-lót-ō-mi; dissection or destruction of the fœtal head, in cases of ineffectual labor.

Cephalotribe, Séf-a-lō-trīb; an instrument employed in cephalotomy.

Cera Alba, Sē-rɑ Al'bɑ; white wax; yellow wax bleached by exposure to sunlight.

Cera Flava, — Flā-vɑ; beeswax; yellow wax.

Cerasus Lauro-cerasus, Sē-rá-sus —; the cherry laurel tree; a synonym for *Prunus Lauro-cerasus*.

Cerasus Virginiana, — Vɛr-jin-i-á-nɑ. Same as *Prunus serotina*.

Cerate, Sē-rat; mixture of oil or lard with wax, spermaceti, or resin; usually medicated.

Ceratocele, Sī-rát-ω-sīl; hernia of the cornea.
Ceratonyxis, Sī-rat-ω-nik-sis; puncturing the cornea in operating for cataract.
Ceratoplastica, Sī-rat-ω-plás-ti-ka; the formation of an artificial cornea. [the cornea.
Ceratotome, Sī-rát-ω-tωm; a knife used for dividing
Ceratotomy, Sī-ra-tót-ω-mi; the process of dividing the cornea.
Ceratum, Sī-rá-tum; a cerate; compounded of wax, or other body, and medicinal constituents.
Cereus Grandiflorus, Sí-rī-us Gran-di-fló-rus; a West Indian cactus plant, used in heart diseases; synonym for *Cactus grandiflora.*
Cerchnus, Sérk-nus; a wheezing kind of respiration.
Cerebelitis, Ser-ī-bel-ị-tis; inflammation of the *cerebellum.*
Cerebellum, Ser-ī-bél-um; the smaller portion of the brain, overlying the fourth ventricle, in the lower and back part of the cranium.
Cerebral; Sér-í-bral; relating to or like brain.
Cerebric, Ser-í-brik; applied to a fatty acid in the brain. [of brain.
Cerebriform, Ser-í-bri-fωrm; resembling the nature
Cerebritis Ser-ī-brị-tis; inflammation of the brain.
Cerebro-Spinal; Ser-í-brω-Spị-nal; pertaining to both the brain and the spinal cord.
Cerebrot, Sér-ī-brot; a fatty substance in the brain, containing phosphorus and sulphur.
Cerebrum, Sér-ī-brum; the brain proper, embracing all lying above the cerebellum.
Cerium, Sí-ri-um; a metallic element the oxalate of which is used in medicine.
Ceroma, Sī-ró-ma; a fatty tumor of the brain.
Cerumen, Sī-rú-men; the wax-like secretion of the ear.
Ceruminous, Sī-rú-min-us; having the nature of cerumen.
Cervical, Sér-vi-kal; belonging to the neck.
Cervix, Sér-viks; the neck, especially the back part; and applied to parts that are narrow like a neck.
Cetaceum, Sī-té-ʃī-um; officinal name for spermaceti, the solid crystalline fat found in the head of the sperm whale.

Cetraria Islandica, Sĕ-trá-ri-ɑ Ĭs-lán-di-kɑ; Iceland moss, a lichen found in cold regions.

Cevadilla, Sev-a-díl-ɑ; the seed of *Veratrum sabadilla,* mostly used to furnish veratria.

Chalaza, Ka-lá-zɑ; *Chalazion;* a small tubercle that forms on the eye-lid chiefly.

Chalk, Ꞓək; native carbonate of calcium.

Chalybeate Water, Ka-líb-ĭ-at —; spring water, containing salts of iron in solution.

Chamælirium Luteum, (Gray,) Kam-ĭ-lír-i-um Lú-tĕ-um; false Unicorn plant; used as tonic, and in diseases of the urinary organs; commonly known as *Helonias dioica.*

Chamomile, Kám-ɷ-mįl; the flowers of *Anthemis nobilis;* tonic in their effects.

Chamomile, German; the flower of *Matricaria Chamomilla;* tonic, similar to chamomile. [poison.

Chancre, Σoṅ-kr; a sore resulting from syphilitic

Change of life; the common phrase indicating the disturbance of the female system at the age when the menstrual discharge ceases.

Charcoal, Ꞓɑ́r-kɷl; a form of carbon obtained by burning wood.

Charpie, Σɑr-pĕ; scraped linen, or fiber obtained from old rags.

Chartæ, Kɑ́r-tĕ; paper; used in prescriptions.

Cheiloplastic, Kį-lɷ-plás-tik; relating to the operation of forming an artificial lip.

Cheiloplasty, Kį́-lɷ-plas-ti; the operation of remedying a defective lip by transferring a portion of healthy skin from an adjacent part.

Chelidonium Majus, Kel-i-dṓ-ni-um Má-jus; celandine, a cathartic and diuretic.

Cheloid, Kḗ-lɵd; a skin disease, causing the surface to look like a tortoise.

Chelone Glabra, Kḗ-lɷn Glá-brɑ; a native plant, balmony; tonic and apperient.

Chemical Compound; elements united by chemism.

Chemical Force; chemism, which see.

Chemical Formula; a collection of symbols representing a molecule.

Chemical Symbol; a capital letter, or a capital and small letter, which represent the name and one atom of an element.

Chemism, Kém-izm, the force which holds molecules and atoms together, and can not be overcome mechanically.

Chemistry, Kém-is-tri; the science which treats of the composition of bodies; and the changes they undergo.

Chemosis, Kē-mṓ-sis; inflammation of the conjunctiva, so that the white of the eye protrudes above the cornea.

Chenopodium Anthelminticum, Kē-nọ-pṓ-di-um; An-thel-mín-ti-kum; American wormseed; a common weed, and an efficient anthelmintic.

Cherry-Laurel, Cér-i Ló-rel; *Prunus Lauro-cerasus;* water distilled from the leaves of which contains a small portion of hydrocyanic acid.

Chevestre, Σa-vá-tr; a kind of double roller used in treating fracture or dislocation of the lower jaw.

Chiasma, Ki-áz-ma; a crossed condition of the fibres of the optic nerve.

Chiaster, Ki-ás-ter; a bandage used to stop hemorrhage of the temporal artery.

Chicken Pox; *Varicella;* the common English for an eruption of smooth, transparent circular vesicles.

Chilblain, Cil-blan; a painful inflammation on the fingers, toes, or heels, resulting from exposure to intense cold.

Child-bed Fever. See Puerperal fever.

Chimaphila Umbellata, Ki-máf-i-la Um-bel-á-ta; pipsissewa; a very small evergreen plant.

Chinoidine, Ki-nǿ-din; an amorphous substance obtained from cinchona after separation of the crystallizable salts; used medicinally like quinine.

Chionanthus Virginica, Ki-ọ-nán-thus —; fringe-tree; the bark of which is used for jaundice.

Chiragra, Kį-ra-gra; gout in the joints of the hand.

Chiretta, Kį-rét-a; *Agathotes Chirayta;* a plant of India, used as a tonic.

Chirurgeon, Kį-rúr-jon. Same as surgeon.

Chirurgery, Kį-rúr-jer-i; the practice of surgery.

Chirurgical, Kį-rúr-ji-kal; relating to surgery.

Chliasma, Klį-áz-ma; a moist, tepid fomentation.
Chloasma, Klō-áz-ma; an affection of the skin, causing it to appear a yellowish brown in spots.
Chloral, Klṓ-ral; a colorless liquid, formed by passing chlorine into pure alcohol; applied to chloral hydrate in commerce.
Chloral Hydrate, — Hį́-drat; a combination of chloral and water, which forms a white crystalline solid; used to produce sleep.
Chlorates, Klṓ-rats; salts of chloric acid.
Chloric Acid, an unstable acid containing one atom each of hydrogen and chlorine and three of oxygen.
Chlorides, Klṓ-rįdz; compounds of chlorine with an element.
Chlorine, Klṓ-rin; a non-metallic element. [water.
Chlorine Water; an officinal solution of chlorine in
Chlorinated Lime; bleaching powder; chloride of lime, a mixture of hypochlorite and chloride of calcium.
Chlorodyn, Klṓ-rō-dín; name applied to a mixture of chloroform, alcohol, morphia, and other strong medicinal substances; used for colic.
Chloroform, Klṓ-rō-form; a colorless volatile liquid; made by distilling alcohol with chlorinated lime; the most valuable anæsthetic.
Chlorometer, Klō-róm-ē-ter; an instrument for measuring the quantity of chlorine in combination with water or a base.
Chlorosis, Klō-rṓ-sis; green sickness, or disease caused in young females by the suppression of the menses.
Choke Damp; Cōk Damp; the miner's term for such non-respirable gases, especially carbonic acid gas, as accumulate in under ground mines. [of ox-gall.
Cholate of Sodium, Kṓ-lat of Sṓ-di-um; a constituent
Cholagogue, Kól-a-gog; a medicine that produces the discharge of bile.
Cholecystitis, Kol-ē-sis-tį́-tis; inflammation of the gall bladder.
Choleic, Kol-ḗ-ik; relating to bile.
Cholein, Kol-ḗ-in; the peculiar principle of bile.

Cholera, Kól-ĕ-ra; a flow of bile; name of a virulent disease, in which vomiting and purging of bile, with painful griping, accompanied with cramps, are the striking features.
Cholera Infantum, — In-fán-tum; "summer complaint" in children; vomiting and purging, the discharges green, and often mixed with slime and blood.
Cholera Morbus, — Mór-bus, violent bilious vomiting and purging, sometimes accompanied with spasms.
Cholericus, Kol-ér-i-kus; relating to cholera, or bilious.
Choleroid, Kol-er-óđ; like cholera.
Cholerophobia, Kol-er-ω-fώ-bi-a; dread, or apprehension of cholera.
Cholerophone, Kol-er-ω-fώ-nĕ; the peculiar weak and whispering voice of patients having the cholera.
Cholesteatoma, Kol-es-tĕ-a-tώ-ma; a species of fatty tumor, composed chiefly of crystals of cholesterin.
Cholesteræmia, Kol-es-ter-ĕ-mi-a; a morbid accumulation of cholesterin in the blood.
Cholesterin, Kol-és-ter-in; *Cholerina;* a pearl-like substance, of which biliary calculi are chiefly formed.
Cholic, Kól-ik; bilious, relating to bile.
Chololithic, Kol-ω-lĭŧ-ik; belonging to the biliary calculi, or gall-stone.
Chololithus, Kω-lól-i-ŧus; a biliary calculi, or gall-stone.
Cholosis, Kω-lώ-sis; (*pl. Choloses*); biliary diseases.
Chondralgia, Kon-drál-ji-a; rheumatic pain in the cartilages. [cornea, etc.
Chondrin, Kón-drin; gelatine procured from cartilages,
Chondrogen, Kón-drω-jen; the base, or pure substance of cartilage.
Chondroglossus, Kon-drω-glós-us; a small muscular fibre, extending from the cartilage of the *os hyoides* to the tongue.
Chondroma, Kon-drώ-ma; a growth of cartilage.
Chondrosis, Kon-drώ-sis; formation of cartilage. [lage.
Chondrotomy, Kon-drót-ω-mi; the dividing of a carti-
Chondrus Crispus, Kón-drus Krís-pus; Irish moss; an alga, or sea weed, obtained principally from the coast of Ireland.

Chorda Tympani, Kór-da Tim-pán-i; one branch of the seventh pair of nerves.
Chorda Ventriculi, — Ven-trík-u-li; "nerve of the stomach;" the plexus of the pneumogastric nerve.
Chordæ Tendineæ, Kór-dē; Ten-dín-i-ē; cords connecting with the valves of the heart.
Chordæ Vocales, Kór-dē Vo-ká-lēz; vocal ligaments.
Chordapsus, Kor-dáp-sus; a violent spasmodic cholic, the large intestines seeming to twist into knots.
Chordee, Kór-dē; a painful erection, and downward curvature of the penis in gonorrhea.
Chorea, Ko-rē-a; St Vitus' dance, manifested by involuntary twitching of the muscles and limbs.
Choreic, Ko-rē-ik; pertaining to chorea. [fœtus.
Chorion, Kó-ri-on; the external membrane of the
Chorium, Kó-ri-um; the skin; the internal lining of the outer coating of the skin; also termed *Chorion*.
Choroid, Kó-roid; like the chorion, applied to several membranes in the brain, and the inner tunic of the eye.
Choroid Plexus; — Plék-sus; a fold of thin membrane, near the latteral ventricles of the brain.
Chromates, Kró-mats; salts of chromic acid.
Chromic Acid, Kró-mik As'id; a brilliant crimson crystalline acid of chromium, used as a caustic.
Chronic, Krón-ik; of long continuance, as compared with acute.
Chronothermal. Kro-no-thér-mal; time and temperature, representing the idea that all diseases have periodic alternations of chill and heat.
Chrotic, Krót-ik; relating to the skin.
Chrysophanic Acid, Kris-o-fán-ik —; a yellow vegetable acid, obtained from rhubarb root and Goa powder; used for skin diseases.
Chyle, Kil; the milk-like fluid in the thoracic duct and lacteal vessels, from which the blood is formed.
Chyliferous, Ki-líf-er-us; carrying or bearing chyle.
Chylification, Ki-lif-i-ká-shon; the process that converts the chyme into chyle.
Chylopoietic, Ki-lo-poi-ét-ik; concerned in the formation of chyle.
Chylosis, Ki-ló-sis. Same as Chylification.

Chyluria, Kị-lṻ-ri-a; the passage of chyle with urine.

Chyme, Kịm; food in the process of digestion, after it has left the stomach.

Chymification, Kịm-i-fi-ká-ʃon; the change of food into chyme.

Cicatricula, Sik-a-trík-ụ-la; a small scar.

Cicatrix, Sík-a-triks; the seam or scar of a healed cut, sore, or ulcer,

Cicatrization, Sik-a-tri-zá-ʃon; the healing of a sore, and formation of a cicatrix.

Cicatrize, Sík-a-trịz; to form a scar, in healing.

Cicely Sweet, Sís-i-li Swēt; *Osmorrhiza longistylis*, the root of which is aromatic.

Cicuta Maculata, Si-kṻ-ta Mak-ụ-lá-ta; water hemlock, a native poisonous plant, narcotic; but seldom used in medicine.

Cicuta Virosa, — Vi-ró-sa; the poisonous water hemlock of Europe.

Cilia, Síl-i-a; the eye-lashes; applied also to minute vibrating hairs on certain animals.

Ciliary, Síl-i-a-ri; relating to the eye-lashes.

Cilium, Síl-i-um; the edge of the eye-lid, out of which the hairs grow.

Cilosis, Si-ló-sis; spasmodic movements of the eye-lids.

Cimex Lectularius, Sị-meks Lek-tụ-lá-ri-us; the common bed-bug, used homœopathically.

Cimicifuga Racemosa, Sim-i-si-fṻ-ga Ra-sē-mó-sa; black cohosh, used in uterine diseases; synonym for Macrotys racemosa.

Cimicifugin, Sim-i-si-fṻ-jin; macrotin, a resinous substance obtained from the root of *Cimicifuga racemosa*.

Cinchona, Sin-kó-na; an extensive genus of South American trees, which yield the many different varieties of Peruvian bark.

Cinchonia, Sin-kó-ni-a; an alkaloid from cinchona bark.

Cinchonidia, Sin-ko-níd-i-a; an alkaloid from cinchona, an anti-periodic.

Cinnabar, Sín-a-bạr; native sulphide of mercury.

Cinnamomum Zeylanicum, Sin-a-mó-mum Ze-lán-i-kum; a small tree of India, which yields Ceylon cinnamon bark.

Cinquefoil, Sín-kwē-fœl; *Potentilla Canadensis*, five-finger, a native creeping herb.
Cionitis, Si-ω-nį-tis; inflammation of the uvula.
Cionotomy Si-ω-nót-ω-mi; cutting away part of the uvula, when too long.
Circulation, Sɛr-kų-lá-ʃon; the flowing of the blood from the heart through the arteries and veins, to the surface, thence back to the heart.
Circulus, Sɛ́r-kų-lus; a ring, or circle; applied to any part of the body that is circular.
Circumagentes, Sɛr-kum-a-jén-tēz; the oblique muscles of the eye.
Circumcision, Sɛr-kum-sí-ʒon; the operation of cutting off a part of the prepuce.
Circumflex, Sɛ́r-kum-fleks; rounded, or curved; applied to various arteries and veins.
Cirrhonosus Sir-on-ώ-sus; yellow appearance of the pleura, peritoneum, etc., in the fœtus.
Cirrhosis, Sir-ώ-sis; used to describe the tuberculated condition of the liver; also to a disease of the kidneys.
Cirsocele, Sɛ́r-sω-sēl; enlargement of the spermatic vein.
Cirsomphalos, Sɛr-sóm-fa-los; a varicose condition of the navel.
Cirsophthalmia, Sɛr-sof-ŧál-mi-ɑ; varicose affection of the parts of the eye.
Cirsos, Sɛ́r-sos; the varix, a dilated vein.
Cirsotomy, Sɛr-sót-ω-mi; the remov∂l of the varix.
Cissampelos Pareira, Sis-ám-pē-los Pɑ-rá-rɑ; a Brazilian climbing plant, that yields pareira brava root.
Cistus Canadensis, Sís-tus Kan-a-dén-sis; rock-rose; synonym for *Helianthemum Canadense*.
Citrates, Sít-rats; salts of citric acid.
Citric Acid, Sít-rik As'id; a common vegetable acid, obtained from the juice of lemons and limes.
Citrine Ointment, Sít-rin Ʊnt-ment; ointment of nitrate of mercury.
Citrullus Colocynthis, Si-trúl-us Kol-ω-sín-ŧis; a plant of Africa, that produces the colocynth apple.
Citrullus Vulgaris, — Vul-gá-ris; water-melon, the seed of which are diuretic.

Citrus, Sį-trus; a genus of southern trees, which yield oranges, lemons, limes, and bergamot oil.

Cl., symbol for the element chlorine.

Clap, Klap; the vulgar term for gonorrhœa.

Clarification, Klar-i-fi-ká-ʃon; the purifying or filtering a liquid.

Clavate, Kláv-at; club-shaped, or something like a club.

Clavicle, Kláv-i-kl; literally, a key; the collar-bone.

Clavicular, Kla-vík-ų-lar; relating to the clavicle, or collar-bone.

Claviculate, Kla-vík-ų-lat; possessed of clavicles, as [man and ape.

Claviform, Kláv-i-form; shaped like a club.

Clavus, Klá-vus; a nail or spike, but applied to a round horny cutaneous growth, on the angular parts of the toes; also to a pain in the head, as if a nail were being driven into it.

Cleavers, Klēv-erz; a common annual weed, *Galium* [*Aparine*.

Cleido, Klį-dœ; a prefix, signifying connection with the clavicle.

Cleisagra, Klįs-a-gra; gouty pain in the clavicle.

Clematis Virginica, Klém-a-tis Vɛr-jín-i-ka; virgin's bower, used as a diuretic and sudorific.

Climacter, Klį-mák-ter; a stair or step, as in the supposed seven stages or periods of human life.

Climacteric, Klį-mák-ter-ik; applied to any stage in human life indicated by the periodic seven years when the body was supposed by the ancients to be peculiarly sensitive to change.

Climacteric Disease; the morbid symptoms that generally occur in advanced life, usually about the time of the grand climacteric, namely, at nine times seven, or sixty-three.

Clinic, Klín-ik; (Fr. *Clinique*,) a school, or lecture, where the science of medicine is taught by the practical treatment of patients.

Clinical, Klín-ik-al; relating to a bed, as that of a patient under treatment.

Clinoid, Klį-nœd; like a bed, certain processes of the sphenoid bone.

Cliseometer, Klis-ē-óm-ē-ter; an instrument for measuring the angle of the female pelvis with the body

Clitoris, Klít-ѡ-ris; a small glandiform body, anterior to the vulva, resembling the structure of the male penis.
Clitorismus, Klit-ѡ-rís-mus; a morbid enlargement of the clitoris.
Clitoritis, Klit-ѡ-rį-tis: inflammation of the clitoris.
Clonic, Klón-ik; spasmodic; alternating rigidity and relaxation, as in epilepsy.
Clover, Red; *Trifolium pratense,* from the blossoms of which an extract is made, that is used in making an ointment for dressing ulcers.
Cloves, Klѡvz; the dried flower-buds of *Caryophyllus aromaticus;* aromatic and stimulant.
Cloven Spine, Klṓ-ven Spįn. Same as *Schistorrhachis.*
Club Foot. See *Talipes.*
Club-Moss. *Lycopodium clavatum.*
Clysters, Klís-terz; *Enemata;* injections into the rectum.
Cnicus Benedictus, Knį-kus Ben-ĕ-dik-tus: blessed thistle; a tonic; synonym for *Centaurea benedicta.*
Coagulable, Kѡ-ág-ų-la-bl; possessing the property of coagulation.
Coagulation, Kѡ-ag-ų-lá-ʃon; the thickening of animal or vegetable fluids by the action of acid or heat.
Coagulum, Kѡ-ág-ų-lum; the jelly-like substance produced by the action of acid or heat on blood, milk, etc.
Coaptation, Kѡ-ap-tá-ʃon; accurate adjustment of the ends of a fractured bone.
Coarctation, Kѡ-qrk-tá-ʃon; the straightening and pressing together of strictures of the intestines and urethra.
Coated, Kṓt-ed: covered with a layer of any substance; the condition of the tongue in fever, or when the stomach is deranged.
Cobweb, Kób-web: the web of the common house-spider, used as an anti-periodic.
Coca, Kṓ-ka: *Erythroxyon Coca,* the leaves of which are used as a stimulant.
Cocculus Indicus, Kók-ų-lus In'di-kus: a climbing plant of the East Indies, the source of fish-berries.
Cocculus Palmatus,—Pal-má-tus: an African vine, *Calumba* or *Columbo,* the root of which affords a mild tonic, without astringency.

Coccus Cacti, Kók-us Kák-tī; small insects found on the cactus plants of Mexico; cochineal.
Coccyodynia, Kok-si-ō-dín-i-a; pain in the coccyx, especially in women.
Coccyx, Kók-siks; the lowest point of the vertebral column, triangular in form.
Cochineal, Kóç-i-nēl; the dried female insects of the *Coccus Cacti;* used for coloring purposes, the source of carmine.
Cochlea, Kók-lē-a; a spiral cavity of the internal ear.
Cochleare, Kok-lē-ār; a shell or a spoon; used in prescriptions for a spoonful.
Cochlearia Armoracia, Kok-lē-á-ri-a Ar-mō-rá-ʃi-a; the horse-radish plant, a native of Europe, the root of which is a stimulant. (*Nasturtium Armoracia.*—Fries.)
Cochlearia Officinalis; scurvy grass; a stimulant and diuretic.
Cocoa, Kō-kō-a; the fruit of *Theobroma Cacao.*
Cocoa Butter. See Cacao Butter.
Coco-nut Oil; a fixed oil, expressed from coco-nuts, used in ointments.
Coction; Kók-ʃon; the process of digestion.
Codeia, Kō-dē-ya; an alkaloid obtained from opium.
Cod-liver Oil, Kód-liv-er Oil; an oil obtained from the fresh livers of the cod-fish, (*Gadus Morrhua,*) and much used as a remedy in consumption.
Cœcum, Sē-kum. Same as *Cæcum.*
Cœlia, Sē-li-a; hollow; the lower portion of the belly; also the stomach.
Cœliac, Sē-li-ak; belonging to the belly; applied to an artery and vein of the abdomen.
Cœliac Passion; a chronic flux, in which the discharges are but half digested.
Cœliac Plexus, — Plék-sus. Same as *Solar plexus.* [which see.
Cœliaca, Sē-lī-a-ka; diseases of the digestive organs; medicines that act on these organs.
Cœlialgia, Sē-li-ál-ji-a; pain in the belly or stomach.
Cœnæsthesis, Sen-es-thē-sis; the sensation or general consciousness of existence.
Coffea, Kóf-ē-a; the seed of *Caffea Arabica;* used medicinally in nervous diseases; and the source of caffein.

Cohosh, Black, Kó-hoʃ, —; *Cimicifuga racemosa;*
" **Blue;** *Caulophyllum thalictroides.*
" **White;** *Actæa alba;* for the descriptions of which see the several words.

Coitus, Kó-i-tus; coition, the act of coming together in procreation; chemically, the mixture of substances in close union.

Colchicin, Kól-çi-sin; an alkaloid, or neutral substance; the active principle of colchicum.

Colchicum Autumnale, Kól-çi-kum Θ-tum-ná-lē; a bulbous plant of Europe, the seed and corm, or root, of which is extensively used to stimulate the secretions, and as a sedative to the nervous system.

Cold, Kωld; the usual term for catarrh, or cough.

Cold Cream; a mild ointment, mostly used as a lip-salve.

Colic, Kól-ik; sharp pains in the colon, or abdomen.

Colica Biliosa, Kól-i-kα Bil-i-ó-sα; bilious colic, resulting from an excess of bile in the intestines.

Colica Calculosa, — Kal-kų-ló-sα, colic resulting from calculi in the intestines.

Colica Meconialis, — Mē-kω-ni-á-lis; colic resulting from the failure of infants to pass the meconium, or original contents of the bowels.

Colica Pictorum, — Pik-tó-rum; painter's colic, sometimes called lead colic.

Coliformus, Kol-i-fór-mus; like a sieve, and descriptive of the ethmoid bone.

Colitis, Kω-lį-tis; inflammation of the mucous membrane of the colon.

Collagen, Kól-a-jen; the principal element of bone, cartilage, tendon, etc., from which glue and gelatine are produced.

Collapse, Ko-láps; great prostration of the vital power; the cold stage of fevers.

Collar Bone, Kól-αr-Bωn; the clavicle.

Colliculus, Ko-lík-ų-lus; slight protuberances in the animal organization.

Colliculus Nervi Optici. — Nér-vį Op'ti-kį; a small eminence on the retina where the optic nerve expands.

Colliculus Seminalis, — Sem-i-ná-lis; the crest of the urethra.

Colliquamentum, Kol-ik-wa-mén-tum; the rudiments, or elements, of the embryo, in generation.

Collinsonia Canadensis, Kol-in-sṓ-ni-ɑ Kan-a-dén-sis; stone-root, used in throat diseases.

Colliquative, Ko-lík-wa-tiv; melting; an excessive discharge, or evacuation.

Collodion, Ko-lṓ-di-on; an officinal solution of gun cotton, used to form an artificial film, impervious to moisture and atmosphere.

Colloids, Kól-ɵdz; uncrystallizable substances, of low diffusibility, such as gum and gelatine.

Collodium, Ko-lṓ-di-um. See Collodion.

Collonema, Kol-ɷ-nḗ-mɑ; a soft tumor, containing a clear greyish matter like gelatine.

Collum, Kól-um; the neck, and applied to any part resembling a neck.

Collutorium, Kol-ɥ-tṓ-ri-um; a wash or gargle, for the mouth or throat.

Collyrium, Ko-lír-i-um; a wash for the eyes.

Coloboma Iridis, Kol-ɷ-bṓ-mɑ Ir'i-dis; descriptive of fissures in the iris.

Colocynth, Kól-ɷ-sinŧ; the pulp of the fruit of *Citrullus Colocynthis*, a powerful cathartic.

Colocynthin, Kol-ɷ-sín-ŧin; the bitter purgative principle of the colocynth fruit.

Colon, Kṓ-lon; the second part of the large intestine, extending from the *cœcum* to the *rectum*.

Colostration, Kɷ-los-trá-ʃon; diseases of the infant resulting from the use of the first milk of the mother.

Colostric, Kɷ-lós-trik: relating to the *Colostrum*.

Colostric Fluid; the first impure milk of the mother, usually called "green milk."

Colostrum, Kɷ-lós-trum; a substance in the earliest secretion of milk, that gives it a greenish color.

Colotomy, Kɷ-lót-ɷ-mi; making an incision into the colon.

Colpocele, Kól-pɷ-sēl; hernia of the vagina.

Colt's-Foot, Kɷlt's-Fut; *Tussilago Farfara*, a little naturalized plant found in clayey soil.

Columbo, Kɷ-lúm-bɷ; a valuable tonic. See *Calumba*.

Columbo American. See *Frasera Carolinensis*.

Columna, Kω-lúm-nɑ; a column; parts resembling a column.

Columna Nasi, — Ná-sį; "column of the nose," or the dividing wall of the nose.

Columna Oris, — Ω'ris; the uvula.

Columna Vertebralis, — Vɛr-tē-brá-lis; the spinal column.

Columnæ Carneæ, Kω-lúm-nē Kɋr-nē-ē; muscular projections in the heart.

Columnar, Kω-lúm-nɑr; relating to a column, or projection.

Coma, Kώ-mɑ; lethargy or stupor, occurring in disease.

Coma-Vigil, Kώ-mɑ-Víj-il; lethargy in typhus fever, accompanied with watchful muttering.

Comatose, Kώ-ma-tωs; a state of complete stupor in congestive fevers.

Combustion, Kom-búst-yon; chemical changes evolving heat and light.

Comfrey, Kóm-fri, or Kúm-fri; *Symphytum officinale*, a common garden herb, native of Europe.

Comminuted, Kóm-in-ų-ted; broken into several pieces, as the comminuted fracture of a bone.

Commissura, Kom-i-ʃų́-rɑ; the angular union of parts, as the mouth and eyelids, a suture or joint.

Communicans, Ko-mų́-ni-kans; applied to diseases that may be communicated from one person to another.

Communicantes Arteriæ, Ko-mų-ni-kán-tēz Ar-tē-ri-ē; communicating arteries, of which there are two in the cranium.

Comparative Anatomy; the dissection of the lower animals and vegetables, to illustrate the principles of organization that are common to any class or division.

Compatible, Kom-pát-i-bl; medicines that may be taken together, or near each other as to time, without interference in their action.

Complicated Fracture, Kóm-pli-ka-ted Frák-tųr; the dislocation of a joint in conjunction with a fracture.

Compounds, Kóm-pɤndz; bodies from which two or more essentially different substances can be obtained.

Compound Fracture; a case in which the end of the fractured bone lacerates the integuments, causing an external wound.

Complexus, Kóm-pleks-us; applied to a muscle of the back of the neck that is complicated with the tendons.

Compress, Kóm-pres; a piece of folded linen, or other material, wet or dry, used to lay over a part for treatment.

Compression, Kom-pré-ʃon; a diseased or abnormal condition of a part, usually the brain, caused by something pressing upon it.

Compressor, Kom-prés-or; name of a muscle which presses parts together.

Compressor Prostatæ, — Pros-tá-tē; fibres of the muscles that hold the prostate gland.

Comptonia Asplenifolia, Komp-tṓ-ni-a As-plen-i-fṓ-li-a; sweet fern, tonic and astringent.

Conarium, Kō-ná-ri-um; like a cone, a name given the pineal gland. [glands of the neck.

Concatenate, Kon-kát-ē-nat; linked together, as the

Concentration, Kon-sen-trá-ʃon; strengthening a fluid by the evaporation of the water it contains.

Conception, Kon-sép-ʃon; the impregnation of the ovum in the female by the semen in the male.

Concha, Kóŋ-ka; a shell, the hollow portion of the external ear.

Conchæ Narium, Kóŋ-kē Ná-ri-um; the arched portion of the ethnoid bone, and the spongy bones of the nose.

Conchus, Kóŋ-kus; a shell; the cranium; applied to the cavities of the eye.

Concoction, Kon-kók-ʃon; the change that food undergoes in the stomach. [a solid.

Concrete, Kon-krét; consolidated, as from a liquid to

Concussion, Kon-kú-ʃon; a shock, by a fall or blow, as upon the brain or other organ.

Condensation, Kon-den-sá-ʃon; reducing the bulk of a body, as by converting gas into liquids, and liquids into solids.

Condenser, Kon-dén-ser; an instrument for condensing gas, vapor or air.

Condimenta, Kon-di-mén-ta; spices, etc., taken with food to give it flavor, or promote digestion.

Condyle Kón-dil; a knot or round prominence on the end of a bone in a joint. [like.

Condyloid; Kón-di-loid; resembling a condyle; **wart-**

Condyloma, Kon-di-ló-ma; a hard tumor, or wart-like tubercle, about the anus or pudenda.

Confections, Kon-fék-ʃonz; medicinal substances incorporated with sweet substances, of the consistence of solid extracts.

Confluent, Kón-flu-ent; applied to eruptions where the pustules become so numerous as to run together.

Congelation, Kon-je-lá-ʃon; hardening by freezing solidification.

Congenital, Kon-jén-i-tal; existing at the time of birth.

Congeries, Kon-jé-ri-ez; a mass of small bodies lumped together.

Congestion, Kon-jést-yon; distention of vessels; engorgements of parts.

Congestive, Kon-jés-tiv; tending to produce congestion

Conglobate, Kon-gló-bat; gathered, or formed, into a ball, as the glands of the axilla, and mesentery gland

Conglomerate, Kon-glóm-er-at; to heap together; to blend into one mass; applied to various glands, as the salivary, pancreatic, etc.

Conglutinate, Kon-glú-tin-at; to unite, as by glue; to heal.

Congressus, Kon-grés-us; coitus; the act of procreation

Coni Vasculosi, Kó-ni Vas-ku-ló-si; conical vessels that ascend from the testes.

Conia, Kó-ni-a; *Conine;* a volatile alkaloid, from *Conium maculatum.*

Conium Maculatum, Kó-ni-um Mak-u-lá-tum; hemlock, the leaves and seed of which are used as a narcotic and sedative; poisonous in over-doses.

Conjunctiva, Kon-juŋk-tí-va; the external coating of the eye-ball, and the lining of the eye-lids.

Conjunctivitis, Kon-juŋk-ti-ví-tis; inflammation of the conjunctiva.

Connate, Kón-at; congenital; existing from birth.

Conoid, Kó-nod; cone-like, as the pineal gland.

Conoid Ligament, — Líg-a-ment; a ligament connecting the coracoid process with the clavicle.

Consensus, Kon-sén-sus; sympathy; the relation between certain organs.

Conservancy, Kon-sérv-an-si; preservation, as the prevention of decay in the excreta, with the view of preserving health.

Constipation, Kon-sti-pá-ʃon; costiveness; inaction of the bowels.

Constitutional, Kon-sti-tų-ʃon-al; hereditary, or acquired through the natural growth of the individual.

Constrictive, Kon-strík-tiv; astringent; drawing or holding together.

Constrictor, Kon-strík-tor; applied to muscles that bind together.

Constrictor Ani, — Ȧ'nį; the *Sphincter Ani*.

Constrictor Oris, Ȯ'ris; the *Orbicularis Oris*.

Constrictores Pharyngis, Kon-strik-tó-rēz Fa-rín-jis; muscles that connect with the pharynx.

Constringentia, Kon-strin-jén-ʃi-a; same as astringents; medicines that check the secretions.

Consumption, Kon-súm-ʃon; wasting of the body, especially in tuberculous phthisis.

Contagion, Kon-tá-jon; the dissemination of disease by contact, or inhalation of affluvia from one affected with a contagious disease.

Contagious, Kon-tá-jus; of the nature of diseases that are produced by contagion.

Continuity, Kon-ti-nų́-i-ti; direct connection, without interruption.

Continuity, Solution of; separation by fracture, or cut, of parts before joined.

Contra, Kón-tra; opposite; over against.

Contra-Fissura, — Fi-ʃų́-ra; a fracture on the opposite side to that on which the blow is given producing it.

Contra Indicate; to indicate that a certain medicine should not be used.

Contractile, Kon-trák-til; having the quality of returning to its normal position, after restraint is removed; it is voluntary, as in the hands and tongue, and involuntary as in the heart and stomach.

Contraction, Kon-trák-ʃon; shortening, as of a fibre or muscle.

Contractura, Kon-trak-tų́-ra; a disease terminating in rigidity of the flexor muscles, as rheumatism.

Contusion, Kon-tú-ʒon; a bruise; an injury caused by collision with any hard body, without severing the integuments.

Convalescence, Kon-va-lés-ens; the period following disease and preceding restoration to health.

Convallaria Multiflora, Kon-va-lá-ri-ɑ Mul-ti-fló-rɑ; synonym for *Polygonatum giganteum*.

Convoluta Ossa, Kon-vω-lų́-tɑ Os'ɑ; descriptive of the convexity of the bones of the nose.

Convolution, Kon-vω-lų́-ʃon; a folding or winding substance, as parts of the intestines.

Convolvulus Panduratus, Kon-vól-vų-lus Pan-dų-rá-tus; synonym for *Ipomœa pandurata*.

Convolvulus Scammonia, — Ska-mώ-ni-ɑ; a twining herbaceous vine of Southern Europe, the source of scammony.

Copaiba, Kω-pá-bɑ; (*Copaiva*,) the thickened juice of several species of *Copaifera*, much used in diseases of the mucous membranes.

Copaifera, Kω-pa-íf-er-ɑ; an extensive genus of South American trees, which yield copaiba.

Copper, Kóp-er; *Cuprum*, a metallic element.

Copperas, Kóp-er-as; impure sulphate of iron; green vitriol; ferrous sulphate.

Copragogus, Kop-ra-gώ-gus; (*pl. Copragoga;*) a purgative.

Coprolite, Kóp-rω-lịt; (*Coprolith;*) fœces that become hardened in the bowels.

Coprostasis, Kω-prós-ta-sis; costiveness.

Coptis Trifolia, Kóp-tis Krị-fώ-li-ɑ; gold-thread, the root of which is a bitter tonic.

Copulation, Kop-ų-lá-ʃon; coitus; the act resulting in generation.

Cor, Kor; (*gen. cordis;*) the heart.

Coracoid, Kór-a-kød; like a crow's beak in form; applied to a process of the scapula.

Coracoid Ligament, a small ligament stretching across the notch of the scapula to the coracoid process.

Coracoid Process; a projection on the upper part of the scapula.

Corallorhiza Odontorhiza, Kor-al-ω-rị́-zɑ Ω-don-tω-rị́-zɑ; coral, the crawley root; a leafless orchidaceous plant.

Coral Root, Kór-al Rɷt; the root of *Corallorhiza odontorhiza*, a diaphoretic.

Cordate, Kér-dat; shaped like a heart.

Cordial, Kér-di-al; a mildly stimulating medicine.

Core, Kɷr; the inner part, as the hard center of a boil, or felon; the pupil of the eye.

Corectomia, Kor-ek-tɷ́-mi-ɑ; an operation for the formation of an artificial pupil of the eye.

Corencleisis, Kor-en-klį́-sis; producing an artificial pupil, by the use of part of the iris.

Coreplastica, Kor-ē-plás-ti-kɑ; the general operation for producing an artificial pupil.

Coriander Seed; Kɷ-ri-án-der Sēd; the aromatic fruit of the *Coriandrum sativum*, a cultivated plant, native of Italy.

Corium, Kɷ́-ri-um; the true skin; leather.

Cormus, Kér-mus; a corm; the body of a tree, or bulb of a plant.

Corn, Kérn; a horny growth on the joints of the toes, caused by pressing or rubbing.

Cornea, Kér-nē-ɑ; a circular transparent substance, constituting the anterior part of the eye-ball.

Cornea Opaca, — ɷ-pá-kɑ; the hard coating of the [eye.

Corneitis, Ker-nē-į́-tis; inflammation of the cornea.

Corniculate, Ker-ník-ų-lat; bearing horns, or parts resembling horns.

Corniculum, Ker-ník-ų-lum; a small horny protuberance upon the arytinoid cartilage.

Cornu, Kér-nų; a horn; a horny kind of wart.

Cornu Ammonis, — A-mɷ́-nis; applied to the appearance of the cerebrum, when cut transversely.

Cornus Florida, Kér-nus Flór-i-dɑ; the dog-wood tree, the bark of which is used as a tonic and anti-periodic.

Cornus Sericea, — Sē-rí-ʃē-ɑ; swamp dog-wood, the bark of which is tonic and astringent.

Cornu Ustum, Kér-nų Us'tum; burnt horn.

Corona, Ko-rɷ́-nɑ; a crown; any eminence of bone or other matter.

Corona Veneris, — Vén-ē-ris; syphilitic blotches around the forhead, like a crown.

Coronal Suture, Ko-rṓ-nal Sū́-tụr; the suture uniting the frontal and parietal bones of the cranium.
Coronary, Kór-ọ-na-ri; applied to arteries and veins of the heart, and to ligaments which encircle parts like a crown.
Corone, Ko-rṓ-nē; the process of the lower jaw-bone, resembling in form a crow's beak.
Coronoid, Kór-ọ-nọd; like a crow's beak, as the process of the ulna, jaw-bone, etc.
Corpora, Kór-pọ-ra; plural of *corpus*, body; applied to various prominences in the physical system.
Corpora Albicantia, — Al-bi-kán-ʃi-a; two small elevations at the base of the brain; called, also, mammilary tubercles, on account of their resemblance to nipples.
Corpora Cavernosa, — Kav-er-nṓ-sa; the *crura*, or legs, of the penis, and the corresponding parts of the clitoris.
Corpora Geniculata, — Jen-ik-ụ-lá-ta; the two tubercles on the inferior portion of the optic *thalami*.
Corpora Mammillaria, — Mam-i-lá-ri-a. See *Corpora Albicantia*.
Corpora Olivaria, Ol-i-vá-ri-a; elevations of the medulla oblongata.
Corpora Pyramidalia — Pir-am-i-dá-li-a; the two anterior elevations of the medulla oblongata.
Corpora Quadrigemina, — Kwod-ri-jém-i-na; bodies found under the pineal gland.
Corpora Restiformia, — Res-ti-fór-mi-a; the posterior elevations that connect the medulla oblongata to the cerebellum.
Corpora Striata, — Strị-á-ta; two striped bodies in the lateral ventricles of the brain.
Corpus, Kór-pus; a body.
Corpus Callosum, — Ka-lṓ-sum; a white substance separating the hemispheres of the brain.
Corpus Cavernosum, — Kav-er-nṓ-sum; a spongy structure in the penis.
Corpus Cinereum, Si-nḗ-rē-um; an oval body of grey matter on each hemisphere of the cerebellum.
Corpus Fimbriatum, — Fim-bri-á-tum; a fringe-like band at the angles of the lateral ventricles of the brain.

Corpus Glandulosum, — Glan-dų-lṓ-sum; a sponge-like substance surrounding the orifice of the urethra.

Corpus Mucosum, Mų-kṓ-sum; a fluid between the cuticle and cutis, that gives color to the skin.

Corpus Pampiniforme, — Pam-pin-i-fór-mĕ; the plexus of the spermatic vein.

Corpus Spongiosum Penis, (or **Urethræ;**) a dark red substance around these parts.

Corpus Varicosum, — Var-i-kṓ-sum; the spermatic plexus.

Corpuscle, Kór-pus-l; an atom, or minute body.

Corpuscular, Kor-pús-kų-lar; belonging to, or like, a corpuscle.

Corrigens, Kór-i-jenz; part of a prescription designed to modify other ingredients.

Corroborant, Ko-rób-ō-rant; strengthening, as an invigorating cordial.

Corrosive, Ko-rṓ-siv; eating, or destroying, especially the texture of a living body.

Corrosive Sublimate, Ko-rṓ-siv Súb-li-mat; bichloride of mercury, mercuric chloride; a poisonous compound of chlorine and mercury.

Corrugator, Kór-ų-ga-tor; descriptive of a muscle that wrinkles the part it acts upon.

Cortex, Kór-teks· the bark, or outermost covering.

Cortex Cerebri, — Sér-ĕ-brį; the greyish substance covering the cerebrum and cerebellum.

Cortical, Kór-ti-kal; pertaining to, or like bark.

Corydalis Formosa, Kor-i-dá-lis For-mṓ-sa; turkey corn, a synonym for *Dicentra Canadensis*.

Cosmetic, Koz-mét-ik; a medicine for external application, to beautify the skin, by removing freckles, blotches, etc.

Costa, Kós-ta; a rib, of which there are twelve on each side of the human organization.

Costal, Kós-tal; relating to the ribs.

Cotton Root; Kót-n Rūt; the root of *Gossypium herbaceum;* a valuable parturient and emmenagogue.

Cotula, Kō-tṹ-la. See *Maruta Cotula.*

Cotyledon Umbilicus, Kot-i-lĕ́-don Um-bi-lį́-kus; a plant of Europe, that grows in old walls, the leaves of which are emollient, externally applied; internally, used for epilepsy, calculus and dropsy.

Cotyloid Cavity, Kót-i-lœd Káv-i-ti; the cup-like cavity that holds the head of the thigh-bone.
Couch Grass, Kuç Gras; *Triticum repens;* used as a diuretic and aperient.
Counter-Indication. See Contra Indication.
Counter-Irritation, Kŏn-ter-Ir-i-tá-ʃon; the application of a blister on one part, for the purpose of exciting irritation and relieving another part.
Counter-Extension; holding a broken limb towards the body, while the outer end is being drawn from it.
Coup de Sang, Ku-dɛ-Soṅ; sudden congestion, without hemorrhage. [heat.
Coup de Soleil, — Sɷ-lál; sun-stroke; prostration from
Court-Plaster, Kɷrt-Plɑ́s-ter; a thin adhesive plaster.
Courses, Kɷ́rs-ez; popular term for the menses.
Cowhage, Kŏ-hej; the hair of cowhage pods, (*Mucuna pruriens;*) used as a mechanical irritation to expel worms.
Coxa, Kóks-ɑ; the haunch or hip-joint.
Coxalgia, Koks-ál-ji-ɑ; pain in the hip-joint.
Cramp, Kramp; an involuntary contraction of a muscle.
Crampbark, Krámp-bɑrk; Viburnum Opulus; a native shrub, the bark of which is used as an anti-spasmodic.
Cranesbill, Kránz-bil; the root of *Geranium maculatum;* a powerful astringent.
Cranial, Krá-ni-al; relating to the skull or cranium.
Craniology, Kra-ni-ól-ɷ-ji; the science of phrenology, as indicated by the size and shape of the skull.
Cranium, Krá-ni-um; the skull that contains the brain, composed of eight bones.
Craquement Pulmonaire, Krɑ́k-moṅ Púl-mɷ-nɑr; a peculiar rattling sound, at the top of the lungs, in the beginning of consumption.
Crassamentum, Kras-a-mén-tum: a clot, or coagulum, nearly solid, formed by venous blood after its extraction. [rhiza.
Crawley Root, Kré-li Rut. See *Corallorhiza odonto-*
Cream of Tartar, Krēm ov Tɑ́r-tɑr; bitartrate of potassium, purified tartar, or argol.
Creasote, or Kreasote, Krḗ-a-sɷt: an oily substance, prepared by the destructive distillation of wood, an antiseptic.

Creatin, or **Creatine**, Kré-a-tin; a neutral body obtained from animal muscle.

Cremaster, Krē-más-ter; the suspensory muscle of the testes.

Crenate, Kré-nat; notched, or scolloped.

Crenulated, Krén-u-la-ted; having small notches or scollops.

Crepitant, Krép-i-tant; rattling.

Crepitation, Krep-i-tá-ʃon; a rattling sound, as in the pressure of the cellular tissue where air is collected, also the grating together of fractured ends of a bone.

Crepitus, Krép-i-tus; the discharge of gas or wind from the bowels; also, same as crepitation.

Creta, Kré-ta; chalk; native carbonate of lime.

Creta Præparata, — Prep-a-rá-ta; prepared, or washed chalk.

Cretinism, Kré-tin-izm; an endemic disease in mountainous countries, attended with goitre, debility, deformity, and idiocy.

Cricoid, Krį-kơd; like a ring, applied to one of the cartilages of the larynx.

Crisis, Krį-sis; the turning point of a disease, when the patient either begins to improve or get worse.

Crista, Krís-ta; a crest; applied to parts resembling a crest, and to an excrescence around the anus.

Crista Galli, — Gál-ı; the process on the ethnoid bone.

Critical, Krít-i-kal; applied to peculiar manifestations of disease, supposed to indicate a crisis; also, to periods of life when changes in the constitution and habits take place.

Critical Age; the time in the life of women when their menses become irregular or cease, during which they are liable to contract serious illness.

Crocus of Antimony, Kró-kus of An'ti-mo-ni; a compound formed by deflagrating a mixture of tersulphuret of antimony and nitrate of potassium.

Crocus Sativus, — Sa-tį-vus; a showy bulbous plant of Europe that yields saffron.

Cross-Birth, Kros-Berþ; a popular phrase applied to unusual or irregular delivery.

Crotaphe, Krót-a-fē; headache, accompanied with throbbing in the temples, and a thumping in the ears.

Crotchet, Króç-et; an instrument for the artificial removal of the fœtus.

Croton Eleuteria, Krō-ton El-ų-tē-ri-a; a shrub of the West Indies, which yields cascarilla bark.

Croton Oil; a powerful cathartic, expressed from the seed of *Croton Tiglium;* applied externally as a liniment, to produce inflammation.

Croton Tiglium, — Tíg-li-um; a small tree of India, the source of croton oil.

Croup, Krup; inflammation of the trachea, accompanied with difficult breathing, a cough, and expectoration.

Crowfoot, Krō-fut; the *Ranunculus bulbosus.*

Crucial, Krú-ʃal; like a cross; applied to ligaments, incisions, etc.

Crucible, Krú-si-bl; a vessel, used by chemists, for fusing substances by great heat.

Crudity, Krú-di-ti; raw material, undigested food.

Crusis, Krú-sis; a scrofulous swelling of the neck.

Crura, Krú-ra; plural of *crus;* legs.

Crura Cerebelli, — Ser-ē-bél-ị; legs, or limbs, of the cerebellum; cords that stretch along each hemisphere of the cerebellum.

Crura Cerebri, — Sér-ē-brị; two groups of fibres connecting with the inferior surface of each hemisphere of the cerebrum.

Crura Diaphragmatis, — Dị-a-frág-ma-tis; addenda below the main tendon of the diaphragm.

Cruræus, Kru-rē-us; a muscle of the leg; belonging to the legs.

Crural Arch, Krú-ral Arç; Fallopius' or Poupart's ligament, the thick part of a tendon stretching from the ilium to the spine of the *os pubis.*

Crus, Krus; the leg; used in the plural to describe various projections.

Crypta, Kríp-ta; a small mucous follicle, or gland.

Cryptorchis, Krip-tór-kis; a person whose testicles are not in the scrotum.

Crystalline Lens, Krís-ta-lịn Lenz; double convex lens in the forepart of the eye.

Crystallization, Kris-tal-i-zá-ʃon; the process of passing from a liquid to a solid state.

Crystalloides, Krís-ta-lœdz; crystalline substances of great diffusibility, such as salt.

Cu.; symbol for the element *Cuprum*, (copper.)

Cubebs, Kú-bebz; the dried berries of the *Piper Cubeba*, used in diseases of the urinary organs, and the smoke from which is inhaled as a remedy for bronchial affections.

Cubitæus, Ku-bi-té-us; relating to the forearm.

Cubitus, Kú-bi-tus; the fore-arm, from the elbow to the wrist.

Cucurbita Pepo, Ku-kúr-bi-ta; the pumpkin, the seed of which forms an emulsion, recommended for tape-worm; also used Homœopathically.

Cucurbita Citrullus, — Si-trúl-us; synonym for *Citrullus vulgaris*.

Cucurbitula, Ku-kur-bit-u-la; a cupping glass.

Cucurbitula Sicca, — Sík-a; a glass used for dry-cupping.

Cudbear, Kúd-bar; a coloring matter obtained from several lichens.

Cul-de-Sac, Kul-dε-Sak; a bag, or tube closed at one end.

Culver's Root, Kúl-ver'z Rut; black rook, the root of *Veronica Virginica*, a native plant.

Cumin Seed, Kú-min Sēd; the aromatic fruit of the *Cuminum Cyminum*, a European plant.

Cupola, Kú-po-la; the extremity of the cochlea.

Cupping, Kúp-iŋ; the extracting of blood by cupping glasses.

Cuprum, Kú-prum; officinal name for copper.

Curaria, Ku-rá-ri-a; a powerful poison, obtained from a South American plant; recommended in lock-jaw, and as an antidote to strychnia poisoning.

Curatio, Ku-rá-ʃi-o; treatment of disease.

Curcuma Longa, Kur-kú-ma Lóŋ-ga; a plant, native of the East Indies, the root of which abounds in a yellow coloring matter; turmeric.

Cusparia, Kus-pá-ri-a; synonym for *Galipea officinalis;* the angustura tree.

Cuspidatus, Kus-pi-dá-tus; in the plural applied to pointed teeth.

Cutaneous, Ku-tá-nē-us; belonging to the skin.

Cutaneous Absorption; the function of the skin by which matter applied to it is absorbed.
Cutaneus Musculus; a thin muscle of the neck.
Cuticle, Kų-ti-kl; the epidermis; the scarf-skin.
Cutis Kų-tis; the skin, including the inner as well as outer coating.
Cutis Anserina, — An-ser-į-na; the condition of the skin when, from cold or other cause, the papillæ stand out from the surface.
Cuttle-Fish Bone, Kút-l-Fiʃ Bɷn; a shell-like substance found in the back of the cuttle fish.
Cyanates, Sį-an-ats; salts of cyanic acid.
Cyanides, Sį-an-įdz; compounds of cyanogen.
Cyanogen, Sį-án-ɷ-jen; a compound body (Cy.;) the acidulous radical of hydrocyanic acid and other cyanides.
Cyanopathia, Sį-an-ɷ-pá-ŧi-a; the "blue disease," or *Cyanosis*.
Cyanosis, Sį-an-ó-sis; the condition of the blood, indicated by the blueness of the skin, resulting from malformation of the heart, which fails to keep separate the venous and arterial currents.
Cynanche, Si-nán-kē; any disease of the throat.
Cynanche Laryngia, — La-rín-ji-a; the croup.
Cynanche Maligna, — Ma-líg-na; putrid sore-throat, as in scarlatina. [mumps.
Cynanche Parotidea, — Par-ɷ-tíd-ē-a ; parotitis, the
Cynanche Pharingea, — Far-ín-jē-a; pharyngitis, inflammation of the pharynx.
Cynanche Strepitoria, Stridula, Suffocativa, Trachealis; different names for croup.
Cynanche Tonsillaris, — Ton-sil-á-ris; the quinsy.
Cynanche Ulcerosa, — Ul-ser-ó-sa; malignant sore-throat.
Cynanthropia, Sin-an-ŧró-pi-a; a species of melancholia in which the victim imagines himself a dog and imitates its bark.
Cynolissa, Sin-ɷ-lís-a; hydrophobia; canine madness.
Cyrtosis, Sɛr-tó-sis; *Cyrtonosis;* recurvature of the spine.
Cystalgia, Sis-tál-ji-a; a painful disease of the bladder.

Cystic, Sís-tik; relating to the bladder, or to the gall-bladder.

Cystic Duct; the duct that connects the gall-bladder with the hepatic duct.

Cystifelleotomy, Sis-ti-fel-ĕ-ót-ω-mi; the operation of removing calculi from the gall-bladder.

Cystin, or **Cystic Oxide**; a rare substance found in urinary calculus.

Cystirrhagia, Sis-ti-rá-ji-a; a discharge from the bladder, of blood or mucus.

Cystirrhœa, Sis-ti-rĕ-a; a catarrhal discharge from the bladder.

Cystis, Sís-tis; a sac, or bladder, in which any morbid matter is held.

Cystitis, Sis-tį-tis; inflammation of the urinary bladder.

Cystitome, Sís-ti-tωm; an instrument for opening a sac or capsule.

Cystocele, Sís-tω-sĕl; hernia of the bladder.

Cystodynia, Sis-tω-dín-i-a; pain in the bladder.

Cystoid, Sís-tœd; like a cyst or bladder.

Cystolithiasis, Sis-tω-li-ŧį-a-sis; "the gravel," or calculus in the urinary bladder.

Cystolithus, Sis-tól-i-ŧus; urinary calculus.

Cystoplasty, Sís-tω-plas-ti; the treatment of fistulous openings in the bladder by uniting a flap taken from some adjoining part.

Cystoplegia, Sis-tω-plĕ-ji-a; paralysis of the bladder.

Cystoptosis, Sis-top-tώ-sis; hernia of the internal coating of the bladder into the urethra.

Cystospastic, Sis-tω-spás-tik: spasm of the bladder.

Cystotome, Sís-tω-tωm; a knife used in opening the bladder.

Cystotomy, Sis-tót-ω-mi; the operation of cutting into the bladder.

Cytisin, Sít-i-sin: a vegetable principle derived from the seeds of the tree *Cytisus Laburnum*, having emetic properties.

Cytisus, Sít-i-sus; the broom plant, synonym for *Sarothamœ Scoparius*.

Cytoblast, Sít-ω-blast: the elementary cell-germs of all animal and vegetable tissues.

D

D.; abbreviation for *Dosis*, a dose.

Dacryo-, Dák-ri-ω; a prefix, relating to tears.

Dacryocyst; Dák-ri-ω-sist; the sac that contains the tears.

Dacryocystitis, Dak-ri-ω-sis-tį-tis; inflammation of the tear-sac.

Dacryolite, Dák-ri-ω-lįt; a calculous formation in the tear-duct.

Dacryoma, Dak-ri-ώ-mα; an obstruction in the lachrymal orifices, causing an over-flow of tears.

Dæmonomania, Dē-mon-ω-má-ni-α; a kind of hallucination, in which the victim fancies himself possessed by a devil.

Dandelion, Dán-dē-lį-on; *Taraxacum Dens-leonis*; a common weed, the root of which is diuretic and tonic.

Daphne Mezereum, Dáf-nē Me-zḗ-rē-um; a British shrub which yields mezereon bark.

Datura Stramonium, Da-tų́-rα Stra-mώ-ni-um; Jamestown weed, or thorn-apple, the seed and leaves of which are narcotic, and in over-doses poisonous.

Daturin, Da-tų́-rin; an alkaloid obtained from *Datura Stramonium*.

Daucus Carota, Dό-kus Ka-rώ-tα; the wild carrot.

Deadly Nightshade; the common name for *Atropa Belladonna*, native of Europe.

Debility, Dē-bíl-i-ti; feebleness, either of body or mind.

Decantation, Dē-kan-tá-ʃon; pouring off the supernatant liquid, as in the washing of precipitates.

Decidua, Dē-síd-ų-α; the chorion, or membrane, cast from the uterus after parturition.

Decidua Reflexa, — Rē-fléks-α; so much of the decidua as surrounds the ovum.

Decidua Vera, — Vḗ-rα; the part of the decidua that lines the uterus.

Decoction, Dē-kók-ʃon; the process of extracting soluble materials from vegetable substances by means of boiling water.

Decollation, Dē-kol-á-ʃon; the removal of a head of a child in delivery, to save the life of the mother.

Decubitus, Dē-kų́-bi-tus; lying down; the peculiar manner in which it is done being sometimes regarded as a symptom of disease.

Decussation, Dē-kus-á-ʃon; the crossing of parts, as the optic nerves.

Decussorium, Dē-kus-ώ-ri-um; an instrument used in trephining the skull.

Defecation, Def-ē-ká-ʃon; clarification; the discharges of the fæces.

Defectio, Dē-fék-ʃi-ω; a failure in strength or resolution.

Deflagration, Def-la-grá-ʃon; a rapid combustion by chemical means.

Defloration, Def-lω-rá-ʃon; loss of signs of virginity in the female.

Defluxion, Dē-flúk-ʃon; the outward flowing of liquids and humors.

Deformation, Dē-fər-má-ʃon; the unnatural growth of any part of the body.

Degeneration, Dē-jen-er-á-ʃon; decay or unhealthy change in the system.

Deglutition, Deg-lų-tí-ʃon; the operation of swallowing a liquid.

Dehiscence, Dē-hís-ens; the bursting open of capsules, pimples, etc.

Dejection, Dē-jék-ʃon; the discharging of the bowels; prostration; depression.

Deligation, Del-i-gá-ʃon; the process of bandaging.

Deliquescence, Del-i-kwés-ens; melting, or dissolving, as some salts, by absorbing the air.

Deliquium, Dē-lík-wi-um; falling, or fainting.

Delirium, Dē-lír-i-um; insanity; wandering, and incoherent in mind.

Delirium Tremens, — Tré-menz; insanity resulting from drunkenness; *mania a potu.*

Delitescence, Del-i-tés-ens; the quick subsidence of inflammation.

Delphinin, Del-fín-in; an alkaloid obtained from the seed of *Delphinium Staphisagria.*

Delphinium Consolida, Del-fín-i-um Kon-sól-i-da; the larkspur, the seeds of which are diuretic.

Delphinium Staphisagria, — Staf-i-sá-gri-a; a plant of Europe that yields stavesacre seed.

Deltoid, Dél-tœd; a triangular muscle that covers the shoulder joint.

Dementia, Dē-mén-ʃi-a; loss of mind.

Demulcent, Dē-múl-sent; mulcilaginous; softening in its effects.

Dengue, Dén-ga; a species of fever, accompanied with pains along the thighs and legs.

Dens, Dens; a tooth; hence dental, relating to teeth.

Dentagra, Den-tá-gra; the head-ache; also the name of a kind of forceps, for extracting teeth.

Dentata, Den-tá-ta; the second of the cervical vertebra, which has a tooth-like projection.

Dentes Cuspidati, Dén-tēz Kus-pi-dá-tị; two pointed teeth in each jaw, the upper ones generally called the eye-teeth.

Dentes Incisores, — In-sị-sṓ-rēz; the four front teeth, called incisors because of their biting functions.

Dentes Molares, — Mō-lá-rēz; the ten grinders in each jaw.

Dentes Sapientia, — Sa-pi-én-ʃi-a; the four rear grinding teeth; also called wisdom teeth.

Dentrifice, Dén-tri-fis; tooth-powder; preparation for cleaning the teeth.

Dentine, or **Dentin**, Dén-tin; the bony inner substance of the teeth.

Dentition, Den-tí-ʃon; the process by which the teeth cut through the gum, in making their first appearance.

Dentium Cortex, Dén-ʃi-um Kór-teks; the enamel that constitutes the coating of the teeth.

Denudation, Dē-nų-dá-ʃon; the exposing, or laying bare of any part.

Deobstruent, Dē- b-strų-ent; medicines that tend to relieve obstructions.

Deodorization, Dē-ō-dor-i-zá-ʃon; neutralizing any foul effluvia by chemical agents.

Deoxidation, Dē-oks-i-dá-ʃon; causing the oxygen to leave any substance.

Dephlegmation, Dē-fleg-má-ʃon; the removal of water from liquid chemicals.

Depilatory, Dē-pil-a-tō-ri; a preparation for removing hair from any part.

Depletion, Dē-plé-ʃon; process of reducing or emptying blood-vessels, by bleeding or evacuating remedies.
Depletory, Dép-lē-tω-ri; producing or aiding depletion.
Deplumation, Dē-plų-má-ʃon; the shedding of the eye-lashes from disease.
Deposit, Dē-póz-it; the act of placing a thing down; also, the substance released from a liquid in which it has been held suspended.
Depressed, Dē-prést; cast down; dispirited.
Depression, Dē-pré-ʃon; dejection; lowness of spirits.
Depressor, Dē-prés-or; a muscle that presses or holds down.
Depressor Anguli Oris, — Aŋ'gų-lį Ω'ris; a muscle that depresses the corner of the mouth.
Deprimens Oculi, Dép-ri-menz Ok'ų-lį; the muscle of the eye that draws down the ball.
Depurantia, Dep-ų-rán-ʃi-ɑ; medicines that are supposed to purify the blood.
Depuration, Dep-ų-rá-ʃon; purifying; the removal of impurities from liquids.
Derivative, Dē-rív-a-tiv; revulsive remedies; counter-irritants, such as blisters.
Derma, Dér-mɑ; the skin.
Dermatalgia, Der-ma-tál-ji-ɑ; pain in the skin; neuralgia of the skin.
Dermatotomy, Der-ma-tót-ω-mi; dissection or cutting of the skin.
Dermoid, Dér-mσd; relating to, or like the skin.
Desiccation, Des-i-ká-ʃon; the process of making dry.
Desiccative, Dē-sík-a-tiv; tending to make dry.
Desmitis, Des-mį-tis; the inflammation of a ligament.
Desmodynia, Des-mω-dín-i-ɑ; pain in the ligament.
Desmoid, Dés-mσd; resembling a ligament, as fibres arranged in bundles. [fluid.
Despumation, Des-pų-má-ʃon; the clarification of a
Desquamation, Des-kwa-má-ʃon; exfoliation, the removal of scales from the skin or bone.
Desudatio, Des-ų-dá-ʃi-ω; sweating; moist eruptions in children.

Detergent, Dē-tér-jent; a cleansing remedy, for wounds and ulcers.

Determination, Dē-ter-min-á-ʃon; excessive flow of blood to any part. [a loud noise.

Detonation, Det-ω-ná-ʃon; a sudden explosion, with

Detritus, Dē-trį-tus; an action that washes and separates parts; the waste substances of such washing.

Detrusor Urinæ, Dē-trú-sor Yu-rį-nē; the muscular fibres, constituting the coat of the bladder, which expel the urine.

Deutoxide, Dų-tóks-id; a substance in the second degree of oxidation.

Dextrin, Déks-trin; British gum, a substance formed from starch by the action of sulphuric acid or diastase.

Dextroglucose, Deks-trω-glų́-kωs; glucose, so called because it turns the plane of polarization of a ray of light to the right.

Di.; a prefix signifying twice; as the oxide believed to contain two atoms of oxygen is the dioxide.

Dia, Dį-α; a prefix, signifying through; also, sometimes, a separation.

Diabetes, Dį-a-bé-tēz; an excessive flow of urine, containing sugar or dextrine. [cauterization.

Diacaustic, Dį-a-kás-tik; a double convex lens, used for

Diachylon, Dį-a-kį-lon; lead plaster.

Diacrisis, Dį-ák-ri-sis; the diagnosis of a disease.

Diæretic, Dį-e-rét-ik; the power of dividing; dissolving; corrosive.

Diæresis, Dį-ér-ē-sis; the division of a part into two sections, as by a wound or ulcer.

Diagnosis, Dį-ag-nó-sis; the science of distinguishing one disease from another by symptoms.

Dialyzed Iron, Dį-al-įzd Ɨ'urn; a solution of oxide of iron, from which the crystalline salts have been mostly separated by dialysis, used as a tasteless substitute for tincture of chloride of iron.

Dialysis, Dį-ál-i-sis; weakness of the limbs, as if by loss of muscle. (*Chem.*) To separate crystalloids from colloids by means of a membrane, such as parchment or bladder.

Diaphoresis, Dį-a-fω-ré-sis; profuse perspiration.

Diaphoretic, Dị-a-fō-rét-ik; having the power to produce perspiration.

Diaphragm, Dí-a-fram; the midriff; a large muscle that separates the thorax and abdomen.

Diaphragmalgia, Dị-a-frag-mál-ji-a; pain in the diaphragm.

Diaphragmatic, Dị-a-frag-mát-ik; relating to the diaphragm.

Diaphragmitis, Dị-a-frag-mí-tis; inflammation of the diaphragm.

Diaphysis, Dị-áf-i-sis; the middle part of a long bone.

Diarius, Dị-á-ri-us; for one day; ephemeral.

Diarrhœa, Dị-a-ré-a; too frequent passages from the bowels.

Diarrhœa Carnosa, — Kar-nó-sa; passages from the bowels in which flesh-like matter is discharged.

Diarthrosis, Dị-ar-thró-sis; a freely movable articulation.

Diastase, Dí-a-stas; a nitrogenous substance formed in germinating grain, said to give the therapeutical value to malt preparations.

Diastasis, Dị-ás-ta-sis; the separation of bones by force, but without fracture.

Diastole, Dị-ás-tō-lē; the periodic expansion of the heart and arteries.

Diathermanous, Dị-a-thér-man-us; admitting of the free distribution of heat.

Diathesis, Dị-áth-ē-sis; habit, or physical disposition.

Dicentra Canadensis, Dị-sén-tra Kan-a-dén-sis; turkey-corn; an alterative and tonic, commonly known as *Corydalis formosa*.

Dicrotic, Dị-krót-ik; description of the pulse when it seems to have a double beat.

Didymi, Díd-i-mị; twins, or pairs; especially the testicles.

Didymus, Díd-i-mus; two and two; applied to one of the testes.

Dies, Dị-ēz; a day, used in writing prescriptions.

Diet, Dí-et; food; especially healthful food for invalids.

Dietetic, Dị-ē-tét-ik; relating to the taking of food.

Digastric, Dị-gás-trik; two-bellied; also a muscle attached to the *os hyoides*.

Digerens, Díj-er-enz; digestive; medicines that favor the secretion of healthy pus.

Digestion, Di-jést-yon; the conversion of food into chyle.

Digitalin, Díj-it-a-lin; an active principle of foxglove.

Digitalis Purpurea, Dij-i-tá-lis Pur-pṳ́-rē-ɑ; fox-glove, a European plant, the leaves of which are much used as a narcotic and diuretic; poisonous in overdoses.

Digitus, Díj-i-tus; (pl. *Digiti;*) a finger.

Digitus Pedis, — Pḗ-dis; "finger of the foot;" a toe.

Dil.; abbreviation for *Dilue,* "to dilute," to reduce in strength.

Dilatation, Dil-a-tá-ʃon; expansion, enlargement, as of the heart, eye, etc.

Dilator, Dį-lá-tor; name of muscles that dilate different parts; also, an instrument for dilating or opening wounds, etc.

Dill Seed, Dil-Sēd; the fruit of *Anethum graveolens,* an umbelliferous and aromatic plant of Europe.

Dimorphism, Dį-mór-fizm; the property that some substances have of crystallizing in two distinct forms.

Dimorphous, Dį-mór-fus; dissimilarity of form.

Dinical, Dín-i-kal; relating to giddiness; medicines for the cure of giddiness.

Dinus, Dį́-nus; vertigo; giddiness.

Dinner Pills; the name of pills composed of aloes and mastic.

Dioscorea Villosa, Dį-os-kω-rḗ-ɑ Vi-lώ-sɑ; the wild yam, an indigenous remedy used in bilious colic.

Diosma, Dį-ós-mɑ; former name for *Barosma;* the plant that yields buchu leaves.

Diospyros Virginiana, Dį-ós-pi-ros Vɛr-jin-i-á-nɑ; the persimmon tree, the bark and unripe fruit of which is used as an astringent.

Dioxide, Dį-óks-id; "an oxide in which two atoms of oxygen are combined with one of an element."

Diphtheria, Dip-ϑḗ-ri-ɑ; a disease of the throat, in which the glands are inflamed and a false membrane is formed, that is difficult to remove.

Diphtheritis, Dip-ϑē-rį́-tis; a form of *Pharingitis,* or sore throat.

Diploe, Díp-lω-ē; a spongy texture in tubular bones; also, the osseous tissue between the tables of the skull.

Diploma, Di-plώ-mɑ; a parchment that confers collegiate honors, professional or literary.

Diplopia, Di-plώ-pi-ɑ; double-vision, resulting from a diseased condition of the optic nerves.

Dipsomania, Dip-sω-má-ni-α; the unnatural thirst of drunkards.

Dipsosis, Dip-sώ-sis; morbid and excessive thirst.

Dipterix Odorata, Díp-tĕ-riks Ω-dω-ré-tα; a leguminous tree or Brazil, the source of tonka beans.

Dirca Palustris, Dér-kα Pa-lús-tris; leather-wood, a native shrub, the bark of which is used as a sudorific.

Director, Di-rék-tor; a grooved instrument for guiding the surgical knife.

Discuss, Dis-kús; to dissipate; to effect the dissolution of tumors, etc.

Discutient, Dis-kų́-ʃent; a remedy for effecting the resolution of tumors.

Disease, Dis-éz; a morbid condition; any derangement of the natural functions of the organized being.

Disinfectants, Dis-in-fék-tants; agents that neutralize the cause of infection.

Dislocation, Dis-lω-ká-ʃon; displacement of the parts of a joint.

Disorganization, Dis-er-gan-i-zá-ʃon; the destruction of an organ; dissolution of an organized body.

Dispensary, Dis-pén-sa-ri; a room or building where medicines are prepared and dispensed, usually for the benefit of the poor.

Dissection, Di-sék-ʃon; the examination of any organism, by cutting it up into minute parts.

Distal, Dís-tal; part of a nerve, or muscle, which is most distant from its origin, or from a fixed point.

Distilled Water; Dis-tíld Wé-ter; water freed from fixed constituents, by condensation of vapor.

Distoma Hepaticum, Dís-tω-mα Hĕ-pát-i-kum; the fluke, a worm rarely found in the liver and gall-bladder of men, but often in those of sheep and goats.

Distortor Oris, Dis-tér-tor Ω'ris; one of the muscles of the cheek.

Distrix, Dís-triks; a disease of the hair that causes it to split at the end.

Diuresis, Dį-ų-ré-sis; an unwonted flow of urine.

Diuretic, Dį-ų-rét-ik; relating to, or that which causes an increased flow of urine.

Div,; abbreviation for "divide;" used in prescriptions.
Divarication, Di-var-i-ká-ʃon; bifurcation, or dividing into two, as in splitting an artery or nerve.
Diverticulum, Dį-ver-tík-ų-lum; a pouch-like process branching out from any principal passage.
Divulsion, Di-vúl-ʃon; any forcible separation or bruising of a part.
Dock, Yellow; *Rumex crispus;* a common weed, the root of which is used in scrofula.
Dogbane, Dóg-ban; the common name for plants of the genus *Apocynum.*
Dog-Fennel, Dog-Fén-el; the common name for *Maruta Cotula.*
Dog-Grass. See *Triticum repens.* [tive plant.
Dog's-Tooth Violet; *Erythronium Americanum;* a na-
Dogwood; Dóg-wɯd; *Cornus florida;* a small indigenous tree, also known as box-wood.
Doli Capex, Dώ-lį Ká-peks; used with reference to a criminal who pleads insanity as an excuse for his acts.
Dolor, Dώ-lor; (pl. *Dolores;*) pain.
Dolorous, Dώ-lor-us; painful; lugubrius.
Donovan's Solution, Dón-ω-van'z Sω-lų́-ʃon; a solution of iodides of arsenic and mercury.
Dorema Ammoniacum, Dω-rḗ-ma Am-ω-nį-a-kum; an umbelliferous plant of Persia, which yields gum ammoniac.
Dorsal, Dór-sal; pertaining to the back, twelve of the vertebræ being distinguished as dorsal vertebræ.
Dorsum. Dór-sum; the back; also, the posterior part of any member.
Dose, Dωs; "give;" the amount of medicine required to be given at once, in order to produce the desired effect.
Dossil, Dós-il; lint prepared in a roll, for introduction into a wound.
Douche, Dɯʃ; a dash of water applied quickly upon the head or any part of the body.
Douve, Dɯv; the French name of an intestinal worm, known in English as the fluke.
Dover's Powder, Dώ-ver'z Pŏ́-der; a compound powder of ipecac, an officinal preparation.

Drachm, Dram; in weight, sixty grains; a teaspoonfull of fluid measure.

Dracontium Fœtidum, Dra-kón-ʃi-um Fét-i-dum; synonym for the *Symplocarpus fœtidus*, the skunk cabbage.

Dragon Root, Drá-gon Rꝏt; the common name for *Arisæma triphyllum.*

Dragon's Blood; a reddish resin exuded from the surface of the fruit of *Calamus draco.*

Drastic, Drás-tik; "active," "brisk;" applied to purgatives that are prompt and violent in their action.

Dripping Sheet Bath; given by means of a wet sheet, with which the whole body, standing or lying, is enveloped and then rubbed.

Drivelling, Drív-el-iŋ; the involuntary flow of saliva, in infancy, old age, and idiocy.

Dropsy, Dróp-si; (contracted from *Hydrops*, water;) a morbid effusion of water into any of the cavities, as the belly, chest, joints, skull, etc.

Drosera Rotundifolia, Drós-er-ɑ Rꝏ-tun-di-fꝏ́-li-ɑ; the sun-dew, a little marsh plant, used for asthma or coughs.

Drug, Drug; a medicinal plant or other substance, in its simple state; also, latterly applied to all medicines.

Dry-Cupping; applying cupping glasses without scarifying the skin, for the purpose of causing a revulsion of blood from any other part.

Duct of Steno, Dukt ov Stĕ́-nꝏ; an excretory duct connected with the parotid gland.

Duct of Wharton, — Hwór-ton; an excretory duct connected with the submaxilary gland.

Ducts of Bellini,— Be-lĕ́-nĕ; the orifices of the urinary canals of the kidneys.

Ductus ad Nasum, Dúk-tus ad Nā́-sum; the lachrymal duct, extending from the lachrymal sac to the nose.

Ductus Aquosi, — A-kwꝏ́-sį; the lymphatic or watery ducts.

Ductus Arteriosus, — Ar-tĕ-ri-ꝏ́-sus; the blood vessels connecting the aorta and the pulmonary artery, in the fœtal circulation.

Ductus Communis Choledochus, — Kom-ụ́-nis Kol-éd-ɷ-kus; the union of the cystic and hepatic ducts, that convey the bile to the duodenum.
Ductus Cysticus, — Sís-ti-kus; the vessel that connects the gall-bladder with the hepatic duct.
Ductus Ejaculatorius, — Ĕ-jak-ụ-la-tɷ́-ri-us; a short duct in the prostate gland, that carries the semen into the urethra.
Ductus Hepaticus, — Hĕ-pát-i-kus. See *Ductus Communis*, etc.
Ductus Lachrymalis. See *Ductus ad Nasum.*
Ductus Lymphaticus Dexter, — Lim-fát-i-kus Déks-ter; a duct on the right side of the thorax, that opens into the right jugular vein.
Ductus Pancreaticus, — Pan-krĕ-át-i-kus; duct that connects with the gall-duct near its junction with the duodenum.
Ductus Venosus, — Vĕ-nɷ́-sus; a blood vessel that communicates between the *vena porta* and the ascending *vena cava* in the fœtus.
Dulcamara, Dul-ka-má-rɑ. See *Solanum Dulcamara.*
Duodenum, Dụ-ɷ-dĕ́-num; the first division of the small intestines, in which the biliary and pancreatic secretions flow.
Dura Mater, Dụ́-rɑ Má-ter; the external membrane of the brain.
Dwarf Elder; *Aralia hispida,* the bark of which is used as a diaphoretic.
Dyads, Dị́-adz; elements whose atoms have two combining units.
Dynamia, Di-ná-mi-ɑ; vital power; strength.
Dynamic, Di-nám ik; belonging to vital power or force.
Dysentery, Dís-en-ter-i; a disease of the bowels, in which frequent mucous and bloody discharges take place, accompanied with fever and griping.
Dysmenorrhœa, Dis-men-ɷ-rĕ́-ɑ; difficult and sometimes painful menstruation.
Dysopsia, Dis-óp-si-ɑ; impaired and painful vision.
Dyspnœa, Disp-nĕ́-ɑ; difficult breathing; the first stage of asphyxia or suffocation.
Dysosmia, Dis-ós-mi-ɑ; imperfect sense of smell.
Dyspepsia, Dis-pép-si-ɑ; indigestion; impaired power of digestion.

Dysphagia, Dis-fá-ji-a; difficulty of swallowing.
Dysphonia, Dis-fó-ni-a; difficulty in using the power of speech.
Dysphoria, Dis-fó-ri-a; disquietude; restlessness; *ennui*.
Dysuria, Dis-ú-ri-a; impeded and painful urination.

E

Earth-Bath, Ert-Bath; a remedial means, consisting of the application of hot earth or sand to the body of the patient.
Eau, O; the French word for water.
Ebullition, Eb-ul-í-ʃon; the act of boiling.
Eburnation, Eb-ur-ná-ʃon; an unusual deposit of phosphate of lime on the cartilages of the joints.
Ecbolic, Ek-ból-ik; medicines that tend to hasten parturition.
Ecchymoma, Ek-i-mó-ma; a blue swelling of the leg, often following parturition.
Ecchymosis, Ek-i-mó-sis; the effusion of blood beneath the cuticle.
Eccoprotic, Ek-o-prót-ik; a mild purgative medicine.
Eccrinology, Ek-ri-nól-o-ji; the philosophy of the secretions.
Eccritica, Ek-rít-i-ka; diseases of the function of secretion.
Eccyesis, Ek-si-é-sis; extra-uterine growth of a fœtus.
Echinate, Ek′i-nat; covered with prickles.
Eclampsy, Ek-lámp-si; a kind of epilepsy in which the patient seems surrounded with flashes of light.
Eclectic, Ek-lék-tik; the name of an ancient as well as modern school of medicine; the doctrine of choosing and using the best thing for the purpose, wherever found.
Ecphlysis, Ek-flí-sis; a vesicular eruption, limited to the surface.
Ecphronia, Ek-fró-ni-a; melancholy, bordering on insanity.

Ecphyma. Ek-fį-ma; a cutaneous excrescence.
Ecpyesis, Ek-pi-ē-sis; a term applied to several suppurating skin diseases, as *impetigo*, *ecthyma*, *scabies*.
Ecstasy, Ek'sta-si; a trance, in which want of sensibility, and voluntary motion, with pulsation and breathing unaffected, are the principal characteristics.
Ecthyma, Ek-tį-ma; an irritable eruption, but without fever.
Ectopia, Ek-tṓ-pi-a; a luxation, or protrusion.
Ectozoon, Ek-tō-zṓ-on; insects that infest the surface of the body, as lice.
Ectropium, Ek-trṓ-pi-um; the eversion of the eyelids.
Ectrotic, Ek-trót-ik; treatment designed to prevent the development of disease. [ters.
Eczema, Ek-zē-ma; an eruption of small smarting blis-
Edulcoration, Ē-dul-kō-rā́-ʃon; sweetening; also, a process for separating substances, one of which is readily soluble and the other is not.
Edulcorator, Ē-dul-kō-rā́-tor; an instrument for applying a sweetened liquid to another substance.
Efferent, Ef'er-ent; carrying out of, or from; applied to vessels that carry fluids from glands, etc.
Efflorescence, Ef-lō-rés-ens; crystalline substances, which yield a portion of their water of crystallization upon exposure to atmosphere.
Effluvium, Ef-lū́-vi-um; an exhalation from animal or vegetable matter, generally in a decaying condition.
Effusion, E-fū́-ʒon; the out-flowing of a liquid from its natural vessel into another; or an overflow upon surrounding parts. [ter.
Egestus, Ē-jés-tus; (pl. *Egesta;*) excrementitious mat-
Ejaculator, Ē-jak-ū-lā́-tor; that which throws out; applied to a muscle of the penis.
Elaterin, Ē-lát-er-in; the active principle of *Elaterium*.
Elaterium, El-a-tē-ri-um; a powerful purgative, obtained from the juice of the fruit of *Momordica Elaterium*, or squirting cucumber.
Elbow, El'bō; the angle, or joint, at the upper end of the fore-arm.
Elder, El'der; *Sambucus Canadensis;* the dried flowers, of which are used as a sudorific.

Elecampane, El-ē-kam-pán; *Inula Helenium*, a common naturalized plant, native of Europe.

Electricity, E-lek-tris-i-ti; the fluid, or property, developed by friction in rubbing amber, glass, sealing-wax, etc.; of late years frequently used as a stimulant in rheumatism, paralysis, dyspepsia, etc.

Electro-Magnetism; a kind of magnetism evolved by electrical currents; galvanic electricity.

Electrolysis, Ī-lek-tról-i-sis; decomposition superinduced by electricity.

Electroscope, Ī-lék-trō-skōp; an instrument for measuring the presence of electricity in a body.

Electro-Vital Currents; two currents, supposed to be of an electrical nature, that exist in animal organizations, one external and the other internal.

Elements, El'ē-ments; those substances which cannot be separated into two or more different substances.

Elements, Metallic; such elements as gold, silver, etc.

Elements, Non-metallic; an arbitrary division of the elements, including chlorine, iodine, oxygen, etc. In chemical characteristics there is considerable uniformity, but it is difficult to draw an exact line between them and the metallic elements.

Elemi, El'ē-mį; a resinous substance, supposed to be obtained from *Canarium commune*, used in the composition of plasters.

Elephantiasis, El-ē-fan-tį-a-sis; a disease of the Arabs and Greeks, whose principal features are swelled legs and face, tubercles, loss of hair and sense of feeling.

Elettaria Cardamomum, El-e-tá-ri-a Kqr-da-mó-mum; a plant of the mountainous portions of India, which yields cardamom.

Elixirs, Ī-líks-erz; unofficinal preparations, in which medicines are made palatable by the presence of sugar, spices and alcohol; cordials.

Elixir of Vitriol; aromatic sulphuric acid.

Elm, Elm; *Ulmus fulva*; slippery elm, a common indigenous tree, the bark of which is used as a demulcent.

Elutriation, Ī-lų-tri-á-ʃon; decantation; the reduction of ores, and other substances, to powder, and then floating away the lighter portions by water.

Elytritis, El-i-trį-tis; inflammation of the vagina.

Elytroplasty, El-i-trɷ-plás-ti; the process of closing a vaginal fistula with a flap from the labia.

Elytroptosis, El-i-tróp-tɷ-sis; a dropping down, or inversion, of the vagina.

Emansio Mensium, Ŀ-mán-ʃi-ɷ Mén-ʃi-um; retention of the *catamenia*.

Emasculate, Ŀ-más-kų-lat; impotent; destitute of virility.

Emasculation, Ŀ-mas-kų-lá-ʃon; the act by which impotency is effected; castration.

Embalming Em-bɋm-iŋ; the preserving of a dead body, by means of ointments, and antiseptics.

Embolia, Em-bɷ́-li-ɑ; (*Embolus;*) the obstruction of a vein or artery by a clot of blood.

Embrocation, Em-brɷ-ká-ʃon; a liniment, or medicated fluid for rubbing any part.

Embryo, Em'bri-ɷ; the earliest stage in which animal organization may be discerned in the ovum; also applied to a vegetable germ; in the human being, limited to the fifth month of gestation.

Embryogeny, Em-bri-ój-en-i; the growth or production of an embryo.

Embryology, Em-bri-ól-ɷ-ji; a desoription of the fœtus, or embryo.

Embryotomy, Em-bri-ót-ɷ-mi; the destruction or dismemberment of the fœtus *in utero*, in order to effect its delivery, when it cannot be accomplished otherwise.

Embryulcia, Em-bri-úl-ʃi-ɑ; the removal of a lifeless fœtus, generally by instruments.

Emesis, Em'ɓ-sis; vomiting; the act of relieving the stomach.

Emetic, Ŀ-mét-ik; a substance that provokes vomiting.

Emetia, (or **Emetin**), E-mɓ-ʃi-ɑ; an alkaloid obtained from ipecac root, a violent emetic.

Emmenagogue, Em-én-a-gog; a substance having the power of promoting the menstrual discharge.

Emmenia, Em-ɓ-ni-ɑ; the menses.

Emollient, Ŀ-mól-i-ent; having the power of softening or soothing.

Empathema, Em-pa-ɫɓ-mɑ; furious passion, violent excitement.

Emphlysis, Em'fli-sis; a vescular eruption, such as in the thrush, cow-pox, etc.

Emphyma, Em-fį-ma; a tumor having its origin below the skin.

Emphysema, Em-fi-sé-ma; the inflation of the skin by the existence of air or gas beneath it.

Empiric, Em-pír-ik; one whose practice of medicine is based on observation and experience, and not in accordance with scientific theory.

Empirical, Em-pír-i-kal; experimental; unscientific.

Empiricism, Em-pír-i-sizm; a practical familiarity with medicines and the treatment of diseases, without a thorough theoretical knowledge of the same.

Emplastra, Em-plás-tra; medicated mixtures, usually of resins and lead plaster, adhesive at the temperature of the body.

Empresma, Em-prés-ma; internal visceral inflammation.

Empyema, Em-pi-é-ma; an accumulation of pus in the thoracic cavity.

Empyesis, Em-pi-é-sis; suppuration; any development of pimples filled with a purulent fluid.

Empyocele, Em′pi-ω-sēl; the existence of pus within the scrotum.

Emulgent, Ē-múl-jent; straining, or drawing through; applied to the office of the kidneys, in straining the urine.

Emulsin, Ē-múl-sin; a substance existing in almonds, by the influence of which bitter almond oil is formed.

Emulsion, Ē-múl-ʃon; suspended particles of finely divided resins or oils, prepared by trituration with water, usually in connection with mucilage, or yelk of egg.

Emunctory, Ē-múŋk-tω-ri; applied to vessels or outlets of excretion.

Enæorema, En-ē-ω-ré-ma; floating *nubecula* in the urine.

Enamel, En-ám-el; the white hard coating of the teeth.

Enanthesis, En-an-θé-sis; a rash, as in measles, scarlet fever, etc.

Enarthrosis, En-ar-θrω-sis; a ball-and-socket joint.

Encanthis, En-kán-θis; the angle of the eye; applied to any excrescence appearing in that locality.

Encephalitis, En-sef-a-lį-tis; inflammation of the brain.

Encephalocele, En-séf-a-lo-sēl; hernia of the brain, through some unnatural fissure of the skull.

Encephaloid, En-séf-a-lơd; similar in appearance to the brain.

Encephalon, En-séf-a-lon; the brain, as a whole, comprising the *cerebrum*, *cerebellum*, *medulla oblongata*, and the contiguous membranes.

Enchondroma, En-kon-drṓ-ma; a tumor, or cartilaginous growth upon the bones.

Encysted, En-sís-ted; enclosed within a sac.

Endemic, En-dém-ik; a disease that prevails within a certain district.

Endermic, En-dḗr-mik; (*Endermatic;*) the application of medicine by rubbing into the skin.

Endocardial, En-do-kár-di-al; within the heart.

Endocarditis, En-do-kar-dí-tis; inflammation of the lining membrane of the heart.

Endocardium, En-do-kár-di-um; the membrane that lines the heart.

Endogastritis, En-do-gas-trí-tis; inflammation of the membrane that lines the stomach.

Endogenous, En-dój-en-us; that which increases by internal growth.

Endolymph, En'do-limf; a watery fluid in the labarynth of the ear.

Endosperm, En'do-sperm; the albumen stored between the integuments and the embryo, for the purpose of nutriment.

Enema, En'ē-ma; a liquid preparation to be injected into the rectum; officinal in the B. P.

Enepidermic, En-ep-i-dḗr-mik; indicating the application of blisters, plasters, poultices, etc., to the skin.

Engorgement, En-górj-ment; the congestion of blood, or other fluids, in the vessels of circulation.

Enostosis, En-os-tṓ-sis; a kind of tumor that sometimes appears in the medullary cavity of a bone.

Ens, Ens; "being;" denoting, in chemistry, any substance that is supposed to embody all the virtues of the materials from which it is composed.

Ensiform Cartilage, En'si-form Kár-ti-laj; the end of the sternum or breast-bone.

Entasis, En'ta-sis; spasms, cramps, lock-jaw.

Entera, En'tē-rɑ; the intestines, or bowels.

Enteralgia, En-ter-ál-ji-ɑ; colic; spasmodic pains in the bowels.

Enteric, En-tér-ik; relating to the bowels.

Enteritis, En-ter-ị-tis; inflammation of the bowels.

Enterocele, En'ter-ω-sēl; hernia or rupture of an intestine.

Enteralithiasis, En-ter-al-i-ŧị-a-sis; the formation of concretions in the intestines.

Enterolithus, En-ter-ól-i-ŧus; the growth of any kind of concretion in the bowels or stomach.

Enterology, En-ter-ól-ω-ji; the physiological laws relating to the intestines.

Enterorrhæa, En-ter-ω-ré-ɑ; excessive mucous secretion of the intestines.

Enteroscheocele, E-ter-ós-kē-ω-sēl; hernia of the scrotum.

Enterotomy, En-ter-ót-ω-mi; any cutting, or surgical treatment of the intestines.

Enterozoon, En-ter-ω-zώ-on; animal life inside the intestines.

Enthetic, En-ŧét-ik; the character of a disease resulting from morbific virus having been implanted in the system.

Entozoon, En-tω-zώ-on; a species of animal life that exists within another, as the common intestinal worm and the tape-worm.

Entropium, En-trώ-pi-um; an inversion of the eyelids and eyelashes towards the eye-ball.

Enucleate, Ē-nų́-kli-at; descriptive of a tumor taken from its place of growth like a seed from its hull.

Enuresis, En-ų-ré-sis; incontinence of urine.

Epanetus, Ep-án-ē-tus remittent, as several kinds of fevers.

Ependema, Ē-pén-dē-mɑ; lining membranes of the cavities of the brain.

Ephemera, Ē-fém-er-ɑ; a fever that runs for but one day.

phemeral, Ē-fém-er-al; lasting for but one day.

Ephialtes, Ef-i-ál-tēz; nightmare; a horribly oppressive dream.

phidrosis, Ef-i-drώ-sis; a profuse and unnatural perspiration.

Epibranchial, Ep-i-bráŋ-ki-al; relating to the upper part of the branchial arch.

Epicanthus, Ep-i-kán-ŧus; a fold of skin in the corner of the eye. [of the skin.

Epichrosis, Ep-i-krṓ-sis; a spotted or discolored state

Epicolic, Ep-i-kól-ik; over the direction of the colon.

Epicondyle, Ep-i-kón-dil; the outer protuberance of the lower end of the *os humeri.*

Epicranial, Ep-i-krā́-ni-al; situated on the skull.

Epicranium, Ep-i-krā́-ni-um; the scalp, or integument covering the skull.

Epicranius, Ep-i-krā́-ni-us; the *occipito frontalis,* or muscle of the forhead.

Epidemic, Ep-i-dém-ik; applied to a disease that prevails over a large district. [demic.

Epidemy, Ep′i-dem-i; a disease that has become epi-

Epidermic, Ep-i-dḗr-mik; relating to the epidermis.

Epidermis, Ep-i-dḗr-mis; the outer nonvascular layer of the skin.

Epididymis, Ep-i-díd-i-mis ; the convoluted portion of the efferent duct of the testicle.

Epigæa Repens, Ep-i-jḗ-ɑ Rḗ-penz ; the trailing arbutus, used as a diuretic. [trium.

Epigastralgia, Ep-i-gas-trál-ji-ɑ; pain in the epigas-

Epigastric, Ep-i-gás-trik; of the nature of the epigastrium.

Epigastrium, Ep-i-gás-tri-um; the upper region of the abdomen, below the sternum, and between the costal cartilages.

Epigenesis, Ep-i-jén-ē-sis; the theory that the embryo is the actual product of both sexes; instead of the idea that the male furnishes the germ and the female the nourishment, or the other theory that the germ exists in the female, and is only endowed with life by the male.

Epiglottic, Ep-i-glót-ik; relating to the epiglottis.

Epiglottis, Ep-i-glót-is; the cartilaginous lid which lies above the glottis, at the root of the tongue.

Epilepsy, Ep′i-lep-si; (*Epilepsia,*) generally known as "the falling sickness;" a sudden convulsion, during which the patient falls, unconscious, and froths at the mouth.

Epileptic, Ep-i-lép-tik; relating to epilepsy.

Epileptoid, Ep-i-lép-tœd; similar to epilepsy.

Epilobium Angustifolium, Ep-i-ló-bi-um An-gus-ti-fó-li-um; the willow-herb, astringent and slightly tonic.

Epinyctis, Ep-i-ník-tis; a rash that appears on the skin at night, but disappears in the day time.

Epiphegus Virginiana, Ep-i-fé-gus Vɛr-jin-i-á-nɑ; a leafless parasite, on the root of beech trees, usually called beech-drops; cancer-root; synonymous with *Orobanche Virginiana*.

Epiphora, E-píf-ɷ-rɑ; an excessive secretion of tears; also, an overflow of tears on account of an obstruction in the lachrymal duct.

Epiphysis, E-píf-i-sis; the growth of bone upon the extremities of long bones.

Epiplocele, Ep-íp-lɷ-sēl; hernia where part of the omentum protrudes.

Epiploic, Ep-i-pló-ik; relating to the omentum.

Epiploitis, Ep-i-plɷ-ị-tis; inflammation of the epiploon, or omentum.

Epiplomerocele, Ep-ip-lɷ-mér-ɷ-sēl; femoral hernia, the omentum protruding near the thigh.

Epiplomphalocele, Ep-ip-lóm-fal-ɷ-sēl; hernia in which the protrusion is at the navel.

Epiploon, Ep-íp-lɷ-on; the omentum, or second covering of the viscera of the abdomen.

Epiploscheocele, Ep-i-plós-kē-ɷ-sēl; hernia in which part of the omentum enters the scrotum.

Epischesis, E-pís-kē-sis; suppression of the excretions.

Epispadias, Ep-i-spá-di-as; a preternatural opening of the penis, terminating the urethra on the upper side of it.

Epispastic, Ep-i-spás-tik; any medical substance that applied to the skin, causes inflammation.

Epistaphylinus, Ep-i-staf-i-lị-nus; relating to the [uvula.

Episternal, Ep-i-stér-nal; over or upon the sternum.

Epithelial, Ep-i-thē-li-al; relating to the epithelium.

Epithelium, Ep-i-thé-li-um; the thin cuticle that covers the lips, nipples, etc., that are destitute of the ordinary skin.

Epizoon, Ep-i-zṓ-on. Same as *Ectozoon*, which see.
Epizootic, Ep-i-zɷ-ót-ik; applied to any disease that prevails extensively among horses or cattle.
Epsom Salts; sulphate of magnesium, a well known cathartic.
Epulis, Ep-ų́-lis; a hard swelling on the gums.
Epulotic, Ep-ų-lót-ik; having a tendency to cicatrize, or heal over.
Equation, Chemical; Ɩ-kwá-ʃon, Kém-i-kal; chemical reactions represented by a collection of symbols and formulæ.
Equinia, Ɩ-kwį́-ni-ɑ; the glanders in horses.
Equisetum Hyemale, Ek-wi-sɛ́-tum Hį-ɛ-má-lɛ; the scouring rush, an astringent, used by Homœopathists.
Equivalent, Ɩ-kwív-a-lent; the amount of one element necessary to displace another in combination.
Erechthites Hieracifolia, Ɩ-rek-ŧį́-tɛz Hį-er-a-si-fṓ-li-ɑ; fireweed, the distilled oil of which is used in colic.
Erethism, Er'ɛ-ŧizm; unusual irritability preceding certain accute diseases.
Erethismus, Er-ɛ-ŧís-mus; applied to the morbid condition resulting from sunstroke.
Ergot, Ɛr'got; spurred or blasted rye, a fungus growth of rye, (*Secale cereale;*) mostly used to produce contraction of the uterus.
Ergotin, Ɛr'gɷ-tin; the active principle of ergot.
Erigeron Canadense, Er-íj-er-on Kan-a-dén-sɛ; Canada fleabane, a diuretic and astringent.
Erigeron Philadelphicum; fleabane, a diuretic.
Erodent, Ɩ-rṓ-dent; gnawing, or eating away.
Erosion, Ɩ-rṓ-ʒon; consumption by ulceration.
Erotomania, Er-ɷ-tɷ-má-ni-ɑ; a mild insanity resulting from love.
Eructation, Ɩ-ruk-tá-ʃon; belching; the expulsion of wind from the stomach, through the mouth.
Eruption, Ɩ-rúp-ʃon; pimples or pustules on the skin.
Eryngium Yuccæfolium, Er-ín-ji-um Yuk-ɛ-fṓ-li-um; (*E. aquaticum;*) the button snakeroot, the root of which is diaphoretic and expectorant.
Erysipelas, Er-i-síp-ɛ-las; St. Anthony's fire, redness and inflammation of the skin with fever.

Erysipelatus, Er-i-síp-i-la-tus; relating to, or resembling erysipelas.

Erythema, Er-i-tħ́-ma; a simple rash, or redness without fever or vesication.

Erythrogen, Er-íth-ro-jen; the coloring matter, or principle, in blood, that forms the red color.

Erythroid, Er-íth-rod; having a red color.

Erythronium Americanum, Er-íth-ró-ni-um Am-er-i-ká-num; dog's-tooth violet, the bulb of which is recommended for scrofula.

Erythrosis, Er-i-thró-sis ; a plethoric condition, the blood being rich in fibrin, and of a bright red color.

Erythroxylon Coca, Er-i-thróks-i-lon Kó-ka; a shrub of South America which yields Coca leaves.

Eschar, Es'kar; the hard and dark slough resulting from the use of caustic.

Escharotic, Es-kar-ót-ik; a caustic, used for destroying flesh.

Esogastritis, Es-o-gas-trí-tis; inflammation of the membrane of the stomach.

Esophagus, E-sóf-a-gus; the gullet, that extends from the pharynx to the cardiac orifice of the stomach.

Esoteric, Es-o-tér-ik; within; used with reference to internal changes in the physical organization.

Essential Oils, Es-én-shal Oilz; volatile oils obtained by distillation in contact with water.

Essera, Es'e-ra; a rash; any mild cutaneous eruption.

Ether, E'ther; oxide of ethyl, a volatile inflammable liquid, obtained by the action of sulphuric acid upon alcohol; and usually called sulphuric ether.

Ethereal Oil, E-thé-re-al Oil; (or Light Oil of Wine,) a product of the action of sulphuric acid upon alcohol.

Ethers, E'therz; bodies which have the same relation to alcohols that metallic oxides have to their hydrates.

Etherization, E-ther-i-zá-shon; the inhalation of ether, to render insensible to pain.

Ethiops Mineral, E'thi-ops Mín-er-al; a mixture of sulphide of mercury and sulphur, obtained by trituration.

Ethmoid Bone, Eth-moid Bon; a bone of the skull having several small holes in it.

Ethnology, Eth-nól-o-ji; the science that treats of the resemblances and differences of the various races of men.

Ethyl, Eŏ'il; a theoretical basylous radical, from which stand ordinary alcohol is a salt of ethyl.
Ethylic Alcohol, — Al'kœ-hol; ordinary alcohol, accepted as the hydrate of ethyl.
Eucalyptus Globulus, Yu-ka-líp-tus Glób-ų-lus; an Australian tree, the leaves of which are used in fevers.
Eudiometer, Yu-di-óm-ĕ-ter; an instrument for measuring the purity of air, gas, etc.
Eugenia Pimenta, Yu-jḗ-ni-a Pi-mén-ta; a tree of the West Indies, the source of allspice.
Eunuch, Yú-nuk; a man from whom the genital organs have been removed.
Euonymus Atropurpureus, Yu-ón-i-mus A-trœ-pur-pų́-rĕ-us; wahoo; burning bush, the bark of which is used as a tonic.
Eupatorium, Yu-pa-tœ́-ri-um; a large genus of native herbs, possessing tonic and bitter principles.
Eupatorium Ageratoides, — A-jer-a-tœ-į-dĕz; the white snake-root.
Eupatorium Purpureum, — Pur-pų́-rĕ-um; queen of the meadow, used in urinary disorders.
Eupatorium Perfoliatum, — Pɛr-fœ-li-á-tum; boneset; thoroughwort; used as a tonic.
Euphorbia, Yu-fér-bi-a; a large genus of plants with milky juice, possessing acrid and caustic properties.
Euphorbia Corollata, — Kor-o-lá-ta; flowering spurge, a native plant, emetic and cathartic.
Euphorbia Hypericifolia, — Hį-per-i-si-fœ́-li-a; an indigenous weed, used in diarrhœa.
Euphorbia Ipecacuanha; — Ip-ĕ-kak-ų-án-a; American ipecac, a reliable emetic.
Euphorbium, Yu-fér-bi-um; a resinous substance obtained from several African Euphorbias, and used as an emetic and active cathartic.
Euphrasia Officinalis, Yu-frá-ʒi-a —; eyebright; used in diseases of the mucous membrane.
Euplastic, Yu-plás-tik; a supposed quality of matter in the animal organization that renews the tissues of the body.
Eustachian Tube, Yu-stá-ki-an Tųb; the canal leading from the soft palate to the internal ear.

Eustachian Valve, — Valv; a fold of the membrane of the heart, in front of the inferior *vena cava.*

Evacuant, Ḗ-vák-ụ-ant; having the power of promoting the evacuation of the bowels.

Evening Primrose, Ḗv'niŋ Prím-rōz; *Œnothera biennis;* a common native plant, used in cutaneous diseases.

Evacuation, Ḗ-vak-ụ-á-ʃon; the act of effecting the discharge of the bowels; the excrement discharged.

Evolution, Ev-ō-lụ́-ʃon; turning, or unfolding.

Evolution, Spontaneous, — Spon-tá-nē-us; a movement of the fœtus, in arm presentations, so that the breech descends.

Exacerbation, Eks-as-er-bá-ʃon; the increase of force or violence.

Exæresis, Eks-ér-ē-sis; the removal of a part, in surgery.

Exania, Eks-á-ni-a; the prolapsus, or depression of the anus.

Exanthema, Eks-an-thḗ-ma; a rash, or any cutaneous eruption.

Exanthematica, Eks-an-thē-mát-i-ka; applied to eruptive fevers generally.

Excipient, Ek-síp-i-ent; any substance used for disguising the nauseous qualities of medicine.

Excision, Ek-sí-ʒon; the cutting out of any part.

Excito-Motory, Ek-sị-tō-Mṓ-tor-i; the power possessed by the spinal nerves of transmitting impressions to the spinal marrow, which is reflected to the starting point.

Excoriation, Eks-kō-ri-á-ʃon; abrasion of the skin.

Excrement, Eks'krē-ment; the fœces, or discharge of the bowels.

Excrementitious, Eks-krē-men-tí-ʃus; possessing the nature of excrement.

Excrescence, Eks-krés-ens; any unnatural growth or matter adhering to the body.

Excretion, Eks-krḗ-ʃon; any waste or useless matter thrown off.

Excretory, Eks'krē-tō-ri; having the power of throwing off; relating to excretions, as excretory ducts.

Exfœtation, Eks-fē-tá-ʃon; extra uterine or imperfect fœtation.

:xfoliation, Eks-fo-li-á-ʃon; the scaling off of dead bone or flesh from the living.
:xhalation, Eks-ha-lá-ʃon; the process of evaporating water or moisture, as from the body.
:xhibit, Eks-íb-it; medically, to administer a remedy.
:xocardial, Eks-o-kár-di-al; external to, or outside the heart.
:xoccipital, Eks-ok-síp-i-tal; applied to the condyloid process of the occipital bone.
:xogenous, Eks-ój-en-us; growing from without; applied to processes of bone that shoot out from the main body.
:xogonium Purga, Eks-o-gó-ni-um Púr-ga; synonym for *Ipomœa Jalapa.*
:xomphalus, Eks-óm-fa-lus; umbilical hernia, occurring mostly in infants.
:xophthalmia, Eks-of-thál-mi-a; swelling and projection of the eyeball.
:xostosis, Eks-os-tó-sis; the enlargement of a bone, by the growth of extraneous matter upon it.
:xoteric, Eks-o-tér-ik; changes that take place in the organization from external causes.
:xpectorant, Eks-pék-to-rant; promoting the discharge of mucus from the lungs.
:xpectoration, Ek-spek-to-rá-ʃon; the discharge of mucous matter from the lungs, by coughing or spitting.
:xpiration, Eks-pi-rá-ʃon; the outward breathing of air from the lungs.
:xploration, Eks-plo-rá-ʃon; the examination of a patient with reference to physical signs of disease, as by inspection of parts, auscultation, percussion, etc.
:xpressed Oils, Eks-prést Ōlz; oils obtained by pressure, as linseed oil.
:xpulsion, Eks-púl-ʃon; the act of emptying the bowels or bladder, delivery of a fœtus, etc.
:xpulsive, Eks-púl-siv; that which presses out, as the action causing pains in child-birth.
:xsanguineous, Ek-san-gwín-ē-us; destitute of blood.
:xsiccation, Ek-si-ká-ʃon; drying of moist bodies by heat, or by absorption.

Exstrophy, Ek'strɑ-fi; displacement of a part, or organ; a cogenital malformation.

Extension, Eks-tén-ʃon; the straightening out of a limb, by pulling in the direction from the trunk.

Extensor, Eks-tén-sor; applied to muscles that stretch outward: *E. brevis digitorum pedis*, a muscle in the back of the foot, that extends the first four toes; *E. communis digitorum pedis*, a muscle in the forepart of the leg that extends the last four toes; *E. digitorum communis*, a muscle of the forearm that extends all the fingers; *E. proprius policis pedis*, a muscle in the forepart of the leg that extends the great toe.

Extirpation, Eks-ter-pá-ʃon; the removal or cutting away of a part.

Extract, Fluid, Eks'trakt, Flụ́-id; solution of the medicinal principles of plants, made by exhausting the proper part of the plant with an appropiate menstruum and evaporating to a specific bulk.

Extract, Solid; essentially a fluid extract evaporated to a consistence proper for forming pills.

Extra Uterine, Eks'trɑ Yú-ter-in; applied to irregular or imperfect fœtation, in which the fœtus is found outside the uterus.

Extravasation, Eks-trav-a-sá-ʃon; the effusion of blood or other fluid, into other than its own proper cavities.

Extroversion, Eks-trɑ-vér-ʃon; the malformation of a part, by its appearing inside out.

Exudation, Eks-ụ-dá-ʃon; the sweating or soaking out of a liquid through the membrane that contains it.

Eye, Ɨ; the organ of sight.

Eyebright, Ɨ'brịt; *Euphrasia officinalis*, which see.

F

F., or **Ft.**; (*fiat;*) make, or let there be made.

Face Ague, Fás Ā´gū; neuralgia; pain in the nerve of the face.

Facial, Fá-ʃal; relating to the face.

Facial Nerve, — Nɛrv; the hard portion of the seventh pair of nerves.

Facial Vein, — Vān; a vein that begins at the top of the forehead, and crosses the face diagonally to the internal jugular vein.

Facies Rubra, Fá-ʃi-ēz Rú-bra; redness in the face.

Faculty, Fák-ul-ti; (*Med.*) the professors and lecturers on medical science.

Fæces, Fé-sēz; excretions from the anus.

Fæcula, Fék-ū-la. See *Fecula.*

Fahrenheit's Thermometer, Fár-en-hīt's Ther-móm-ē-ter; it marks freezing at 32°, and boiling at 212°; other scales differ, but this is generally in use in the United States.

Falciform Process, Fál-si-fɘrm Pro´ses; a scythe-shaped process that separates the hemispheres of the brain.

Falling Sickness. See *Epilepsy.*

Fallopian Ligament, Fa-lṓ-pi-an Líg-a-ment; the round ligament of the uterus, first described by the anatomist Fallopius.

Fallopian Tubes; two canals extending from the ovaries to the uterus.

False Bittersweet, Fɘls Bít-er-swēt; *Celastrus scandens*, a native climbing shrub.

False Membrane, — Mém-bran; resulting from inflammation in croup, diptheria, etc.

False Ribs, Fɘls Ribz; the five inferior ribs.

False Unicorn, — Yú-ni-kɘrn; *Chamælirium luteum*, an indigenous plant.

Falx Cerebelli, Falks Ser-ē-bél-ī; the part of the *dura mater* which separates the lobes of the *cerebellum*.

Falx Cerebri, — Sér-ē-brī. Same as *Falciform Process*, which see.

Farcy, Fär-si; *Equinia*, or the glanders, a disease of horses, sometimes communicated to men.

Farina Tritici, Fa-rī-na Trít-i-sī; wheat flour.

Fascia, Fáʃ-i-a; a bandage, or ligament; the expansion of muscles.

Fascia Cribriformis, — Krib-ri-fór-mis; a cellular web stretched over the inguinal glands.

Fascia Iliaca, — I-lī-a-ka; a fascia that covers the iliac and psoac muscles.

Fascia Lata, — Lá-ta; a tendinous band covering the upper part of the thigh.

Fascia Spiralis, — Spī-rá-lis; the roller or bandage that is wound round a limb.

Fascia Superficialis, — Sų-per-fi-ʃi-á-lis; a membrane that extends over the abdomen, and down in front of the thighs.

Fascia Transversalis, — Trans-ver-sá-lis; a cellular membrane outside the peritoneum, lining the transversalis muscle.

Fasciate, Fáʃ-i-at; flattened, or broadened like a band.

Fasciation, Faʃ-i-á-ʃon; applying a bandage to a wounded part.

Fascicular, Fa-sík-ų-lar; bound together; clustered in bundles.

Fasciculus, Fa-sík-ų-lus; a small bundle of fibres or muscles.

Fasciola Hepatica, Fa-sī-ϖ-la Hē-pát-i-ka; the *distoma*, or fluke worm.

Fat Acids, Fat As′idz; those acids which enter into the composition of fats, as oleic acids.

Fauces, Fé-sēz; the cavity in the back of the mouth.

Faux, Fɵks; (pl. *fauces;*) the opening of the pharynx.

Favus, Fá-vus; honey-comb; a pustule resembling honey-comb.

Fe.; Fē; symbol for ferrum.

Febrifuge, Féb-ri-fųj; a remedy for abating the violence of fevers.

Febrile, Féb-ril; feverish; belonging to fever.

Febris, Fé-bris; (pl. *febres;*) a fever.

Fecula, Fék-ų-la; starch; deposit of the vegetable juices.

Feculent, Fék-ų-lent; having the nature of dregs.

Fecundation, Fē-kun-dá-ʃon; impregnating; making fruitful.

Fel Bovinum, Fel Bɷ-vį-num; ox-gall, used in cases where there is a deficient biliary secretion.

Fellifluus, Fel-íf-lų-us; flowing with bile.

Felon, Fél-on; a deep and painful abscess, generally on the fingers, arising beneath the periosteum.

Femoral, Fém-or-al; belonging to the thigh.

Femorocele, Fém-or-ɷ-sēl; *hernia cruralis;* rupture or tumor of the leg.

Femur, Fé-mur; the thigh; the long tubular bone of the thigh.

Fenestra, Fē-nés-tra; a window, or opening; applied to two openings of the tympanum of the ear.

Fennel Seed, Fén-el Sēd; the aromatic fruit of the *Fœniculum vulgare*, used as a carminative.

Fenugreek, Fén-ų-grēk; the seed of *Trigonella Fœnum-græcum*, mostly used in horse and cattle powders.

Fermentation, Fɛr-men-tá-ʃon; the decomposition of organic substances with production of alcohol.

Ferric Salts, Fér-ik Sɵlts; those which contain less metal than ferrous salts, as Ferric Sulphate, the higher of the two sulphates.

Ferrous Salts, Fér-us Sɵlts; those which contain the largest relative proportion of metal; as Ferrous Sulphate, the lower of the two sulphates.

Ferriferous, Fer-íf-er-us; containing, or having the nature of iron.

Ferrum, Fér-um; the metal iron.

Ferula Assafœtida, Fér-ų-la As-a-fét-i-da; synonym for *Narthex Assafœtida.*

Fever, Fé-ver; a form of disease that involves the general system, in which increased heat and pulse, thirst, and debility are prominent indications.

Fever-root; *Triosteum perfoliatum*, a native plant, the root of which is a mild cathartic.

Feverfew, Fé-ver-fų; *Pyrethrum parthenium*, a garden herb, used as a tonic; *Leucanthenum Parthenium Gordon.*

Fibre, Fį-ber; minute filaments or threads, animal or vegetable, composing the structure.

Fibril, Fį-bril; the diminutive of *fibre*, applied to the extremely attenuated threads composing muscular organization.

Fibrin, Fį-brin; a whitish compound substance existing in both vegetable and animal organizations.

Fibro-Cartilage, Fį-brō Kąr-ti-lej; a membranous substance at the base of the ear, and of which the rings of the trachea are formed.

Fibula, Fíb-ų-la; the smaller of the long bones extending from the knee to the ankle.

Ficus Carica, Fį-kus Kár-i-ka; the fig tree.

Figwort, Fíg-wurt; *Scrophularia nodosa*, a native plant of Europe, but now a common weed of the United States, used in blood diseases.

Filaria, Fil-á-ri-a; the thread-like worm that infests the eyes of horses.

Filix Mas, Fį-liks Mas; the male fern, *Aspidium Filix mas;* the root of which is used for the expulsion of tape-worms. [filter.

Filtrate, Fíl-trat; the liquid which passes through the

Filtration, Fil-trá-ʃon; separating impurities from a fluid, by straining.

Filtrum, Fíl-trum; a filter.

Fimbria, Fím-bri-a; a fringe; the fringe-like extremities of the Fallopian tubes.

Fire-Damp, Fįr-Damp; an explosive gas, found in mines, composed chiefly of light carburetted hydrogen.

Fireweed, Fįr-wēd; *Erechthites hieracifolia;* a common weed, largely used in preparing volatile oil, valuable in liniments.

First Intention, Fɛrst In-tén-ʃon; union of a wound by adhesion without suppuration.

Fish Berries, Fiʃ Bér-iz; the fruit of *Cocculus Indicus*, a narcotic poison, mostly used to stupefy fish.

Fissura Longitudinalis, Fi-ʃų́-ra Lon-ji-tų-di-ná-lis; a deep fissure on the median line of the brain.

Fissura Sylvii, — Síl-vi-į; the fissures between the anterior and middle lobes of the cerebrum.

Fissura Umbilicalis, — Um-bil-i-ká-lis; the fissure in which the umbilical vein lies in the fœtus.

Fissure, Fíʃ-ųr; a groove; a crack in a bone.

Fistula, Fís-tų-la; an ulcer, or opening, from an internal part of the body, that is difficult to heal.

Fistula in Ano, — in Ȩ'nω; an ulcer in the cellular walls of the anus.

Five-Finger; a common name for *Potentilla Canadensis;* cinquefoil.

Five-flowered Gentian, — Jén-ʃan; *Gentiana quinqueflora*, used as a tonic.

Flag, Blue. See *Iris versicolor.*

Flag, Sweet. See *Acorus Calamus.*

Flatulence, Flát-ų-lens; wind or gas in the stomach and bowels, caused by fermentation.

Flatus, Flá-tus; flatulence, etc., same as above.

Flax, Flaks; *Linum usitatissimum*, the seed of which are demulcent, and ground are used to form poultices; they also yield linseed oil.

Fleabane, Flē-ban; *Erigeron Philadelphicum*, a common [weed.

Fleabane, Canada; *Erigeron Canadense*, a weed, diuretic and astringent.

Fleam, Flēm; a large lancet, used for bleeding horses.

Flesh-colored Asclepias, As-klē-pi-as; *Asclepias incarnata*, white Indian hemp, a native plant found on the banks of streams.

Flexor, Fléks-or; applied to numerous muscles that bend joints; *Flexor longus digitorum pedis*, a muscle rising on the tibia and extending to the last four toes, which it bends; *F. longis policis*, a muscle that bends the thumb; *F. longus policis pedis*, a muscle that bends the great toe.

Floating Ribs, Flōt-iŋ Ribz; the last two of the false ribs, not united with the others.

Floccillation, Flók-si-lá-ʃon; the thoughtless picking at the bed-clothes by a patient, a dangerous symptom.

Flocci Volitantes, Flók-sį Vol-i-tán-tēz; small objects apparently flying before the eyes, in impaired vision.

Flocculus, Flók-ų-lus; one of the lobes of the cerebellum.

Flooding, Flúd-iŋ; uterine hemorrhage, especially at the time of parturition.

Flores, Fló-rēz; flowers of plants, but also applied to such minerals as take a pulverized form by sublimation.

Flowering Spurge, Flő-er-iŋ Spurj; *Euphorbia corollata.*

Flowers of Sulphur, Flő-erz ov Súl-fur; sublimed sulphur, obtained by rapid condensation of sulphur vapor; often improperly written Flour of Sulphur.

Fluid Extracts, Flú-id Eks'trakts; solutions of the medicinal principle of plants in alcohol and mixtures of alcohol, glycerine, and water.

Fluid, Magnesia, Flú-id Mag-nē-ʒi-a; a solution of carbonate of magnesium in carbonic acid water; used as a laxative.

Flux, Fluks; to flow; an excessive discharge of diluted matter from the bowels.

Fluxion, Flúk-ʃon; fusion; the concentration of blood to any organ.

Fœniculum Vulgare, Fē-ník-ų-lum Vul-gá-rē; an umbelliferous plant of Europe, which yields fennel.

Fœtal, Fé-tal; pertaining to the fœtus.

Fœticide, Fé-ti-sīd; the unlawful destruction of the *fœtus in utero.*

Fœtation, Fē-tá-ʃon; pregnancy.

Fœtor, Fé-tor; a rank, putrid smell.

Fœtus, Fé-tus; the child, five months from conception till time of birth.

Follicle, Fól-i-kl; a small bag or cavity.

Folliculate, Fol-ík-ų-let; having follicles.

Fomentation, Fo-men-tá-ʃon; application of hot cloths, with or without medicinal preparations.

Fomes, Fó-mēz; (pl. *Fomites,*) woollen clothing, or other porous substances capable of carrying contagious effluvia.

Fons Pulsatilis, Fons Pul-sá-til-is; the front fontanel, so named because arterial pulsation may be there felt for years after birth.

Fontanel, Fón-tan-el; the spaces in the skulls of infants between the frontal and parietal bones.

Fonticulus, Fon-tík-ų-lus; a place of issue, or artificial ulcer.

Foramen, For-á-men; a small hole or opening.

Foramen Cæcum, — Sé-kum; the cavity at the base of the spine of the frontal bone; also, the follicle at the root of the tongue.

Foramen Magnum Occipitis, — Mág-num Ok-síp-i-tis; the large opening of the occipital bone.

Foramen Monroe, — Mon-rṓ; the opening by which each lateral ventricle of the brain communicates with the third ventricle.

Foramen Ovale, — Ō-vá-lē; the opening in the partition between the right and left auricles of the fœtus.

Foramen Winslow, — Wínz-lō; the passage through which the smaller sac of the peritoneum communicates with the sac of the omentum.

Foramen Rotundum, — Rō-tún-dum; the aperture of the internal ear.

Force, Chemical. See *Chemism.*

Fore-Arm, Fōr-Ārm; the part of the arm between the elbow and wrist.

Formates, Fór-mats; salts of formic acid.

Formic Acid, Fór-mik As′id; an acid found in ants and the leaves of the stinging-nettle.

Formula, Fór-mu-la; (See Chemical Formula); also applied to prescriptions and receipts.

Fornix, Fór-niks; a whitish substance of the brain.

Fossa, Fós-a; a shallow groove, or sinus.

Fossa Hyaloidea, — Hi-a-lō-í-dē-a; the cavity in which the crystalline lens is set.

Fossa Innominata, — In-nom-i-ná-ta; the depression between the helix and the anthelix of the ear.

Fourchette, Fur-ʃét; a small fold connecting the labia of the vulva in the female.

Fousel Oil, Fú-sel Ōl. See Fusel Oil.

Foveate, Fṓ-vē-at; pitted; having little depressions.

Foveolate, Fṓ-vē-ō-lat; characterized by small depressions.

Fowler's Solution, Fóu-ler'z Sō-lú-ʃon; an alkaline solution of arsenious acid.

Foxglove, Fóks-gluv; *Digitalis purpurea;* a fine flowering plant of Europe; the leaves a valuable sedative and diuretic.

Fractura, Frak-tú-ra; a fracture or break in a bone. It may be *comminuted,* crushed in several pieces; *compound,* when the bone protrudes through the integuments: or *simple,* divided without laceration of the flesh.

Fræna Epiglottidis, Frē-na Ep-i-glót-i-dis; a membrane that unites the epiglottis to the *os hoides* and tongue.

Frænum Labiorum, Frē-rum Lab-i-ō-rum; the lower membrane uniting the labia of the vulva.

Frænum Linguæ, — Liŋ-gwē; a membrane under the base of the tongue.

Fragilitas Ossium, Fra-jíl-i-tas Os'i-um; unnatural brittleness of the bones.

Frasera Carolinensis, Fra-zē-ra Kar-ō-lį-nén-sis; American Columbo; an indigenous plant, the root of which is tonic; synonym for *Frasera Walteri*.

Fraxinus, Frák-si-nus; the generic name for the different species of ash trees.

Fraxinus Ornus, — Θr'nus; the flowering ash, a tree of Sicily, the source of manna.

Fremitus, Frém-i-tus; vibration; an irregular movement of the muscular system.

Friction, Frík-ʃon; a rapid rubbing of the skin, with a towel, or brush, which stimulates the circulation of the blood to the surface.

Fringe-Tree, Frinj Trē; *Chionanthus Virginica*, a small tree, native of the southern states.

Frons, Frons; the forehead, between the eyebrows and hair of the head.

Frostwort, Frost-wurt; *Helianthemum Canadense*, an indigenous plant, used for the scrofula.

Fucus Vesiculosus, Fų́-kus Ve-sik-ų-lṓ-sus; bladder-wrack; recommended as anti-fat.

Fuming Sulphuric Acid, Fų́-miŋ Sul-fų́-rik As'id; Nordhausen sulphuric Acid, made by distillation of sulphate of iron.

Fumitory, Fų́-mi-tō-ri; *Fumaria officinalis*, a European plant, naturalized in the United States, and used as a tonic and alterative.

Fundament, Fún-da-ment; the bottom; the anus.

Fungus, Fúŋ-gus; (pl. *fungi;*) a cellular excrescence over wounds and ulcers; proud flesh.

Fungus Hæmatodes, — Hem-a-tṓ-dēz; Medullary sarcoma, or soft cancer; malignant, and generally fatal.

Fused Nitrate of Silver; lunar caustic.

Fusel Oil Fú-sel Ōl; an oily liquid substance in the distillation of alcoholic liquors, chiefly amylic alcohol, and used in preparing artifical valerianic acid.
Fustic, Fús-tik; a yellow dye-wood, obtained from *Morus tinctoria.*

G

Gadus Morrhua, Gá-dus Mór-ω-a; the cod-fish. See Cod-liver Oil.
Galactagogue, Ga-lák-ta-gog; that which causes a flow of milk.
Galactia, Ga-lák-ʃi-a; a defective or excessive flow of milk.
Galactin, Ga-lák-tin; the principle of milk that causes coagulation.
Galactirrhœa, Ga-lak-ti-ré-a; a morbid and unusual flow of milk.
Galactocele, Ga-lák-tω-sēl; a swelling that contains a milk-like fluid.
Galactometer, Gal-ak-tóm-ē-ter; an instrument for testing the quality of milk.
Galangal, Ga-láŋ-gal; the root of *Maranta Galanga,* used as a stimulant.
Galbanum, Gál-ba-num; an exudation from an umbelliferous plant of Persia, used as a stimulant and antispasmodic.
Galea, Gál-ē-a; a kind of headache; a bandage for the head.
Galena, Ga-lé-na; native sulphuret of lead.
Galenic, Ga-lén-ik; according to Galen, a distinguished physician, noted for the non-chemical use of drugs.
Galipea Officinalis, Ga-li-pé-a Of-i-si-ná-lis; a tree of the West Indies and South America, the source of Angustura bark.
Galipot, Gál-i-pot; white resin, obtained from a species of pine trees.
Galium Aparine, Gál-i-um Ap-a-rí-nē; cleavers; goose-grass; used as a diuretic.

Gall, Gel; the secretion of the liver; purified ox-gall.

Gall-bladder; Gél-blad-er; the receptacle of bile under the right lobe of the liver.

Gall-Duct; the duct that connects the gall-bladder with the liver, or hepatic duct.

Gall-Stone, Gel-Stωn; biliary concretions that form in the gall-bladder or ducts.

Gallic Acid, Gál-ik As'id; a vegetable acid, always made from tannic acid.

Gallicus Morbus, Gál-i-kus Mér-bus; sometimes used as a synonym for Syphilis.

Gallipot, Gál-i-pot; an earthen pot, used to contain ointments.

Galls, Gelz; morbid growths on the dyer's oak, (*Quercus infectoria,*) caused by the punctures of insects; they are very astringent, and are the source of gallic and tannic acids.

Galvanic Moxa, Gal-ván-ik Mók-sɑ; the employment of electricity for producing the effects of cauterization.

Gamboge, Gam-bώj; a yellow gum resin, the concrete juice of *Garcinia Morella;* an active cathartic.

Gambogic Acid, or **Cambogic Acid**; the resinous purgative principle of gamboge.

Gangliform, Gáŋ-gli-ferm; having the appearance of a ganglion.

Ganglion, Gáŋ-gli-on; a knot or enlargement on a tendon or nerve, an encysted tumor similarly located.

Gangrene, Gáŋ-grēn; incipient mortification.

Garcinia Morella, Gɋr-sín-i-ɑ Mω-rél-ɑ; a tree of India, the source of gamboge.

Gargarisma, Gɋr-ga-rís-mɑ; a gargle, or wash for the throat.

Garlic, Gɋ́r-lik; *Allium sativum*, a garden plant, the bulb of which is used as a stimulant.

Gasserian Ganglion, Ga-sē-ri-an Gáŋ-gli-on; enlargement of the fifth pair of nerves.

Gaster, Gás-ter; the stomach, or belly.

Gastremia, Gas-trē-mi-ɑ; congestion, in which the veins of the stomach become engorged.

Gastralgia, Gas-trál-ji-ɑ; pain in the stomach.

Gastric Fever, formerly applied to bilious fever.

Gastric juice; a secretion of the stomach.

Gastricism, Gás-tri-sizm; a theory that derangements of the stomach and bowels are the cause of all diseases.

Gastritis, Gas-trį-tis; inflammation of the stomach.

Gastrocele, Gás-trω-sēl; hernia in which a portion of the stomach protrudes.

Gastrocnemius, Gas-trok-né-mi-us; the chief muscle of the calf of the leg.

Gastrodynia, Gas-trω-dín-i-ɑ; spasms of pain in the [stomach.

Gastroenteritis, Gas-trω-en-ter-į-tis; inflammation of the mucous membrane of the stomach and bowels.

Gastroepiploic, Gas-trω-ep-i-plώ-ik; belonging to the stomach and omentum; applied to arteries, veins, etc., of the stomach.

Gastroid, Gás-trœd; resembling the stomach.

Gastrolithus, Gas-tról-i-thus; calculus, or stone, in the stomach.

Gastromalacia, Gas-trω-ma-lá-ʃi-ɑ; softening of the stomach.

Gastronosos; Gas-trón-ω-sos; derangement of the stom-[ach.

Gastropathy, Gas-tróp-a-thi; affection, or disease, of the stomach.

Gastrotomy, Gas-trót-ω-mi; an incision through the abdomen, for removing a fœtus or tumor.

Gelatin, Jél-a-tin; a pure kind of glue, obtained from bone-cartilage, tendons, etc.

Gelatinous Tissues, Jē-lát-in-us Tíʃ-ųz; such as, when boiled in water, yield a substance resembling gelatine.

Gelsemin, Jél-sem-in; an alkaloid of gelsemium; it is poisonous, and resembles the root in action.

Gelseminic Acid, Jel-sem-ín-ik As'id; acid found in gelsemium, strongly fluorescent when dissolved in an alkaline solution.

Gelsemium Sempervirens, — Sem-per-vį-renz; yellow jasmine, an evergreen twining shrub of the southern states, the fresh root of which is used to control the heart's action and to quiet the nerves.

Gena, Jé-nɑ: the cheek; *Genæ*, the cheeks.

Genetica, Jē-nét-i-kɑ; diseases of the sexual function.

Geneticus, Jē-nét-i-kus; belonging to the generative functions.

Geniculate, Jen-ik-ų-lɑt; bent like the knee.

Geniculum, Jen-ík-ų-lum; a small joint, or knot, as on the knee.

Genitals, Jén-i-talz; the organs of generation.

Genito-Crural, Jén-i-tō-Krú-ral; the nerve rising from the first lumbar, and supplying the spermatic cord and crural arch.

Genu, Jē-nų; (pl. *Genua;*) the knee; the joint between the leg and thigh.

Gentian, Jén-ʃan; the root of *Gentiana lutea*, a mountainous plant of Europe; a valuable tonic.

Gentiana, Jen-ʃi-á-na; a genus of plants possessing tonic and bitter principles. The *Gentiana lutea*, or gentian plant of Europe, and the *Gentiana puberula* and *G. quinqueflora*, (five flowered gentian), of the United States are the species most used.

Genua Valga, Jén-ų-a Vál-ga; the deformity that results in the knees knocking together as one walks.

Geranium Maculatum, Jer-á-ni-um Mak-ų-lá-tum; cranesbill, an indigenous showy plant, the root of which is an astringent.

Geraticus, Jē-rát-i-kus, pertaining to old age; pl. *Geratici*, a class of diseases.

German Chamomile, Jér-man Kám-ō-mịl; the flower of *Matricaria Chamomilla*, tonic in its nature.

Germinal Membrane. See *Blastoderm*.

Gerocomia, Jer-ō-kó-mi-a; the hygiene and medical treatment required for old age. [child *in utero*.

Gestation, Jes-tá-ʃon; pregnancy; the growth of the

Geum Rivale, Jē-um Rị-vá-lē; water avens, the root of which is astringent and slightly tonic.

Gibbiformis, Gib-i-fór-mis; resembling a hump; crookedness or convexity of the spine.

Gibbosity, Gi-bós-i-ti; the condition of having convexity of the spine.

Gillenia Stipulacea, Ji-lē-ni-a Stip-ų-lá-sē-a: Bowman's root; properties similar to those of *G. trifoliata*, and more efficacious.

Gillenia Trifoliata, — Trị-fō-li-á-ta; Indian physic; an indigenous remedy; root emetic and cathartic.

Gimbernat's Ligament, Jim-ber-nat's —; the broad part of Poupart's ligament.

Ginger, Jín-jer; the root of *Zingiber officinale*, an aromatic stimulant.
Gingiva, Jin-jį-va; the gum, or covering of the base of the teeth.
Gingivitis, Jin-ji-vį-tis; inflammation of the gums.
Ginglimus, Jíŋ-gli-mus; a hinge-like joint, as the knee and elbow.
Ginseng, Jín-seŋ; *Aralia quinquefolia*.—Gray; (*Panax quinquefolium*,) a native plant,the root of little medical virtue, mostly used by the Chinese.
Glabbella, Gla-bél-a; the space between the eye-brows.
Glabrous, Glá-brus; smooth; devoid of hair.
Glacial Acetic Acid; acetic acid free from water.
Glacial Phosphoric Acid; a transparent glass-like substance, which should be metaphosphoric acid, but is usually impure.
Gland, Gland; an organ for secreting different fluids [from the blood.
Glanders, Glán-derz; diseases of horses. See Farcy.
Glandula, Glán-dų-la; a small gland.
Glans Clitoridis, Glanz Klit-ór-i-dis; the extreme end of the clitoris.
Glans Penis, — Pē-nis; the extremity of the penis.
Glauber's Salts, Gló-ber'z Selts; sulphate of sodium, a well known horse cathartic.
Glaucoma, Glo-kṓ-ma; (*Glaucosis*,) opacity of the vitreous humor of the eye, causing dimness of vision.
Glaucomatous Glo-kóm-a-tus; affected with glaucoma.
Glechoma Hederacea, Glē-kṓ-ma Hed-er-á-sē-a; synonym for *Nepeta Glechoma*.
Gleet, Glēt; chronic gonorrhœa; a thin matter appearing in ulcerous sores.
Glisson, Capsule of, Glís-on; the fibrous sheath enveloping the vessels of the liver.
Globulin, Glób-ų-lin; the colorless residuum after the red matter has been extracted from the blood.
Globus Hystericus, Glṓ-bus His-tér-i-kus; the sense of choking, in hysteria, caused by the rising of air in the œsophagus.
Globus Major, Glṓ-bus Má-jor; the upper extremity of the epididymis.
Globus Minor, — Mį-nor the lower part of the *epididymis*.

Glomerate, Glóm-er-at; congregated, compacted together.

Glonoine, Glώ-nω-in; nitro-glycerine; a mixture of glycerine, sulphuric acid, and fumigating vitric acid; used by the Homœopathists for headache. [taste.

Glossa, Glós-ɑ; the tongue, which is the chief organ of

Glossagra, Glós-a-grɑ; (*Glossaglia;*) pain in the tongue.

Glossanthrax, Glos-án-ŧraks; carbuncle on the tongue.

Glossitis, Glos-ị-tis; inflammation of the tongue.

Glossocele, Glós-ω-sĕl; involuntary extrusion of the tongue. [form.

Glossoides, Glos-ω-ị-dĕz; resembling the tongue in

Glossology, Glos-ól-ω-ji; the nature and science of the tongue.

Glossolysis, Glos-ól-i-sis; paralysis of the tongue.

Glossomantia, Glos-ω-mán-ʃi-ɑ; prognosis of a disease from the condition of the tongue.

Glosso-Pharyngeal, Glós-ω-Far-ín-jĕ-al; applied to the eighth pair of nerves.

Glossoplegia, Glos-ω-plĕ́-ji-ɑ; paralysis of the tongue.

Glossoscopia, Glos-ω-skώ-pi-ɑ; diagnosis of disease by examination of the tongue.

Glottis, Glót-is; the opening into the wind pipe, or apperture of the larynx.

Glottitis, Glot-ị-tis; inflammation of the glottis.

Glucose, Glɥ-kώs; grape-sugar, which see.

Glucosides, Glɥ́-kω-sịdz; proximate vegetable principles which, under the influence of dilute acids and heat, are decomposed, yielding as one product, glucose.

Glucosuria, Glɥ-kω-sɥ́-ri-ɑ; descriptive of the urine in *diabetes mellitus.*

Glutæus, Glɥ-tĕ́-us; three muscles of the buttocks, viz: *maximus*, *medias*, and *minimus*.

Gluten, Glɥ́-ten; glue; vegetable albumen, or the residue of wheat after the starch has been extracted.

Glutitis, Glɥ-tị-tis; inflammation of the muscles of the buttocks. [stance obtained from fats.

Glycerin, Glís-er-in; (Glyceric Alcohol;) a sweet sub-

Glycerites, Glis-er-ị-tĕz; mostly solutions of medicinal substances in glycerin.

Glycogen, Glík-ɷ-jen; a substance in the liver that may be converted into glucose.

Glycyrrhiza Glabra, Glis-er-į-zα Glá-brα; a leguminous plant of Spain, which yields liquorice root.

Glycyrrhizin, Glis-er-į-zin; a sweet substance found in liquorice root.

Gnaphalium Polycephalum, Na-fá-li-um Pol-i-séf-α-lum; everlasting, cudweed; a native woolly plant, aromatic and slightly astringent.

Gnathalgia, Na-ťál-ji-α; pain in the jaw.

Gnathitis, Na-ťį-tis; inflammation of the jaw.

Gnathoplasty, Náť-ɷ-plas-ti; the transposition of a healthy part of a cheek to repair a wound or disease of another part.

Goa Powder, Gώ-α Pȣ-der; the powder obtained from the decaying fibre of a tree of Brazil, which is largely composed of chrysophanic acid.

Godfrey's Cordial, Gód-fri'z Kǿrd-yal; a solution in domestic use, containing more than a grain of opium to each fluid ounce.

Goitre, Gǿ-ter; bronchocele; enlargement of the thyroid gland.

Gold, Gɷld; an elementary substance, the chloride of which is used in medicine.

Golden Rod, Gώl-den Rod; a common name for an extensive genus of plants of the United States, (*Solidago*), one of the species of which, *S. odora*, is used as a carminative.

Golden Seal, — Sɨl; a common name for *Hydrastis Canadensis;* yellow root.

Goldthread, Gώld-ťred; *Coptis trifolia*, a pretty little indigenous plant.

Gomphosis, Gom-fώ-sis; an articulation of bones like the junction of teeth in their sockets.

Gonacratia, Gon-a-krá-ʃi-α; sexual impotence.

Gonagra, Gón-a-grα; pain, or gout in the knee.

Gonarthritis, Gon-αr-ťrį-tis; inflammation of the knee.

Gonepoiesis, Gon-ɨ-pǿ-ɨ-sis; secretion of the seminal fluid.

Gonocace, Gɷ-nók-a-sɨ; white swelling in the knee.

Gonocele, Gón-ɷ-sɨl; a swelling of the testicle, or spermatic cord; the effusion of semen from rupture of the seminal vesicles.

Gonoid, Gó-nœd; resembling semen.

Gonophysema, Gon-ω-fi-sē-ma; white swelling, or hernia of the knee.

Gonorrhœa, Gon-ω-rē-a; infectious discharge of purulent matter from the generative organs.

Gonorrhœa Balani, — Bál-a-nj; purulent exudation from the inflamed surface of the *glans penis*.

Gonoscheocele, Gω-nós-kē-ω-sēl; swelling of the epididymis, supposed to be from the accumulation of semen.

Gonyocampsis, Gon-i-ω-kámp-sis; curvature at the knee.

Gonyocele, Gon-i-ω-sēl; hernia of the knee; white swelling.

Gonytyle, Gón-i-tįl; thick, or callous skin on the knee.

Goose-Grass, Gus-Gras. See *Galium Aparine*.

Gorget, Gór-get; an instrument for performing the operation of lithotomy.

Gossypium Herbaceum, Gos-íp-i-um Hεr-bá-sē-um; the cotton plant; the fresh bark of the root is used as a parturient.

Goulard's Cerate, Gú-lard'z Sē-rat; cerate of subacetate of lead.

Goulard's Extract; solution of subacetate of lead.

Gout, Gσt; arthritis; painful inflammation of the small joints.

Gout-Stone; a concretion in the gouty joints.

Graafian Follicles, Grą-fi-an Fól-i-klz; small globular bodies, the interior coat enclosing the *ovum*, called the *ovisac*.

Gracilis, Grás-i-lis; a thin muscle of the thigh.

Grains of Paradise; the aromatic seed (not capsules) of a variety of cardamom, *Elettaria Grana Paradisi*.

Granatum, Gran-á-tum. See *Punica Granatum*.

Grando, Grán-dω; a small tumor, or hard swelling on the eye-lid.

Granular, Grán-ų-lar; like a grain in form or nature.

Granulation, Gran-ų-lá-ʃon; the filling up of a wound or tumor, by grain-like formations of new flesh.

Grape Sugar; glucose; a kind of sugar found in many fruits, and also the variety met with in diabetic urine.

Graphioides, Graf-i-ǫ-į-dēz; like a style; the styloid process of the temporal bone.
Graphite, Gráf-įt; a form of carbon, known as blumbago, or black lead.
Gravedo, Gra-vé-dǫ; catarrh, with sense of weight in the forehead.
Gravel, Gráv-el; small calculous formations in the kidneys, that are passed in the urine, with great pain.
Gravel-plant, *Epigœa repens*, trailing arbutus, an indigenous plant used as a diuretic.
Gravid Uterus, Gráv-id Yú-ter-us; the womb during gestation.
Graviditi, Gra-víd-i-ti; the condition of pregnancy.
Greek Valerian, Grēk Va-lé-ri-an; *Polemonium cœruleum*, an English plant.
Green Hellebore, Grēn Hél-ē-bǫr. See *Veratrum viride.*
Green Iodide of Mercury; mercurious iodide, made by rubbing iodine with mercury; used in constitutional syphilis.
Green Vitriol, — Vít-ri-ol; impure sulphate of iron.
Grindelia Robusta, Grin-dé-lí-a Rǫ-bús-ta; a California plant, recommended for asthma.
Grocer's Itch, Gró-ser'z Iç; *Acarus Sacchari*, caused by an animalcule found in sugar.
Ground Ivy, Grȣnd Ī-vi; *Nepeta Glechoma*, a native creeping plant.
Groundsel, Grȣ́nd-sel; common name in Europe for plants of the genus *Senecio*.
Grumous, Grú-mus; curdled, clotted.
Grutum, Grú-tum; a white tubercle in the skin resembling a millet seed.
Guaiac, Gwį-ak; a resin obtained by decoction from the heart wood of *Guaiacum officinale;* used in rheumatism and as an alterative.
Guaiacum Officinale, Gwį-a-kum Of-i-si-ná-lē; a tree of the West Indies the wood of which is used as a stimulant.
Guarana, Gwą-rą́-na; a brownish mass, prepared from the powdered seed of *Paullinia sorbilis;* it contains caffein, and is used in nervous diseases.
Gubernaculum Testis, Gų-ber-nák-ų-lum Tés-tis; a vascular ligament connecting the testicle with the scrotum in the fœtus.

Gum; a constituent of vegetable juices, soluble in water, not in alcohol; familiar as gum Acacia.

Gummi Guttæ, Gúm-i Gút-ē; gamboge, an inodorous substance, obtained from various trees; it is a powerful drastic, hydragogue cathartic, employed in dropsy.

Gum Resins, Gum Réz-inz; concrete vegetable juices of certain plants, such as ammoniacum, containing both resin and gum.

Gum Tree; a name applied to different species of *Eucalypus*.

Gun Cotton; Pyroxylon, an explosive substance obtained from cotton by the action of nitric acid; used to make collodion.

Gurjun Balsam, Gúr-jun Bǿl-sam; a fluorescent oleoresin, resembling copaiba both therapeutically and chemically.

Gustatory Nerve, Gús-ta-tω-ri Nɛrv; the nerve of taste, and general sensibility, a branch of the *inferior maxillary*, that sends out numerous filaments to the tongue.

Gutta Opaca, Gút-ɑ Ω-pá-kɑ; "opake drop;" cataract of the eye, in which the humors are dark.

Gutta Percha, Gút-ɑ Pɛ́r-çɑ; a firm flexible substance obtained from *Isonandra Gutta*, and used in surgical operations as splints, or as collodion after solution in bisulphide of carbon.

Gutta Serena, — Ser-ē-nɑ; amaurosis; paralysis of the retina, causing partial loss of vision.

Guttatim, Gu-tá-tim; drop by drop, as in prescriptions.

Guttur, Gút-ur; the throat, including also the windpipe.

Gynatresia, Jin-a-trē-ʒi-ɑ; imperforation, or absence of the vagina.

Gynecology, Jin-ē-kól-ω-ji; the science of the peculiarities of the female constitution.

Gyniacus, Jin-ī-a-kus; in the plural applied to diseases of women.

Gypsum, Jíp-sum; sulphate of calcium.

Gyri, Jī-rī; the spiral cavities of the internal ear; applied, also, to the convolutions of the brain.

Gymnocladus Canadensis, Jim-nók-la-dus —; the American coffee-tree, the leaves of which are cathartic and contain emetic properties.

H

H.; symbol for the element *Hydrogen.*

Habitat, Háb-i-tat; applied to the locality where a plant or animal exists in a state of nature.

Habromania, Hab-rō-má-ni-a; a kind of delirium in which the patient manifests levity.

Hæma, Hé-ma; a prefix signifying blood.

Hæmacelinosis, Hem-a-sel-i-nó-sis; "blood spot diseases;" purpura.

Hæmadynamometer, Hem-a-din-a-móm-ē-ter; an instrument for measuring the circulation of the blood.

Hæmagogue, Hém-a-gog; a medicine that promotes the menstrual discharge.

Hæmal, Hé-mal; relating to the blood, or to the sanguineous system.

Hæmal Arch, — Arç; the arch formed by the sternum and ribs, with the vertebra as a base.

Hæmaleucina, Hem-a-lu-si-na; the fibrin, or coat of the blood.

Hæmalopia, Hem-a-ló-pi-a; an affection of the eye, causing objects to seem blood-colored.

Hæmasthenosis, Hē-mas-tén-ō-sis; poverty, or weakness of the blood.

Hæmataporrhosis, Hem-a-tap-o-ró-sis; the removal of serum from the blood, as in cholera.

Hæmatemesis, Hem-a-tém-ē-sis; the vomiting of blood from the stomach.

Hæmathermous, Hem-a-thér-mus; warm-blooded.

Hæmatoma, Hem-a-tó-ma; a bloody tumor.

Hæmatica, Hē-mát-i-ka; diseases of the function of the blood; also, applied to medicines for their treatment.

Hæmatin Hém-a-tin; the red coloring matter of blood.

Hæmatocele, Hém-a-tω-sēl; the effusion of blood within one or the other of the tunics of the scrotum.

Hæmatocœlia, Hem-a-tω-sé-li-α; the effusion of blood into the cavity of the peritoneum.

Hæmatocolpus, Hem-a-tω-kól-pus; the escape of blood into, or accumulation of the catamenial discharge in the vagina.

Hæmato-Crystalline, Hém-a-tω-Krís-ta-lin; applied to a crystalline substance in the remains of blood.

Hæmatocystis, Hem-a-tω-sís-tis; the effusion of blood into the bladder.

Hæmatoid, Hém-a-tσd: having a resemblance to blood.

Hæmatometachysis, Hem-a-tω-met-ák-i-sis; the transfusion of blood.

Hæmatorrhœa, Hem-at-ω-ré-α; the moderate, natural flow of blood. [blood.

Hæmatosis, Hem-a-tώ-sis; hæmorrhage, a flow of

Hæmatoxylin, Hem-a-tóks-i-lin; the coloring matter of logwood.

Hæmatoxylon Campechianum, — Kam-pē-çi-á-num; a tree of South America that yields logwood.

Hæmatozoon, Hem-a-tω-zώ-on; an animalcule found in the blood.

Hæmin, or **Hæmine,** Hé-min; a crystalline residuum of dried blood, insoluble by strong acids.

Hæmophthalmus, Hem-of-tál-mus; an effusion of blood into the cavities of the eye. [the lungs.

Hæmoptysis, Hē-móp-ti-sis; discharge of blood from

Hæmorrhage, Hém-ω-rαj; a sudden and free discharge of blood from any cause. [especially to the piles.

Hæmorrhoid, Hém-ω-rσd; a hæmorrhage, but applied

Hæmospasia, Hem-ω-spá-si-α; causing the absence of blood from a considerable surface of the body, as in dry-cupping.

Hæmostasis, Hē-mós-ta-sis: stagnation of the blood.

Hæmotrophy, Hem-ót-rω-fi; excessive nutriment of the blood.

Hair-cap Moss, Hąr-kap Mos; *Polytrichum juniperinum;* a common moss of the United States, used as a diuretic.

Halitus, Hál-i-tus; vapor; applied to the vapor arising from newly drawn blood.

Halo, Há-lo; the circle, or areola that surrounds the nipple of the female breast; also the red circle around pustules.

Haloid Salt, Há-led Selt; a name formerly applied to salts containing two simple radicals, in contradistinction to oxysalts, but now obsolete.

Hamamelis Virginica, Ham-a-mí-lis Ver-jín-i-ka; witch-hazel, a native shrub; an aqueous preparation distilled from the fresh leaves of which is much used by Homœopathists.

Hare-lip, Hár-lip; a congenital fissure in the upper lip.

Hartshorn, Hárts-horn; a name applied to the preparations of ammonia, generally aqua ammonia.

Hay-Fever, Ha-Fí-ver; a peculiarly violent catarrh, occurring regularly every summer with its victims.

Haunch, Hanç; the hips and latteral parts of the pelvis.

Haversian Glands, Ha-vér-ʃi-an Glandz; a fatty substance found in connection with joints.

Haversian Tubes, — Tubz; small channels in the body of bones, containing a kind of marrow.

Hawkweed, Hók-wīd; a common name applied to plants of the genus *Hieracium*, several species of which are used in domestic practice as tonic and as tringent.

Head, Hed; the part of all the higher animals that contains the brain; also, applied to the upper end of bones, muscles, etc.

Heart, Hart; a hollow muscular body, in the center of the circulatory system of the superior grades of animals, whose function it is to give circulation to the blood.

Heart-Burn; the common name for *Cardialgia*.

Heavy Oil of Wine; an etherial oil, used in making Compound Spirit of Ether.

Hebe, Hí-bī; down, or incipient beard; applied to the hair of the pubes, or the age at which it appears.

Hebegynus, Hī-bég-i-nus; having incipient ovaries.

Hebeticus, Hī-bét-i-kus; youthful; the state of puberty.

Hectic Fever, Hék-tik Fē-ver; a fever resulting from habits, or the condition of the body, rather than from miasmatic or external causes, accompanied with night sweats.

Hedeoma Pulegioides, Hed-ē-ó-ma Pu-lē-ji-o-ī-dēz; pennyroyal; a native labiate plant, used as a stimulant and emmenagogue.

Helcodes, Hel-kó-dēz; affected with ulcers.

Helcoid, Hél-koid; similar to an ulcer.

Helcomenia, Hel-ko-mē-ni-a; a catamenial discharge from an ulcer.

Helenium Autumnale, He-lē-ni-um Θ-tum-ná-lē; sneezewort, a native plant.

Helianthemum Canadense, Hē-li-án-thē-mum; frostwort, a native plant.

Helianthus Annuus, Hē-li-án-thus An'u-us; sun-flower, the seeds of which are demulcent and expectorant.

Helix, Hē-liks; the border of the external ear.

Hellebore Hél-ē-bor; (American or Green;) *Veratrum viride.*

Hellebore, Black; *Helleborus niger*, which see.

Hellebore, White. See *Veratrum album.*

Helleborin, He-léb-o-rin; a glucoside found in *Helleborus niger.*

Helleborus Fœtidus, He-léb-o-rus Fét-i-dus; the European bearsfoot; cathartic and anthelmintic.

Helleborus Niger, — Nī-jer; black hellebore, a drastic cathartic; poisonous in over doses.

Helminthagogue, Hel-mín-tha-gog; a vermifuge.

Helminthiasis, Hel-min-thī-a-sis; the breeding of worms in diseased parts.

Helminthic, Hel-mín-thik; pertaining to worms.

Helminthophthisis, Hel-min-thóf-thi-sis; wasting of the system on account of worms.

Helodes, Hē-ló-dēz; a fever in which the sweating is profuse.

Helonias Dioica, Hē-ló-ni-as Dī-o-ī-ka; synonym for *Chamælirium luteum*, which see.

Helopyra, Hē-lóp-i-ra; a marsh or miasmatic fever.

Helos, Hē-los; the name of a tumor resulting from prolapsus or the dropping of the iris.

Hematoxylon. See *Hœmatoxylon.*

Hemeralopia, Hem-er-a-lṓ-pi-a; defective vision, in consequence of which nothing can be seen except in clear daylight.

Hemicrania, Hem-i-krá-ni-a; nervous pain on one side [of the head.

Hemiopsy, Hem-i-óp-si; imperfect vision, by which only the half of objects can be seen.

Hemiplegia, Hem-i-plí-ji-a; paralysis of one side of the body.

Hemisphere, Hém-i-sfīr; half a sphere; in the plural, applied to the two portions of the cerebrum.

Hemlock, Hém-lok; *Conium maculatum,* a poisonous plant of Europe, naturalized in many parts of the United States.

Hemlock Spruce, — Spruus; *Abies Canadensis,* an American evergreen.

Hemp, Hemp; *Cannabis sativa,* which see.

Henbane, Hén-ban; *Hyoscyamus niger,* a poisonous plant of Europe occasionally naturalized in the United States.

Hepar, Hí-par; the liver, whose office it is to secrete the bile.

Hepar Sulphuris, — Sul-fú-ris; sulphuret of lime, used Homœopathically.

Hepatalgia, Hep-a-tál-ji-a; pain in the liver.

Hepatic, Hī-pát-ik; relating to the liver.

Hepatica Triloba; Liverwort; kidney leaf; a small native herb, used as a demulcent.

Hepatitis, Hep-a-tí-tis; inflammation of the liver.

Hepatization, Hep-a-ti-zá-ʃon; a change in which the lungs become like the liver.

Hepatocele, Hép-a-tō-sīl; hernial tumor, in which part of the liver protrudes through the abdominal walls.

Hepatodynia, Hep-a-tō-dín-i-a; hepatalgia, or pain in the liver, that has become chronic.

Hepatogastric, Hep-a-tō-gás-trik; applied to the inferior omentum.

Hepatolithus, Hep-a-tól-i-thus; calculus or stone in [the liver.

Hepatoncus, Hep-a-tón-kus; swelling of the liver.

Hepatophyma, Hep-a-tō-fí-ma; a festering discharge from the liver.

Hepatorrhagia, Hep-a-tœ-rá-ji-a; hepatorrhœa, or bleeding from the liver.

Hermaphrodite, Her-máf-rœ-dīt; having the organs of both sexes partly developed, occurring more frequently in plants than in animal organizations.

Hernia, Hér-ni-a; a rupture; the protrusion of viscera through the walls of the abdomen, or displacement of any part from its natural cavity.

Hernia Cerebri, — Sér-ē-brī; protrusion of brain through a fracture of the skull.

Hernia Cruralis, — Kru-rá-lis; protrusion into the crural canal.

Hernia Humoralis, — Hu-mor-á-lis; swelling and inflammation of the testicle.

Hernia Inguinal, — In-gwī-nal; hernia at the groin; complete when it passes through the abdominal ring, and incomplete when it does not.

Hernia Umbilical, — Um-bíl-i-kal; when a part of the bowels protrude at the navel.

Herniotomy, Her- ni-ót-œ-mi; operation for strangulated hernia.

Herpes, Hér-pēz; tetter; a cutaneous eruption.

Herpes Circinatus, — Ser-sin-á-tus; the ring-worm.

Herpes Exedens, — Eks'ē-dens; a form of tetter that spreads rapidly.

Hesperidin, Hes-pér-i-din;. a hydro-carbon obtained from orange peel.

Heterochronia, Het-er-œ-krœ́-ni-a; a change of some part or tissue, at a time when not anticipated.

Heterologous, Het-er-ól-œ-gus; applied to tumors, ulcers, etc., that differ in nature from the rest of the body.

Heteropathy, Het-er-óp-a-thi; a mode of curing disease by changing the system from one morbid condition to another.

Heuchera Americana, Hu-kē-ra A-mer-i-ká-na; alum-root; an indigenous plant, the root of which is a powerful astringent.

Hg.; symbol for hydrogen.

Hiatus Fallopii, Hī-á-tus Fal-œ́-pi-ī; an opening in the tympanum.

Hibiscus, Hį-bís-kus; a genus of plants possessing demulcent properties.

Hiccough, Hík-up; *Singultus*, a convulsion of the diaphragm and surrounding parts.

Hidroa, Hį-drώ-ɑ; eczema, or heated eruption.

Hidrodes, Hį-drώ-dēz; sweaty.

Hidropedesis, Hį-drop-ē-dē-sis; unusual sweating.

Hieracium Venosum, Hį-er-á-ʃi-um Vē-nώ-sum; hawkweed; a reputed antidote for snake bites.

Hiera Picra, Hį-er-ɑ Pį-krɑ; an old name for a mixture of powdered aloes and canella.

Highmorianum Antrum, Hį-mo-ri-á-num An'trum; *Antrum maxillæ*, a cavity in the superior maxillary bone.

High Cranberry; *Viburnum Opulus*, Cramp-bark, a native shrub.

Hilus Lienalis, Hį-lus Lį-en-á-lis; the part of the spleen that is concave.

Hip; the articulation of the thigh with the pelvis.

Hip-Bath; a half bath, in which the hips and surrounding parts enter the bath tub.

Hip-Joint Disease. See *Caxalgia*.

Hippocampus, Hip-o-kám-pus; (Major and Minor;) two small eminences in the lateral ventricles of the brain.

Hippocoryza, Hip-o-ko-rį-zɑ; an inflammation of the mucous membrane of the nostrils, in horses and cattle.

Hippuric Acid, Hip-ų-rik As'id; a constituent of urine, especially in herbiverous animals; is contained in horses' urine; it is used for preparing benzoic acid.

Hippus, Hip-us; an affection of the eyelid that causes a tendency to wink.

Hippus Pupillæ, — Pų-pil-ē; a morbid condition of the iris, in which there is an alternate dilation and contraction of the pupil.

Hircismus, Hεr-sís-mus; the odor from the human armpit, resembling that of the goat.

Histodialysis, His-to-di-ál-i-sis; the formation of organic texture.

Histogenetic, His-to-jen-ét-ik; relating to the formation of organic texture.

Histology, His-tól-o-ji; anatomy; the science of organized bodies.

Histotomy, His-tót-ɷ-mi; the dissection and analysis of organized bodies.

Hive Syrup, Hiv Sír-up; a popular name for Compound Syrup of Squills.

Hoffman's Anodyne, — An'ɷ-din; a popular name for Compound Spirit of Ether.

Homesickness. (See *Nostalgia.*)

Homœopathy, Hɷ-mē-óp-a-thi; the system of curing disease promulgated originally by Hahnemann, based on the maxim, *similia similibus curantur*, (like cures like;) or, that medicine which in large doses would tend to excite a certain disease, will, in infinitesimal doses, cure such disease.

Homœosis, Hom-ē-ó-sis; the assimilation of different things to one in quality.

Homologue, Hóm-ɷ-log; any part of an animal that corresponds in character with such a part in another animal.

Homology, Hɷ-mól-ɷ-ji; the science which determines the correspondence of parts in the structure of animals.

Homonymous, Hɷ-món-i-mus; that branch of anatomy which determines the correlation of different parts.

Honey, Hún-i; a sweet semi-fluid liquid, secreted by honey-bees, (*Apis mellifica.*)

Hooper's Pills; pills of considerable reputation for the cure of female diseases.

Hooping Cough, Hup-iŋ Kof. (See *Pertussis.*)

Hops; the fruit, or strobiles, of *Humulus Lupulus;* used as a bitter tonic.

Hordeum Distichum, Hór-dē-um Dís-ti-kum; barley, the seed of which is extensively used in the preparation of malt.

Horehound, Hór-hɤnd; *Marrubium vulgare*, a common naturalized plant, used as a tonic and in coughs.

Horridus, Hór-i-dus; a sensation of cold, with shivering.

Horripilation, Hor-i-pi-la-ʃon; a creeping sensation, and feeling as if each hair on the body were stiff; a symptom of fever.

Horse-Chestnut; Hors Ȼés-nut; *Æsculus Hipyocastanum*, an Asiatic tree, the bark of which is said to be antiperiodic.

Horsemint, Hórs-mint; *Monarda punctata*, a native labiate plant, used as a carminative.

Horse-radish; the root of *Cochlearia armoracia*.

Horse-weed; *Ambrosia trifida*, a common coarse weed; stimulant and astringent.

Hor. un. Spatio, (*Horæ unius spatio;*) used in prescriptions, "at the end of an hour."

Hospital Fever; a kind of fever arising from the peculiar condition of hospitals and inmates.

Hospital Gangrene, — Gáŋ-grīn; a highly infectious ulceration, attended with humid gangrene.

Humectation, Hų-mek-tá-ʃon; the making of anything moist.

Humeral, Hų́-mer-al; relating to the arm.

Humerus, Hų́-mer-us; the shoulder, or the arm proper; also the long bone, from the shoulder to the elbow.

Humor, Hų́-mor; any fluid of the body other than the blood.

Humoral Pathology, Hų́-mor-al Pa-ŧól-ɷ-ji; an ancient theory, that attributed the causes of all diseases to the condition of the fluids in the system.

Humulus Lupulus, Hų́-mų-lus Lų-pų́-lus; the hop plant, twining and herbaceous, much cultivated in the United States.

Huxham's Tincture, Húks-am'z Tíŋk-tųr; a popular name for a Compound Tincture of Cinchona.

Hyalitis, Hį-a-lį́-tis. See *Hyaloiditis*.

Hyaloid, Hį́-a-lơd; transparent, like glass; applied to a membrane of the eye.

Hyaloiditis, Hį-a-lơ-dį́-tis; inflammation of the hyaloid membrane.

Hydatid, Hį-dát-id; a small watery tumor; also a species of intestinal worms.

Hydatidoma, Hį-dat-i-dɷ́-ma; a kind of tumor that generates hydatids.

Hydradenitis, Hį-dra-den-į-tis; inflammation of the lymphatic gland.

Hydræma, Hį-drḗ-ma; a condition of the blood that renders the serum transparent.

Hydragogue, Hį́-dra-gog; a medicine that tends to relieve the system of the superfluous secretion of water.

Hydrangea Arborescens, Hi-drán-jē-a Ar-bo-rés-ens; seven barks' hydrangea; a shrub, the root of which is much used for the removal of calculous deposits in the bladder.

Hydrangeitis, Hi-dran-jē-í-tis; inflammation of the lymphatic glands.

Hydrargyrum, Hi-drár-ji-rum; officinal name for the element mercury.

Hydrastia, Hi-drás-ti-a; a white crystalizable alkaloid, found in the root of *Hydrastis Canadensis.*

Hydrastin, Hi-drás-tin; a name often applied to berberin, properly *Hydrastia.*

Hydrastis Canadensis, Hi-drás-tis Kan-a-dén-sis; yellow root, golden seal, yellow puccoon; the root tonic, and used in diseases of the mucous membrane.

Hydrated Peroxide of Iron; known as hydrated oxide of iron, and hydrated sesquioxide of iron; it is the best and most common antidote for poisoning by arsenic. [*Hydrate.*

Hydrate of Chloral, Hí-drat of Kló-ral. See *Chloral*

Hydrate of Potassium; caustic potash.

Hydrates, Hí-drats; salts obtained by displacing one-half the hydrogen of water with an equivalent of another radical.

Hydrencephalocele, Hi-dren-sef-ál-o-sēl; hydrocephalic hernia.

Hydrencephalus, Hi-dren-séf-a-lus; hydrocephalus, or water in the head.

Hydriodic Acid, Hi-dri-ód-ik As'id; a combination of iodine and hydrogen.

Hydrobromic Acid, Hi-dro-bróm-ik; a combination of bromine and hydrogen; bromide of hydrogen.

Hydrocarbons, Hi-dro-kár-bonz; compounds of carbon and hydrogen, embracing volatile oils, paraffins, etc.

Hydrocele, Hí-dro-sēl; dropsy within the testicle.

Hydrocephaloid, Hi-dro-séf-a-lod; similar to hydrocephalus.

Hydrocephalus, Hi-dro-séf-a-lus; dropsy of the brain.

Hydrochloric Acid, Hi-dro-kló-rik As'id; commonly called muriatic acid, and composed of equal volumes of hydrogen and chlorine united by chemism.

Hydrocirsocele, Hį-drœ-sẽr-sœ-sīl; dropsy of the spermatic cord, accompanied with varicose veins.
Hydrocœlia, Hį-drœ-sé-li-a; dropsy of the belly.
Hydrocrania, Hį-drœ-krá-ni-a; dropsy of the brain.
Hydrocyanic Acid, Hį-drœ-si-án-ik As'id; Prussic acid, an extremely poisonous acid, composed of hydrogen and a compound body, cyanogen; is used in diluted form as a remedy in whooping cough.
Hydroderma, Hį-drœ-dẽr-ma; general dropsy of the integuments of the body.
Hydrogen, Hį-drœ-jen; an elementary body, the lightest known substance, entering into numberless combinations, and accepted as the unit for chemical calculations.
Hydrogen Salts; "the commonest salt of any radical whatsoever is a salt of hydrogen."—*Attfield.*
Hydrohæmia, Hį-drœ-hé-mi-a; reduced condition of the blood.
Hydrohystera, Hį-drœ-hís-ter-a. See *Hydrometra.*
Hydromeningitis, Hį-drœ-men-in-jį-tis; dropsy, complicated with inflammation of the brain.
Hodrometra, Hį-dróm-ē-tra; dropsy of the womb.
Hydronephros, Hį-drón-ē-fros; dropsy of the kidneys.
Hydropathy, Hį-dróp-a-thi; a system of curing diseases by the application of water, chiefly externally, at various degrees of temperature.
Hydropericardium. Hį-drœ-per-i-kár-di-um; dropsy of the membranous sac of the heart.
Hydrophobia; Hį-drœ-fó-bi-a; convulsions resulting from the bite of a mad dog or other rabid animal.
Hydrophthalmia, Hį-drof-thál-mi-a; dropsy of the eye.
Hydrops, Hį-drops; the dropsy, a disease in which there is a morbid accumulation of serous fluids in different parts of the system.
Hydrops Articuli, — Ar-tík-ų-lį; dropsy of a joint, generally at the knee.
Hydrops Siccus, — Sík-us; "dry dropsy;" or more properly *tympanites.*
Hydrorchis, Hį-drór-kis; dropsy of the testicle.
Hydrosarca. Hį-drœ-sár-ka; general dropsy in the flesh.

Hydrothorax Hị-drō-thṓ-raks; dropsy in the chest.
Hygeia, Hị-jḗ-yạ; health.
Hygiene, Hḯ-ji-ēn; the art, or means of preserving health.
Hygrology, Hị-grŏl-ō-ji; description of the fluids of the body.
Hygroma, Hị-grṓ-mạ; a tumor that contains a fluid, not pus.
Hymen, Hḯ-men; a semi-circular membrane that extends across the entrance of the vagina.
Hymenitis, Hị-men-ḯ-tis; inflammation of the hymen.
Hymenology, Hị-men-ŏl-ō-ji; description of the membranous system.
Hyoglossus, Hị-ō-glŏs-us; a large muscle connecting the tongue with the neck.
Hyoscyamin, Hị-os-ḯ-am-in; an alkaloid obtained from hyoscyamus.
Hyoscyamus Niger, Hị-os-ḯ-a-mus Nḯ-jer; henbane, a poisonous plant, the seed and leaves of which are used as a narcotic.
Hyper-, Hḯ-per; a prefix, meaning the highest of several; *per-* is generally used.
Hyperæmia, Hị-per-ḗ-mi-ạ; an excessive amount of blood; engorgement of blood vessels.
Hyperæsthesis, Hị-per-es-thḗ-sis; excessive sensibility.
Hyperasthenia, Hị-per-as-thḗ-ni-ạ; loss of strength; great debility.
Hypercatharsis, Hị-per-ka-thạ́r-sis; excessive purging.
Hyperemesis, Hị-per-ém-ē-sis; protracted vomiting.
Hypericum Perforatum, Hị-pér-i-kum Per-fō-rā́-tum; St. John's wort, the leaves of which are used as an astringent, and externally in liniments.
Hypo-, Hip-ō-; a prefix denoting under, thus: the hypophosphites contain less oxygen than the phosphites.
Hypochondriasis, Hip-ō-kon-drḯ-a-sis; low spirits, melancholy tending to insanity.
Hypochondrium, Hip-ō-kŏn-dri-um; the space under the false ribs.
Hypodermic, Hịp-ō-dḗr-mik; used in reference to the application of medicines under the skin, or after it has been removed by blistering.

Hypogastralgia, Hip-ω-gas-trál-ji-a; pain in the lower part of the abdomen.

Hypogastric, Hip-ω-gás-trik; descriptive of glands and a plexus of nerves in the region of the hypogastrium.

Hypogastritis, Hip-ω-gas-trį-tis; partial inflammation of the stomach.

Hypogastrium, Hip-ω-gás-tri-um; the lower part of the abdomen, just above the pubic regions.

Hypogastrocele, Hip-ω-gás-trω-sēl; hernial tumor in the hypogastrium.

Hypoglossal, Hip-ω-glós-al; under the tongue.

Hypoglottis, Hip-ω-glót-is; the under side of the tongue.

Hypohæmia, Hip-ω-hé-mi-a; loss, or deficiency of blood.

Hypophosphorous Acid, Hip-ω-fós-for-us As'id; an acid containing less of oxygen than phosphorous acid, formed when phosphorus is boiled with milk of lime.

Hypopyum, Hip-ó-pi-um; a pus-like fluid in the chamber of the eye.

Hypospadia, Hip-ω-spá-di-a; a malformation of the penis, consisting of an opening into the urethra on the under side.

Hyposthenia, Hip-os-thé-ni-a; loss of strength; general debility.

Hyssopus Officinalis, His-ó-pus —; hyssop; a garden plant, used as a stimulant.

Hystera, His-tē-ra; the womb; applied also to the vulva.

Hysteralgia, His-ter-ál-ji-a; pain in the womb.

Hysteria, His-té-ri-a; a spasmodic affection resulting from uterine irregularity or disease, attended with difficult breathing, palpitation of the heart, etc.

Hysteritis, His-ter-į-tis; inflammation of the womb.

Hysterocele, His-tér-ω-sēl; hernia of the womb.

Hysterodynia, His-ter-ω-dín-i-a; pain in the womb.

Hysterolythus, His-ter-ól-i-thus; calculus in the womb.

Hysteromania, His-ter-ω-má-ni-a; nymphomania, or morbid sexual desire.

Hysteroscirrhus, His-ter-ω-skír-us; incipient cancer of the womb.

Hysterotomy, His-ter-ót-ω-mi; the Cæsarean operation, i.e., the cutting an opening into the womb for the extraction of the child, when necessary.

I

I.; symbol for iodine.

Iamatology, Ī-am-a-tól-ŏ-ji; the science that treats of remedies for diseases.

Iatraleptic, Ī-a-tra-lép-tik; a method of treating disease by external applications and friction.

Iatria, Ī-a-trį-a; the healing art; a cure for disease.

Ice-Poultice, Īs-Pōl-tis; the application of pounded ice, in a bladder or rubber pouch, to inflamed tumors, etc.

Iceland Moss, Īs'land Mos; *Cetraria Islandica*, a mild nutritious tonic.

Ichor, Ī'kor; a thin, acrid discharge from a sore.

Ichoræmia, Ik-or-ē-mi-a; a vitiated condition of the blood.

Ichthyocolla, Ik-thi-ŏ-kól-a; the swimming bladder of fish, consisting of gelatin, and from which isinglass is procured.

Ichthyosis, Ik-thi-ō-sis; "fish-skin disease," in which the skin becomes hard and rough, or scaly.

Icteric, Ik-tér-ik; relating to jaundice.

Icteroid, Ik-ter-oid; resembling the jaundice.

Icterus, Ik'ter-us; jaundice, a bilious disease, attended with yellowness of the skin and eyes.

Ictodes Fœtidus, Ik-tō-dēz Fét-i-dus; skunk cabbage; synonym for *Symplocarpus fœtidus*.

Ictus Solis, Ik'tus Sō-lis; *coup de soleil*, stroke of the sun.

Idiopathic, Id-i-ŏ-páth-ik; relating to primary disease, not symptomatic or sympathetic.

Idiopathy, Id-i-óp-a-thi; original, or spontaneous disease.

Idiosyncrasy, Id-i-ŏ-sín-kra-si; peculiarity of constitution.

Ignatia Bean, Ig-ná-ʃi-a Bēn; the poisonous seed of *Strychnos Ignatia*, having properties similar to *nux vomica*.

Ignis Actualis, Ig'nis Ak-tų-á-lis; "actual fire;" cautery of the flesh by fire, or heated iron.

Ignis Sacer, Ig'nis Sá-ser; erysipelas.

Ignis Sancti Antonii, — Sáŋk-tị An-tṓ-ni-ị; another name for erysipelas.
Ileitis; Il-ē-ị-tis; inflammation of the ilium.
Ileo-Cæcal Valve, Il'ē-ō-Sē'kal Valv; a fold of membrane, that prevents the return of matter to the ilium from the colon. [intestines.
Ileum, Il'ē-um; the third and longest of the smaller
Ilex Paraguaiensis, Ī'leks Par-a-gwa-i-én-sis; Paraguay tea; a shrub of South America, the leaves of which are used as a nervous stimulant.
Ilex Verticillata, — Vεr-ti-sil-á-tɑ; black alder; tonic, alterative and astringent; synonym for *Prinos verticillatus*. [also, the small intestines.
Ilia, Il'i-ɑ; the flanks that enclose the small intestines;
Iliac, Il'i-ak; belonging to, or near the flanks.
Iliac Arteries; — Ar'ter-iz: several divisions of arteries, arising at the bifurcation of the aorta, and diverging to the iliac regions.
Iliac Fossa, — Fós-ɑ; a shallow cavity in the upper surface of the iliac bone.
Iliac Passion, — Pá-ʃon; griping pain, and vomiting of fecal matter, with spasms or peristaltic motion of the intestines.
Iliac Region, — Rē-jon; the sides of the abdomen, between the ribs and hips. [haunch bone.
Ilium, Il'i-um; the superior bone of the pelvis; the
Illicium Anisatum; Il-í-ʃi-um An-i-sá-tum; star-anise, a tree of China, the seed of which contains an aromatic oil very closely resembling oil of anise.
Imperforate, Im-pέr-for-et; congenital closure of natural openings.
Impetigo, Im-pét-i-gō; a humid running tetter.
Imposthume, Im-pós-ŧųm; an abscess.
Impotence, Im'pō-tens; want of power; male sterility.
Impotent, Im'pō-tent; inability of procreation.
Impregnation, Im-preg-ná-ʃon; the act of fecundation.
Inanition, In-an-í-ʃon; exhaustion; emptiness, from inability to take food.
Inappetency, In-áp-ē-ten-si; anorexia; loss of appetite.
Incarnation, In-kɑr-ná-ʃon; the process of granulation, or the growth of flesh.

Incerniculum, In-sɛr-ník-ų-lum; the basin of the kidneys through which the urine is strained.

Incineration, In-sin-er-á-ʃon; the act of burning out carbon and organic compounds in a crucible, the ash alone remaining.

Incisors, In-sį-sorz; the four front cutting teeth.

Incontinence, In-kón-tin-ens; inability to retain the natural evacuations.

Incubation, In-kų-bá-ʃon; the hatching of eggs; the slow development of disease.

Incus, In´kus; a small bone of the internal ear.

Indian Hemp; *Cannabis sativa* var. *Indica;* a powerful narcotic.

Indian Physic; *Gillenia trifoliata;* the root of which is cathartic, and in large doses emetic.

Indian Turnip; common name for *Arisæma triphyllum.*

Indigestion, In-di-jést-yon; when chronic, dyspepsia.

Indigo, In´di-gɷ; a blue coloring matter obtained from *Indigofera tinctoria*, a plant of the East Indies.

Indigo, Wild; *Baptisia tinctoria*, a native plant, used in decoctions as an antiseptic.

Inferior Longitudinal Sinus; a vein of the external membrane of the brain; extending along the lower part of the *falx cerebri.*

Infiltration, In-fil-trá-ʃon; the straining of fluids into the cellular tissues.

Influenza, In-flų-én-za; an epidemic catarrh, attended with depression and distressing fever.

Infundibulum, In-fun-díb-ų-lum; a funnel; applied to three ducts in the kidney, and to a canal connecting with the third ventricle of the brain.

Infusions, In-fų́-ʒonz; liquids obtained by macerating vegetable organic substances, in water that has reached the boiling point.

Inguinal, In´gwi-nal; belonging to the groin.

Inguinal Ligament. See Poupart's ligament.

Inhalation, In-ha-lá-ʃon; a method of applying medicines, by breathing medicated vapors into the lungs and head.

Injection, In-jék-ʃon; the application of water, or medicated liquids, to a cavity or internal part, by means of a syringe.

Inochondritis, In-ɷ-kon-drį-tis; inflammation of cartilages.

Inoculation, In-ok-ɥ-lá-ʃon; the insertion of the virus of a disease into some part of the body, for the purpose of inciting the same disease, but in a mild form.

Inoma, In-ɷ́-mɑ; a species of fibrous tumor.

Inorganic Chemistry, In-ər-gán-ik Kém-is-tri; the chemistry of the mineral kingdom.

Inorganic Compounds, — Kóm-pɤndz; a distinction once drawn between substances found in plants and animals, and those obtained from the mineral or inorganic kingdom.

Inosculation, In-os-kɥ-lá-ʃon; union of the extremities of vessels.

Insalivation, In-sal-i-vá-ʃon; the admixture of saliva with food in eating.

Insomnia, In-sóm-ni-ɑ; sleeplessness; wakefulness.

Inspissation, In-spi-sá-ʃon; boiling down, and thickening, as in making vegetable extracts.

Insufflation, In-suf-lá-ʃon; the act of blowing air into a cavity; inflating the lungs of a new-born child.

Integument, In-tég-ɥ-ment; that which covers anything.

Interarticular, In-ter-ɋr-tík-ɥ-lɑr; between the joints.

Intercellular, In-ter-sél-ɥ-lɑr; intervening between the cells of animal tissue.

Intercostal, In-ter-kós-tal; between the ribs. [tween.

Intercurrent, In-ter-kúr-ent; sporadic; running be-

Intermaxillary, In-ter-máks-il-ɑ-ri; applied to a small osseous body between the maxillary bones.

Intermittent Fever, In-ter-mít-ent Fí-ver; any fever in which the paroxysms of heat intermit and return at regular intervals.

Interne, In-tér-nē; a house physician or surgeon.

Interocular, In-ter-ók-ɥ-lɑr; located between the eyes.

Interosseous, In-ter-ós-ē-us; applied to anything between bones.

Interscapular, In-ter-skáp-ɥ-lɑr; lying between the shoulder blades. [cess.

Interspinal, In-ter-spį-nal; between the spinus pro-

Interstice, In′ter-stis; the space between any two parts.

Intervertebral, In-ter-vĕr-tē-bral; between the vertebræ.

Intestinal, In-tés-tin-al; relating to the intestines.

Intestine, In-tés-tin; the long canal from the stomach to the anus.

Introflexed, In′trō-flekst; bent inwards.

Intumescence, In-tū-més-ens; swelling, or increasing the size of any part.

Introsusception, or **Intussusception**; the falling or sliding of one portion of an intestine into another.

Inula Helenium, In-ū-la Hē-lén-i-um; *Elecampane*, the root used as a tonic.

Invagination, In-vaj-i-ná-ʃon; an operation for hernia by introsusception.

Iodates, Ī′ō-dats; compounds of iodic acid.

Iodic Acid, Ī-ód-ik As′id; a compound in which one atom each of hydrogen and iodine are united with three of oxygen; properly it is *iodate* of *hydrogen*. [element.

Iodides, Ī′ō-dīdz; compounds of iodine with another

Iodine, Ī′ō-dīn; a non-metallic element.

Iodinium, Ī-ō-dín-i-um; officinal name for *iodine*.

Iodism, Ī′ō-dizm; the morbid condition resulting from the continued use of iodine.

Iodoform, Ī-ód-ō-form; a yellow compound, with a strong, disagreeable odor, containing a large amount of iodine.

Ionthus, Ī-ón-thus; down, or incipient beard; also a pimple on the face; acne.

Ipecac, American, Ip′ē-kak —; *Euphorbia Ipecacuanha*, a native plant used as an emetic.

Ipecacuanha, Ip-ē-kak-ū-án-a; ipecac root; the root of *Cephaelis Ipecacuanha;* an emetic, and in small doses, expectorant.

Ipomæa Jalapa, Ip-ō-mē-a Ja-láp-a; a twining vine of Mexico, the root of which is jalap; synonym for *Exogonium purga*.

Iralgia, Ī-rál-ji-a; pain in the iris.

Iridectomy, Ir-i-dék-tō-mi; the operation for cutting out part of the iris.

Iridocele, Ir′i-dō-sēl; hernia, in which part of the iris protrudes.

Iridotomy, Ir-i-dót-ɷ-mi; same as Iridectomy.
Iris, Ī'ris; the circular colored membrane of the eye; also, name of a plant.
Iris Florentina, Ī'ris Flor-en-tī-na; a plant of Italy that yields orris root.
Iris Versicolor, — Vér-si-kul-or; blue flag; an alterative and diuretic, [demulcent.
Irish Moss, Ī'riʃ Mos; *Chondrus crispus;* a nutritive
Iritis, Ī-rī-tis; inflammation of the iris.
Iron, Ī'urn; a metallic element; *Ferrum.*
Iron by Hydrogen; finely divided iron, obtained by decomposition of oxide of iron, heated to redness by means of hydrogen gas.
Iron Weed; *Vernonia fasciculata*, a native weed, the root of which is used as a tonic.
Irritating Plaster, Ir'i-tat-iŋ Plás-ter; a name applied to compound tar plaster, used by Eclectic physicians.
Ischiagra, Is-kī-a-gra; gout in the hip; sciatica.
Ischialgia, Is-ki-ál-ji-a; pain in the ischium. [nerve.
Ischiatitis, Is-ki-a-tī-tis; inflammation of the ischiatic
Ischidrosis, Is-ki-dró-sis; suppression of sweat; want of perspiration.
Ischiocele, Is'ki-ɷ-sēl; hernia in the ischiatic foramen.
Ischiophthisis, Is-ki-óf-ŧi-sis; disease and wasting of the hip-joint.
Ischium, Is'ki-um; the lower bone of the pelvis.
Ischuria, Is-kū-ri-a; retention or suppression of urine.
Isinglass, Ī'ziŋ-glas; a gelatinous substance, obtained from the air-bladders of fish.
Isomorphous Bodies, Ī-sɷ-mér-fus Bód-iz; substances of similar chemical constitution, which replace each other in crystalized compounds and do not alter the geometrical figure.
Isonandra Gutta, Ī-sɷ-nán-dr-a Gút-a; a tree of the East Indies, the source of gutta percha.
Isopathy, Ī-sóp-a-ŧi; a feature of Homœopathy that teaches the use of the virus of any disease, in infinitesimal quantities, to cure the same disease.
Isothermal, Ī-sɷ-ŧér-mal; having the same temperature.

Issue, Iʃ'ų; an artificial ulcer, kept open for the purpose of relieving irritation elsewhere.

Isthmus, Ist'mus; "a neck," and applied to a narrow passage, as that of the fauces.

Itch, Iç; scabies, an infectious eruption. (See, also, Baker's, Bricklayer's and Grocer's Itch.)

Iter, Ɨ'ter: a passage between two or more parts.

Iter ad Infundibulum; the passage between the third ventricle of the brain and the infundibulum.

Iter a Palato ad Aureum; the Eustachian tube.

Iter a Tertio Ad Quartum Ventriculum; the aqueduct of Sylvius, in the brain.

Itis, Ɨ'tis; a suffix, denoting inflammation of a part.

Ivy, American, Ɨ'va; *Ampelopsis quinquefolia*, a native climbing shrub, the leaves of which are used as an alterative.

Ivy, Ground; *Nepeta Glechoma*.

Ivy, Poison: *Rhus Toxicodendron*.

Ivory, Black, Ɨ'vɷ-ri Blak; bone black; animal charcoal.

J

Jaborandi, Jab-or-án-dį; the leaves of *Pilocarpus pinnatus*, used as a diaphoretic and sialagogue.

Jactitation, Jak-ti-tá-ʃon, tossing about, with great restlessness.

Jalap, Jál-ap; the root of *Ipomœa Jalapa*, a well known and reliable cathartic.

Jamaica Ginger, Ja-má-ka Jín-jer; white ginger; ginger root, deprived of the cortical portion, and bleached.

Jamestown Weed, Jámz-tʊn Wēd; *Datura Stramonium;* generally called jimson weed, or thorn-apple.

Janipha Manihot, Ján-i-fa Mán-i-hot; a South American plant, from the root of which tapioca is obtained; the fresh root contains a volatile poison.

Jasmine, Yellow, Jás-min; *Gelsemium sempervirens*.

Jaundice, Jɋn-dis; a bilious disease, attended with yellow skin and eyes. See *Icterus*.

Jeffersonia Diphylla, Jef-er-sṓ-ni-ɑ Dį-fíl-ɑ; twin leaf, an early-flowering indigenous plant.

Jejunum, Jē-jų́-num; empty; the second of the smaller intestines, which is generally empty in the corpse.

Jersey Tea, Jér-zi Tē; an indigenous small shrub; *Ceanothus Americanus*.

Jesuits' Bark; Jéʒ-ų-its' Bɋrk; an old name for cinchona bark.

Jimson Weed, Jím-sun Wēd; Jamestown weed, *Datura Stramonium*.

Jugales, Jų-gá-lēz; the superficial nerves of the cheek bones.

Juglans Cinerea, Jų́-glanz Sin-ĕ-rē-ɑ; butternut tree, the bark of which is a mild cathartic.

Jugular, Jų́-gų-lɑr; belonging to the throat.

Jugular Veins, — Vanz; large veins, internal and external, of the neck, descending to the sheath of the carotid artery. [neck.

Jugulum, Jų́-gų-lum; the throat, or front part of the

Jumentosus, Jų-men-tṓ-sus; descriptive of urine having a rank odor.

Juncus Effusus, Júŋ-kus Ef-ų́-sus; the flowering rush, having aperient virtues.

Juniperus Communis, Jų-níp-er-us Kom-ų́-nis; the juniper tree; the fruit, known as juniper berries, are used as a diuretic, and in the preparation of gin.

Juniperus Sabina, — Sa-bį́-nɑ; a European shrub which yields an essential oil, (oil of savine,) used as a stimulant and irritant.

Juniperus Virginiana, — Vɛr-jin-i-á-nɑ; red cedar, a native tree.

Juvantia, Jų-ván-ʃi-ɑ; aiding, as medicines used to relieve pain or distress, in conjunction with curative remedies.

Juventus, Jų-vén-tus; adolescence.

K

K.; symbol for the element kalium, (*Potassium.*)
Kalium, Ká-li-um; officinal name for the element potassium.
Kameela, or **Kamala**, Ka-mí-la, Ka-má-la; a reddish powder, possessing anthelmintic and cathartic properties, obtained from the fruit of *Rottlera tinctoria.*
Kalmia Latifolia, Kál-mi-a Lat-i-fó-li-a; sheep laurel, a native shrub, the leaves of which are sedative and astringent.
Kelp, Kelp; the ashes of sea-weed, the source of iodine.
Keratome, Kér-a-tom; a hard tumor or swelling.
Keratonyxis; Ker-a-to-níks-is; the operation of inserting a needle through the cornea, for cataract.
Kerectomy, Ker-ék-to-mi; the operation of cutting away the outer layers of the cornea, so as to render it opaque.
Kermes Mineral, Kér-mēz Mín-er-al; oxy-sulphuret of antimony.
Kidney Leaf, Kíd-ni Lēf; *Hepatica triloba.*
Kidneys, Kíd-niz; the two glandular bodies lying in the loins, which secrete the urine.
Kinesipathy, Kin-ē-síp-a-thi; a system of treating disease by exercise, muscular kneading, and friction on the skin; also called Motorpathy.
King's Evil, Kiŋ'z Ē'vil; scrofula, which was so called because it was once supposed it might be cured by the friendly touch of the king.
Kinic Acid, Kį-nik As'id; an acid of cinchona.
Kino, Kį-no; a very astringent extract, the dried juice of *Pterocarpus Marsupium.*
Kleptomania, Klep-to-má-ni-a; the propensity to pilfer various articles by persons not needing them, and able to purchase them; moral insanity.
Koosso, Kú-so; a powerful vermifuge; the dried flowers of *Brayera anthelmintica.*
Krameria Triandra. See *Rhatany.*
Kreosot, Kré-o-sot. See *Creasote.*

L

Labarraque's Solution, Lab-ár-a-ke'z Sω-lų́-ʃon; a disinfecting liquid. Solution of chlorinated sodium.
Labia, Lá-bi-ɑ; the lips.
Labia Majora, — Ma-jώ-rɑ; the outer folds of the vulva.
Labia Minora, — Mi-nώ-rɑ; the inner folds of the vulva.
Labia Pudendi, — Pų-dén-dį; the external lateral protuberances of the vulva.
Labial, Lá-bi-al; pertaining to the lips.
Labium, Lá-bi-um; the lip; often applied to parts resembling a lip.
Labium Leporinum, — Lep-ω-rį-num; the hare lip.
Labor, Lá-bor; parturition; the process of child-birth.
Labrador Tea, Láb-ra-dor Tē. See *Ledum latifolium*.
Labrum, Lá-brum; the extremity of the lips, especially of the upper lip.
Labyrinth, Láb-i-rinϑ; the second cavity of the ear.
Lac, Lak; officinal name in B. P. for cow's milk; also applied to a resinous substance that exudes from certain trees in the East Indies.
Lacerum Foramen, Lás-er-um For-á-men; applied to two jagged openings between the occipital and temporal bones.
Lachesis, Láç-ē-sis; the poison of the serpent *Trigonocephalus Lachesis;* used by Homœopathists.
Lachnanthes Tinctoria, Lak-nán-ϑēz Tiŋk-tώ-ri-ɑ; spirit weed, the root of which is astringent and tonic.
Lachryma, Lák-ri-mɑ; a tear; the limpid secretion of the eyes.
Lachrymal Bone, Lák-ri-mal Bωn; a small thin bone on the inner side of the orbit of the eye.
Lachrymal Caruncle, — Ka-rúŋ-kl; a small reddish eminence in the inner corner of each eye.
Lachrymal Duct, — Dukt; the duct by which the tears are conveyed to the nose.
Lachrymal Gland, — Gland; a glomerate gland of the eye that secretes the tears.

Laciniate, La-sín-i-at; fringed; having a jagged edge.

Lac Sulphur, Lak Súl-fur; a form of sulphur obtained by precipitating sulphur from combination with lime, by means of muriatic acid; hence the name precipitated sulphur.

Lactation, Lak-tá-ʃon; the act of yielding milk to the young.

Lacteal, Lák-tī-al; applied to vessels that absorb the chyle, a milk-like fluid.

Lactescent, Lak-tés-ent; milk-like, or that which yields a milky juice, as some plants.

Lactic Acid, Lák-tik As'id; the acid produced when milk turns sour.

Lactiferous Duct; the main ducts of the mammary glands.

Lactifugus, Lak-tíf-ų-gus; that which checks the secretion and flow of milk.

Lactucarium, Lak-tų-ká-ri-um; the concrete juice of *Lactuca sativa;* a sedative and narcotic.

Lactuca Sativa, Lak-tų́-ka Sa-tį-va; the garden lettuce; the source of *Lactucarium.*

Lacuna, La-kų́-na; applied in the plural to microscopic cavities in the excretory ducts.

Lacuna Orbitæ; — Or'bi-tē; the arch of the orbit of the eye.

Ladies' Slipper, Lá-diz' Slíp-er; *Cypripedium pubescens;* a common native plant.

Lady Webster's Pills; dinner pills, which see.

Lagophthalmia, La-gof-tál-mi-a; a defective shortening of the eyelid, that prevents entire closing of the eye.

Lagostoma. La-gós-tō-ma; the malformation, hare-lip.

Lamina, Lám-in-a; a thin plate or membrane.

Laminated, Lám-in-a-ted; foliated; consisting of layers.

Lampblack, Lámp-blak; a form of carbon in a very fine state of division, once obtained from the soot of lamps.

Lanceolate, Lán-sē-ō-lat; having the shape of a spear.

Lancinating, Lán-sin-a-tiŋ; piercing, like a lance.

Lanugo, Lan-ų́-gō; soft hair, or down.

Laparoscopia, Lap-a-rō-skṓ-pi-a; an examination of the loins with the stethoscope.

Laparotomia, Lap-a-rō-tṓ-mi-a; the making of an incision into the abdomen in the region of the loins.

Lapidescent, Lad-i-dés-ent; stony; like a stone in hardness.

Lappa Officinalis, Láp-a Of-is-i-ná-lis; common burdock; synonym for *Arctium Lappa.*

Laqueus Gutturis, Lák-wĭ-us Gút-ur-is; inflammation of the throat or tonsils.

Larch, Larç; *Larix Europœa;* an evergreen tree of Europe, the bark astringent.

Larkspur, Lárk-spur; a common name for several species of *Delphinium.*

Larval, Lár-val; like a mask; descriptive of the skin when disfigured by certain diseases.

Laryngeal, La-rín-jĭ-al; relating to the larynx.

Laryngismus, Lar-in-jís-mus; spasms of the larynx.

Laryngitis; Lar-in-jí-tis; inflammation of the larynx.

Laryngophthisis, Lar-in-góf-ti-sis; phthisis; laryngeal consumption.

Laryngotomy, Lar-in-gót-o-mi; the operation of making an incision into the larynx.

Larynx, Lár-iŋks; the top of the windpipe, the organ of the voice.

Lateral Sinuses, Lát-er-al Sí-nus-ez; the veins that run along the spine at the back of the head.

Laudanum, Ló-da-num; tincture of opium, twenty-five drops of which are equivelant to one grain of opium.

Laurus, Ló-rus; a genus to which the plants producing camphor, sassafras and cinnamon were formerly referred.

Lavandula Vera, Lav-án-du-la Ví'ra; lavander; an aromatic, labiate shrub of Europe, the flowers of which are used as a stimulant.

Laxation, Laks-á-ʃon; loosening, as of the bowels.

Laxative, Láks-a-tiv; having a slightly purgative quality

Laxator Tympani, Laks-á-tor Tím-pan-i; a muscle of the tympanum

Laxus, Láks-us; loose, applied to animal fiber.

Lead, Led; an elementary substance. (See *Plumbum.*)

Lead Plaster, —Plás-ter; a plaster made from litharge and olive oil.

Ledum Latifolium Lí-dum Lat-i-fó-li-um; Labrador tea; a native northern shrub, the leaves of which are tonic.

Leeches, Lēç-ez; *Hirudo medicinalis*, an aquatic worm, used for extracting blood.
Lemon, Lém-on; the fruit of *Citrus limonium*.
Lenitive, Lén-i-tiv; assuaging, gentle remedies.
Leontice Thalictroides, Lē-on-tį-sē Ŧa-lik-trō-į-dēz; synonym for *Caulophyllum thalictroides*.
Leontodon Taraxacum, Lē-ón-tō-don Ta-ráks-a-kum; synonym for *Taraxacum Dens-leonis*.
Leonurus Cardiaca, Lē-ō-nṹ-rus Kqr-dį-a-ka; mother-wort; an introduced weed, used in domestic practice in female diseases.
Leporinum Labium, Lep-ō-rį-num Lá-bi-um; hair-lip.
Lepriasis, Lep-rį-a-sis; leprosy.
Leprous, Lép-rus; scaly; resembling leprosy.
Leptandra Virginica, Lep-tán-dra Vɛr-jín-i-ka; Culver's root; black root; a synonym for *Veronica Virginica*.
Leptandrin, Lep-tán-drin; a resinous substance obtained from black root, (*Veronica Virginica*.)
Lesion, Lē-ʒon; disease or injury of any part; a cut or wound.
Lethal, Lē-ŧal; fatal; relating to death.
Lethargy, Lŧ-ar-ji; a sleepy stupor; insensibility.
Lettuce Let-us; *Lactuca sativa;* the flowering plants possess narcotic properties.
Leuchæmia, Lų-kē-mi-a; whitish, or almost colorless and thin blood.
Leucoma, Lų-kṓ-ma; opacity of the cornea, a white speck on the eye.
Leucopathia, Lų-kō-pa-ŧį-a; the condition of an African albino, whose skin turns white.
Leucophlegmatic, Lų-kō-fleg-mát-ik; relating to a dropsical and flabby condition of the body.
Leucorrhœa, Lų-kō-rē-a; a white or mucous secretion of the vagina, arising from a morbid state of that locality.
Levant Wormseed, Lē-vánt Wúrm-sēd; the dried flower-heads, (not seeds,) of a Russian species of *Artemisia;* used as a vermifuge.
Levator, Lē-vá-tor; that which elevates; applied to numerous lifting muscles.

Levigation, Lev-i-gá-ʃon; the process of reducing to an impalpable powder.

Leyden Jar, Lá-den Jqr; a glass vessel, coated with tin, used for collecting electricity.

Liatris Spicata, Li-á-tris Spi-ká-tɑ; button snake-root, a native plant, used as a diuretic and tonic.

Liatris Squarrosa, — Skwa-rṓ-sɑ; blazing star; an indigenous showy plant.

Lichen, Líç-en; a tribe of cryptogamic plants; also a cutaneous eruption of pimples. [undigested.

Lientery, Lį-en-ter-i; diarrhœa in which the food passes

Life Root, Lįf Rut; *Senecio aureus;* a native plant, used as a diuretic and in female diseases.

Ligament, Líg-a-ment; an elastic membranous cord, stretching from end to end of movable bones.

Ligamenta Subflava, Lig-a-mén-tɑ Sub-flá-vɑ; the yellow ligaments, which fill the space between the vertebræ.

Ligation, Li-gá-ʃon; securing an artery by ligature.

Ligature, Líg-a-tųr; a small cord, or strong thread, used in surgery in tying arteries or other parts.

Ligusticum Levisticum, Li-gús-ti-kum Lē-vís-ti-kum; lovage, the leaves of which are used as a carminative.

Ligustrum Vulgare, Li-gús-trum Vul-gá-rē; privet; a cultivated shrub, the leaves of which are used in domestic practice as an astringent.

Lilium Candidum, Líl-i-um Kán-di-dum; white lily; the mucilaginous bulb of which is used as a tonic.

Lime, Lįm; (caustic lime,) oxide of calcium, quick lime, obtained by calcining limestone.

Lime Hydrate, — Hį-drat; (slacked lime,) obtained from lime by the action of water. [or defective.

Limosis, Li-mṓ-sis; a morbid appetite, either excessive

Lindera Benzoin, Lín-dē-rɑ Ben-zṓ-in; an aromatic native shrub, the spice bush; synonym for *Benzoin odoriferum.*

Linea Alba, Lín-ē-ɑ Al'bɑ; a whitish tendonous line, extending from the epigastrium to the pubes.

Linea Aspera, — As'per-ɑ; a rough prominence on the posterior surface of the femur, affording attachment to the muscles.

Linea Innominata, Lín-ē-a In-nom-i-ná-ta; a slightly raised line, forming part of the brim of the pelvis.

Lineæ Albicanthes, Lín-e-ē Al-bi-kán-thēz; whitish lines, extending from the navel to the pubes, more prominent in women soon after child-birth.

Lineæ Semilunares, Sem-i-lu-ná-rēz; lines formed by the abrupt termination of the fibers of the abdominal muscles.

Lineæ Transversæ, — Trans-vér-sē; lines which cross the *recti* muscles of the abdomen.

Lineola, Li-nē-o-la; small white lines that may be seen on some female breasts.

Lingual, Líŋ-gwal; relating to the tongue.

Liniment, Lín-i-ment; a liquid preparation used externally.

Linseed Oil, Lín-sēd Oil; a fixed oil, expressed from flax seed, used as an application to burns.

Linum Usitatissimum, Lí-num Yu-si-ta-tís-i-mum; flax; a cultivated plant that yields flax seed.

Lint, Lint; scraped linen, or the prepared fiber of the flax plant, used in dressing wounds.

Liparocele, Lip-ár-o-sēl; a fatty tumor in the *scrotum*.

Lipoma, Li-pó-ma; a fatty encysted tumor.

Liposphyxia, Lip-o-sfíks-i-a; cessation of the pulse.

Lippitude, Líp-i-tud; inflammation of the margin of the eye-lids, from which a humor exudes.

Liquidambar Orientale, Lik-wid-ám-bar O-ri-én-tal; a tree of Russia, the source of storax.

Liquid Storax, Lík-wid Stó-raks. See *Storax*.

Liquor, Lík-or; a solution of medicinal substances in water.

Liquor Amnii, — Am′ni-ī; water that surrounds the *fœtus in utero*.

Liquor Sanguinis, — Sáŋ-gwi-nis; the colorless fluid element of the blood.

Liquorice or **Licorice**, Lík-or-is; the root of *Glycyrrhiza glabra*; the powdered root is extensively used as an excipient for pills, and an extract from the root is used in cough mixtures, and to disguise the taste of bitter medicines.

Liquor Potassæ Arsenitis, — Po-tás-ē Ar-sen-í-tis; a solution of arsenious acid in water, by means of carbonate of potassium. (Fowler's Solution.)

Lithagogue, Lít-a-gog; a medicine for expelling calculi from the bladder or kidneys.
Litharge, Lít-qrj; oxide of lead.
Lithectasy, Lit-ék-ta-si; the operation of removing calculi from the bladder by dilating the urethra.
Lithiasis, Lit-į-a-sis; the formation of urinary calculus; also the growth of small hard tumors on the eyelids.
Lithic Acid, Lít-ik As'id; a name applied to uric acid.
Lithica, Lít-i-ka; medicines for preventing the formation of urinary calculus.
Lithium, Lít-i-um; an elementary substance, salts of which are used in gout and urinary diseases.
Lithoclast, Lít-ω-klast; an instrument for entering the urethra, to reduce calculi in the bladder so that they may be passed out.
Lithometra, Lit-ω-mé-tra; ossification of the uterus.
Lithotomy, Lit-ót-ω-mi; the operation of cutting into the bladder for the removal of calculi.
Lithotripsy, Lít-ω-trip-si; the wearing down, or grinding of calculi, in the bladder, by an instrument.
Lithotrity, Lit-ót-ri-ti; the breaking of calculi in the bladder, for removal.
Litmus, Lít-mus; a blue pigment, prepared from a species of lichen; acids turn the solution red.
Litmus Paper; paper colored with either the blue solution of litmus, or acidulated red solution. The blue paper turns red in the presence of acids; the red turns blue in the presence of alkalies.
Liver, Lív-er; the largest glandular body of animal organization, whose function is to secrete the bile.
Liver, Inflammation of. See *Hepatitis*.
Liverwort, a name commonly applied to *Hepatica triloba*, but properly belonging to cryptogams of the section *Hepaticæ*.
Lobate, Ló-bat; having lobes, as the lungs and liver.
Lobe, Lωb; a division or distinct part of an organ.
Lobelia Cardinalis, Lω-bé-li-a Kqr-di-ná-lis; cardinal flower; a native plant with showy red flowers.
Lobelia Inflata, — In-flá-ta; Indian tobacco, lobelia; a native plant, the leaves and seed of which are used as an emetic, and in small doses expectorant.

Lobulus Accessorius, Lób-ų-lus Ak-ses-ṓ-ri-us; a small lobe on the under side of the liver.

Lobulus Caudatus, — Ke-dá-tus; a tail-shaped lobe of the liver, hanging down from the great lobe.

Lobus Spigelii, Lṓ-bus Spi-jḗ-li- į; the smaller of the principal lobes of the liver.

Locellate, Lo-sél-at; having smaller or secondary cells.

Lochia, Lṓ-ki-a; a flow of cerous liquid from the vagina, after delivery, usually called "cleansings."

Lochiorrhœa, Lṓ-ki-o-rḗ-a; excessive lochial discharge.

Lochoperitonitis, Lo-ko-per-i-to-nį-tis; inflammation of the peritoneum after child-birth.

Locked-Jaw, Lókt-Je. See *Tetanus*.

Logwood, Lóg-wud; the wood of *Hæmatoxylon Campechianum;* extensively used as a dye-wood, and as a mild astringent.

Loimophthalmia, Lo-mof-thál-mi-a; contagious inflammation of the eyes.

Loins, Lonz; the lumbar regions, lower part of the back.

Longing, Lóŋ-iŋ; peculiar and capricious desires of females, generally in regard to food, during pregnancy.

Longissimus, Lon-jís-i-mus; the longest, applied to various muscles.

Longitudinal Sinus, Lon-ji-tų́-di-nal Sį-nus; a canal running lengthwise within the skull, on the upper margin of the *falx cerebri*. **L. S. Inferior**; a similar canal, or vein, along the lower margin of the *falx cerebri*.

Longus Colli, Lóŋ-gus Kól-į; the long muscle of the neck.

Lordosis, Lor-dṓ-sis; curvature of the spine forward.

Lotion, Lṓ-ʃon; a medicated fluid, to be applied externally.

Lovage, Lúv-ej; *Ligusticum levisticum*, an aromatic plant of Europe.

Loxa Bark, Lóks-a Bark; a variety of *Cinchona*.

Loxia, Lóks-i-a; wry-neck; the distortion of the head to one side of the body.

Loxophthalmus, Loks-of-thál-mus; squinting or oblique eyes.

Lumbago, Lum-bá-go; rheumatics in the muscles of the loins.

Lumbar, Lúm-bar; relating to the loins.

Lumbricales, Lum-bri-ká-lēz; four muscles of the hand and foot.

Lunar, Lú-nar; like the moon; applied to a bone of the carpus, on account of its shape.

Lunar Caustic, — Kôs-tik; fused nitrate of silver.

Lungs, Luŋz; the respiratory organs, occupying the thorax.

Lupia, Lú-pi-a; corroding, destructive, as a species of ulcer; also applied to a species of wen.

Lupinosus, Lu-pi-nó-sus; an ulcerous disease of the skin.

Lupulin, Lú-pu-lin; a yellow glandular powder found on hops.

Lupus, Lú-pus; "a wolf;" a malignant ulcer, or cancer, especially on the face.

Luscitas, Lú-si-tas; a defect in which an eye is turned to one side.

Lusus Naturæ, Lú-sus Na-tú-rē; a monster, from deformity.

Luxation, Luks-á-ʃon; dislocation of a bone.

Lycanthropy, Lį-kán-þro-pi; an insanity that leads a man to think himself a wolf.

Lycomania, Lį-ko-má-ni-a. Same as *Lycanthropy*.

Lycopodium, Lį-ko-pó-di-um; a fine yellow powder, the spores of *Lycopodium clavatum*, chiefly used as an excipient in making pills.

Lycopodium Clavatum, — Kla-vá-tum; club-moss, a little evergreen flowerless plant.

Lycopersicum, Lį-ko-pér-si-kum; the tomato; used medicinally by Homœopathists.

Lycorexia, Lį-ko-réks-i-a; *Bulimia;* unnatural, ravenous hunger.

Lycopus Virginicus, Lį-kó-pus Vɛr-jín-i-kus; bugle-weed, a tonic astringent.

Lymph, Limf; a colorless fluid in the lymphatic vessels.

Lymphadenitis, Lim-fa-den-į-tis; inflammation of the lymphatic glands.

Lymphatic, Lim-fát-ik; having the nature of lymph, applied to vessels that convey the lymphatic fluid.

Lypothymia, Lip-o-þím-i-a; grief, or mental affliction.

Lyssa, Lís-a; rage, fury; applied to hydrophobia.

Lyssoides, Lis-o-į-dēz; madness resembling hydrophobia.

M

M.; abbreviation of *manipulus*, "handful;" also of *misce*, "mix," in prescriptions.

Mace, Mes; an aromatic substance, detached from the kernels of the nutmeg tree.

Macerate, Más-er-et; to steep for the purpose of extracting soluble substances.

Macies, Mé-ʃi-ēz; emaciation, or washing away.

Macrocephalia, Mak-ro-se-fé-li-a; macrocephalous, having an abnormally large head.

Macromelia, Mak-ro-mé-li-a; deformity, by excessive size of some member.

Macrotys Racemosa, Ma-krót-iz Ra-sē-mó-sa; a synonym in common use for *Cimicifuga racemosa;* black cohosh.

Macula, Mák-ų-la; a blemish, or spot; *Macula matricis*, "spot from the mother," a prenatal mark on the skin of a child.

Maculous, Mák-ų-lus; abounding in spots.

Madder, Mád-er; a reddish dye-stuff, obtained from the roots of *Rubia tinctorum.*

Magnetism, Mág-net-izm; the property of attraction and repulsion in the load-stone.

Magnesia, Mag-né-ʒi-a; oxide of magnesium.

Magnesia Calcined, — Kál-sįnd; oxide of magnesium obtained by heating the carbonate.

Magnesium, Mag-né-ʒi-um; an elementary substance, salts of which are much used in medicine.

Magnetism, Animal; a theory revived by Mesmer in 1776, attributing all manifestations of life to a kind of magnetic fluid that he supposed pervades all matter.

Magnolia, Mag-nó-li-a; a genus of southern trees, noted for their magnificent flowers; the bark of several species is used as a tonic.

Maiden-Hair, Méd-en Hąr; *Adiantum pedatum;* a native fern, used as an expectorant.

Malacia, Ma-lé-ʃi-a; depraved appetite, as in pregnancy, and in some abnomal conditions.

Malacoma, Mal-a-kō-ma; softening, as happens to the brain, bones, kidneys, etc.
Malar, Mā-lar; belonging to the cheek.
Malaria, Ma-lā-ri-a; miasm; infectious, or noxious effluvia arising from decaying vegetable or animal matter.
Malates, Māl-ats; salts of malic acid and a base.
Male Fern, Mal Fern; *Aspidium Filix-mas*, a European fern, the root of which is used to expel tape worm.
Malic Acid, Māl-ik As'id; an acid found in the juice of rhubarb stalks, unripe apples, goose-berries, etc.
Malignant, Ma-līg-nant; dangerous or pestilential.
Malingering, Ma-līn-jer-iŋ; feigning disease, to avoid military service or punishment.
Malleolar, Ma-lē-o-lar; relating to the artery of the ankle.
Malleolus, Ma-lē-o-lus; the projections of bone forming part of the ankle joint.
Malleus, Māl-ē-us; a small bone of the internal ear, resembling a hammer.
Malpighian Bodies, Mal-pē-ji-an Bód-iz; small corpuscles, or points, found in the kidneys, spleen, and lymphatic gland.
Malt, Molt; barley that has been allowed to germinate, and then baked in a kiln.
Malva, Māl-va; a genus of plants possessing demulcent properties.
Mamma, Mām-a; the female breast, the source of milk.
Mammalia, Mam-ā-li-a; animals which suckle their young.
Mammary Gland, Mām-a-ri Gland; a gland beneath the mamma which secretes the milk.
Mammalaria Mam-a-lā-ri; resembling a breast.
Mammillation, Mam-i-lā-ʃon; small protuberances on a mucous surface of the body.
Mammose, Mām-os; having breasts, or the appearance of breasts.
Mandragora Officinalis, Man-drāg-o-ra Of-i-si-nā-lis; the true mandrake; a plant of the old world, of the natural order *Solanaceæ*.
Mandrake, Mān-drak; a name commonly applied in this country to *Podophyllum peltatum*, but properly belonging to *Mandragora officinalis* of Europe.
Manganese, Mān-ga-nēs; an elementary substance of steel-grey color when crystallized.

Mangifera Indica, Man-gíf-er-a In'di-ka; a tree of India, the bark of which is used as an astringent.
Mania, Má-ni-a; delirium, madness.
Mania a Potu, — a Pó-tų; delirium and nervous derangement from the use of intoxicating drinks.
Manna, Mán-a; a sweetish concrete substance, exuded from the stems of the *Fraxinus ornus*, a well known laxative.
Mannite. Mán-ịt; the sweet principle of manna.
Manubrium, Man-ų́-bri-um; a handle, applied to the upper part of the sternum.
Maranta Arundinacea, Ma-rán-ta A-run-di-ná-sē-a; a plant, native of the West Indies, from the roots of which the nutritious starch known as arrow root is obtained.
Maranta Galanga, Ma-rán-ta Ga-láŋ-ga; an East Indian plant that yields galangal root. [consumption.
Marasmus, Ma-rás-mus; withering, wasting, a kind of
Marble, Mą́r-bl; a native form of carbonate of lime.
Marigold, (Garden,) Má-ri-gold; *Calendula officinalis.*
Marjoram, (Sweet,) Mąr-jó-ram; *Origanum Majorana*, an aromatic garden herb.
Marrubium Vulgare, Ma-rú-bi-um Vul-gá-rē; horehound, the leaves of which are used for coughs.
Marsh-Mallow, Mąrʃ-Mál-o; the demulcent roots of *Althæa officinalis.*
Marsh Rosemary, — Róz-me-ri; *Statice Limonium* var. *Caroliniana*, (Gray;) a native plant, the root of which is astringent.
Marsupium, Mar-sų́-pi-um; a pouch, such as the peritoneum and scrotum.
Maruta Cotula, Ma-rú-ta Kót-ų-la; dog-fennel, mayweed, the dried flowers of which are sometimes used as a tonic.
Masseter, Mas-é-ter; a thick muscle of the lower jaw.
Mastaden, Más-ta-den; the gland of the female breast.
Mastadenitis, Mas-ta-den-ị-tis; inflammation of the mammary gland.
Mastodynia, Mas-to-dín-i-a; pain or neuralgia in the mamma, or female breast.
Mastoid, Más-tod; resembling the mamma, or nipple.

Mastoid Process, — Pró-ses; the projection of the temporal bone.
Mastomenia, Mas-tω-mē-ni-a; shifting of the menstrual discharge to the breasts.
Mastorrhagia, Mas-tω-rá-ji-a; hæmorrhage from the breast.
Masturbation, Mas-tur-bá-ʃon; manual excitement of the genital organs; termed also secret vice.
Materia Medica, Ma-tē-ri-a Méd-i-ka; the branch of medical science which treats of materials used for the cure of diseases.
Mastic, Más-tik; a resin obtained from *Pistacia lentiscus*.
Matico, Ma-tē-kω; the aromatic leaves of *Artanthe elongata*, used in diseases of the mucous membrane.
Matricaria Chamomilla, Mat-ri-ká-ri-a Kam-ω-míl-a; a herb which yields German chamomile flowers.
Matrix, Má-triks; the womb, or mother.
Maxilla, Maks-íl-a; the jaw, either upper or lower.
Maxillary, Máks-il-a-ri; relating to the jaw.
Maxillary Sinus, — Sį-nus; a cavity in the superior or upper jaw-bone.
May-Apple, Má-Ap-l; a common name for *Podophyllum Peltatum*.
Mayweed, Má-wēd. See *Maruta Cotula*.
Mayer's Ointment, Má-er'z Ơnt'ment; an ointment of olive oil, red lead, camphor, etc., used for old sores.
Measles, Mē-zlz; an eruptive and contagious fever.
Meatus, Mē-á-tus; an opening or passage.
Meatus Urinarius, — Yω-ri-ná-ri-us; orifice of the urethra.
Meconate of Morphia, Mē-kó-nat of Mór-fi-a: the natural salt of morphia as it exists in opium.
Meconic Acid, Mē-kón-ik As'id; an acid found in opium.
Meconium, Mē-kó-ni-um; the fæces found in the large intestine of a fœtus, and which passes off after birth.
Median, Mē-di-an; the middle or central portion.
Median Line, an imaginary vertical line, supposed to divide the body into two equal parts.
Median Nerve, — Nεrv; the middle branch of the brachial plexus, in the inner part of the arm.
Mediastinum, Mē-di-as-tį-num; the membranous partition which divides the thorax in two sections.

Medicine, Méd-i-sin; drugs or other material used for their curative effects; also the science of prescribing medicines.

Medicus, Méd-i-kus; a physician; one who attempts to heal diseases.

Meditullium, Med-i-túl-i-um; the juice in the spongy tissues of bones.

Medulla, Mē-dúl-a; marrow of bones; the pith or pulp of vegetables.

Medulla Oblongata, — Ob-loŋ-gá-ta; the base of the brain, or inferior portion of the spinal cord.

Medulla Spinalis, — Spị-ná-lis; the spinal cord or marrow.

Medullary Sarcoma, Méd-ul-a-ri Sar-kó-ma; a tumor that resembles the brain in structure.

Medulosus, Med-ụ-ló-sus; similar to or full of marrow.

Megrim, Mī-grim: a headache that affects but one side, and that near the eye.

Meibomian, Mị-bó-mi-an; small glands of the eyelids.

Mel, Mel; honey, the saccharine secretion of the *Apis mellifica*.

Melæna, Me-lē-na; the black vomit.

Melaleuca Cajeputi, Mel-a-lụ́-ka Kaj-ē-pụ́-tị; a tree of the East Indies, from which oil of cajeput is obtained.

Melanæmia, Mel-a-nē-mi-a; a dark condition of the blood, attended with a feeling of suffocation.

Melancholy, Mél-an-kol-i; a disease that leads to hypochondria, resulting from nervous derangement.

Melanismus, Mel-a-nís-mus; a kind of jaundice in which the skin turns dark.

Melanoma, Mel-a-nó-ma; dark tubercles; black cancer.

Melilotus, Mel-i-ló-tus; sweet clover, three leaved; used Homœopathically.

Melissa Officinalis, Mē-lís-a Of-i-si-ná-lis; a naturalized fragrant herb; lemon-balm.

Melituria, Mel-i-tụ́-ri-a; an excessive flow of urine, having a saccharine character.

Membrana Granulosa, Mem-brá-na Gran-ụ-ló-sa; the lining membrane of the Graafian vesicles of the ovary.

Membrana Limitans, — Lím-i-tans; the membrane which bounds the anterior and posterior surface of the retina.

Membrana Propria, Mem-brá-na Pró-pri-a; the basement membrane by which in the fœtus the pupil is closed.
Membrana Tympani, — Tím-pan-i; the membrane which closes the drum of the ear.
Membrane, Mém-bran; a tissue consisting of interwoven fibers, for covering some part; there are *mucous*, *serous* and *fibrous* membranes, according to their use and location.
Meningeal, Men-ín-jē-al; relating to certain membranes of the spinal cord and brain.
Meninges, Men-ín-jēz; membranes of the brain.
Meningitis, Men-in-jí-tis; inflammation of the membranes of the brain.
Meningium, Men-ín-ji-um; the delicate membrane between the *dura* and *pia mater*.
Meninguria, Men-in-jú-ri-a; the voiding of urine containing membranous matter.
Meniscus, Men-ís-kus; a crescent-like cartilage between the bones of a joint.
Menispermum Canadense, Men-i-spér-mum Kan-a-dén-sē; yellow parilla; a twining native plant, the root used as an alterative.
Menolipsis, Men-o-líp-sis; failure or lessening of the catamenial discharge.
Menoplania, Men-o-plá-ni-a; a catamenial discharge from some other part, at the menstrual period. [menses.
Menorrhagia, Men-o-rá-ji-a; an excessive flow of the
Menorrhagia Alba, — Al'ba; leuchorrhœa, which see.
Menostasia, Men-os-tá-si-a; suppression of the menses.
Mens; the Latin word for mind.
Menses, Mén-sēz; month; hence applied to the monthly discharge from the uterus.
Menstrual, Mén-stru-al; relating to the menses.
Menstruation, Men-stru-á-shon; the monthly flow of the menses, or catamenial discharge.
Menstruum, Mén-stru-um; any liquid that is used for extracting the virtue of a substance; a solvent.
Mensuration, Men-su-rá-shon; measurement of the chest, abdomen, etc., for the purpose of determining their strength and condition.

Menta, Mén-ta; *membrum virile*, the male member of generation.
Mentha Piperita, Mén-ŧa Pip-er-į-ta; peppermint, a labiate plant of Europe, abounding in an aromatic volatile oil.
Mentha Viridis, Mén-ŧa Vi-rį-dis; spearmint, properties similar to peppermint.
Menyanthes Trifoliata, Men-i-án-ŧēz Trį-fō-li-á-ta; bog-bean, recommended as a tonic.
Mephitic, Mē-fit-ik; noxious or suffocating.
Mephitis Mē-fį-tis; a noxious gas or poisonous exhallation.
Mercurial Ointment, Mɛr-kų́-ri-al Ơnt'ment; mercury thoroughly triturated with lard and suet.
Mercurial Pill, — Pil; metallic mercury, triturated with confection of roses until the globules of metal disappear.
Mercurius Vitæ, Mɛr-kų́-ri-us Vį-tē; an old name for precipitated oxychloride of antimony.
Mercuric Salts, Mɛr-kų́-rik Səlts; those compounds in which the acidulous radical is greatest; as, the higher of the chlorides is mercuric chloride.
Mercurialis Perennis, Mɛr-kų-ri-á-lis Per-én-is; dog's mercury, a plant having narcotic properties that act on the brain and spinal marrow. (Homœopathic)
Mercurial Tremor, — Trē-mor; convulsive movements of the muscles of those who have long been exposed to mercurial vapors.
Mercurous Salts, Mɛ́r-kų-rus Səlts; those compounds in which the acidulous radical is in lesser amount, as the lower of the two chlorides is *mercurous chloride*.
Mercury, Mɛ́r-kų-ri; a silver-white element, liquid at ordinary temperature.
Mercury with Chalk; mercury rubbed with chalk until the globules are no longer visible with the naked eye.
Meridrosis, Mer-i-drṓ-sis; partial perspiration, in places.
Merocele, Mér-ō-sēl; femoral hernia, occurring mostly with females.
Meropia, Mē-rṓ-pi-a; partial obscuration of vision.
Mesencephalum, Mes-en-séf-a-lum; the central portion of the brain.

Mesenteric, Mes-en-tér-ik; relating to the mesentery.
Mesenteritis, Mes-en-ter-ị-tis; inflammation of the mesentery.
Mesentery, Més-en-ter-i; the larger fold of the peritoneum, that unites and holds the intestines in place.
Mesial Line, Més-i-al Lịn. Same as *Median Line*.
Mesmerism, Més-mer-izm. Same as *Magnetism, Animal*.
Mesocæcum, Mes-ɷ-sē-kum; the part of the peritoneum to which the cæcum is joined.
Mesocolon, Mes-ɷ-kɷ́-lon; the part of the peritoneum to which the colon is joined.
Mesogastrium, Mes-ɷ-gás-tri-um; middle of the abdomen.
Mesometrium, Mes-ɷ-mē-tri-um; a cellular membrane about the uterus.
Mesorectum, Mes-ɷ-rék-tum; the part of the peritoneum to which the rectum is joined.
Metabasis, Mē-táb-a-sis; change in the character of a disease, or in the symptoms indicating certain remedies.
Metacarpal, Met-a-kɋ́r-pal; relating to the metacarpus.
Metacarpus, Met-a-kɋ́r-pus; the part of the hand between the wrist and fingers.
Metachysis, Mē-ták-i-sis; the operation of transfusing blood from one living body to another.
Metal, Mét-al; an elementary body, solid and opaque, having the properties of fusibility, tenacity, elasticity, etc., in a greater or less degree.
Metalloid, Mét-a-lɷd; resembling metal; non-metallic elements are sometimes so called.
Metaphosphoric Acid, Met-a-fos-fór-ik As'id; ordinary medicinal phosphoric acid, (orthophosphoric,) dedeprived of the elements of water.
Metastasis, Mē-tás-ta-sis; change in the seat of a disease.
Metatarsal, Met-a-tɋ́r-sal; relating to the metatarsus.
Metatarsus Met-a-tɋ́r-sus; the part of the foot between the ankle and toes.
Metatrophia, Met-a-trɷ́-fi-ɑ; unnatural, or imperfect nutrition.
Methogastrosis, Meŧ-ɷ-gas-trɷ́-sis; diseased condition of the stomach caused by alcoholic drinks.
Methomania, Meŧ-ɷ-mā́-ni-ɑ; delirium, or madness from drunkenness.

Methyl, Méth-il; an alcoholic radical, the base of wood spirit. [metopantrum.
Metopantritis, Met-ō-pan-trī-tis; inflammation of the
Metopantrum, Met-ō-pán-trum; the frontal sinus or depression.
Metra, Mé-tra; the womb, or uterus.
Metræmia, Me-tré-mi-a; the expanding or swelling of blood in the womb.
Metralgia, Mē-trál-ji-a; pain in the womb. [the womb.
Metranæmia, Met-ra-né-mi-a; deficiency of blood in
Metritis, Mē-trī-tis; inflammation of the womb. [womb.
Metrodynia, Met-rō-dín-i-a; pain in the uterus or
Metromania, Met-rō-má-ni-a. See *Nymphomania*.
Metrometer, Mē-tróm-ē-ter; an instrument for measuring the size of the womb.
Metroperitonitis, Met-rō-per-i-tō-nī-tis; inflammation of the peritoneum and uterus. [polypus.
Metropolypus, Met-rō-pól-i-pus; the womb affected by
Metrorrhagia, Met-rō-rá-ji-a; hemorrhage of the womb.
Metrorrhexia, Met-rō-réks-i-a; rupture of the uterus.
Metroscope, Mét-rō-skōp; an instrument for introducing into the uterus, by means of which to hear the heart-beats of the fœtus.
Mezereon, Mez-e-ré-on; the bark of *Daphne Mezereum*, used as a vesicant. [or animal.
Miasm, Mī-azm; a morbid gasseous emanation, vegetable
Microcosm, Mī-krō-kozm; a little world; applied to man as an epitome of the great world. [urinate.
Micturition, Mik-tū-rí-ʃon; frequent disposition to
Midriff, Míd-rif; the diaphragm, a large muscle dividing the thorax from the abdominal cavity.
Midwifery, Míd-wīf-er-i; the art, or occupation, of aiding a patient in child-birth.
Miliaria, Míl-i-a-ri; an eruptive fever.
Milk, Milk; the secretion of the mammary glands; cow's milk is officinal in the British Pharmacopœa.
Milk-Fever, — Fé-ver; a feverish condition attending women preceding the secretion of milk. [with water.
Milk of Lime, — Līm; slacked lime made into a paste
Milk Sickness; — Sik-nes; a peculiar endemic disease, attended with trembling.
Milk Crust. See *Porrigo*.

Milk-Weed, Milk-Wēd; a common name for plants of the genus *Asclepias*, especially the *A. Cornuti*.

Mindererus, (Spirits of,) Min-de-rḗ-rus; a solution of acetate of ammonium.

Mineral, Mín-er-al; a metal; any inorganic substance [in the earth.

Mineral, Ethiop's, — Ē'thi-op's. See *Ethiops mineral*.

Mineral, Kermes', — Kér-mēz'; a name once applied to sulphide of antimony.

Minim, Mín-im; the sixtieth part of a fluid drachm, containing 0.91 grains of water.

Misanthropy, Mis-án-thro-pi; a morbid condition that incites hatred of mankind.

Miscarriage, Mis-kár-ej. Same as *Abortion*.

Misogynous, Mis-ój-in-us; dislike of women.

Mistletoe, Mís-l-to; a parasite on trees, (*Phoradendron flavescens*,) used in nervous diseases.

Mistura, Mis-tú-ra; a mixture of two or more things.

Mitchella Repens, Miç-él-a Rḗ-pens; partridge-berry, a small evergreen plant, used as a diuretic.

Mixture, Brown, Míks-tur, Brun; Compound mixture of liquorice.

Mobility, Mo-bíl-i-ti; ability or tendency to move; nervous susceptibility.

Mola, Mó-la; the knee-pan; a molar tooth; also a flesh-like body in the uterus.

Molar, Mó-lar; applied to the grinding teeth.

Molar Glands, — Glandz; two small bodies situated in the cheeks, between the buccinator and masseter muscles, whose orifices open into the mouth opposite the rear molar tooth.

Mole, Mol; a small hard projection anywhere on the skin; also, a fleshy body, or tumor in the uterus.

Molecular Death, Mo-lék-u-lar Deth; death of any small part.

Molecular Weight, — Wat; the sum of the weight of the atoms of a body.

Molecule, Mól-e-kul; the smallest particle of matter that can exist in a free state.

Mollities, Mol-íʃ-i-ēz; softness; preternatural tenderness.

Mollities Cerebri, — Sér-ē-bri; softening of the brain.

Mollities Ossium, — Os'i-um; softening of bones.

Mollusca, Mo-lús-kɑ; one of the four general divisions of animals; they have soft bodies with no skeletons.

Molluscum, Mo-lús-kum; a cutaneous eruption of small tumors resembling mollusks. [substance.

Molybdenum, Mol-ib-dé-num; an elementary metallic

Momordica Elaterium, Mɷ-mɵ́r-di-kɑ El-a-té-ri-um; a European vine, the fruit of which yields elaterium.

Monad, Món-ad; an atom capable of replacing one atom of hydrogen; the most minute of infusorial animals.

Monarda Punctata, Mɷ-nɑ́r-dɑ Puŋk-tɑ́-tɑ; horsemint, a native plant. [nite plant.

Monkshood, Múŋks-hud; a common name for the aco-

Monoblepsis, Mon-ɷ-blép-sis; a condition of vision when objects can only be seen by one eye.

Monomania, Mon-ɷ-mɑ́-ni-ɑ; insanity, but only in regard to one subject.

Monomaniac, Mon-ɷ-mɑ́-ni-ak; a person who is insane on some single subject.

Monorchis, Mɷ-nór-kis; having but one testicle.

Mons Veneris, Mons Vén-er-is; the pubic prominence in women.

Monster, Món-ster; the unnatural formation of a fœtus.

Morbid, Mɵ́r-bid; diseased; relating to disease.

Morbific, Mɵr-bíf-ik; causing disease.

Morbilli, Mɵr-bíl-į; *Rubeola*, the measles.

Morbillous, Mɵr-bíl-us; relating to the measles.

Morbus, Mɵ́r-bus; sickness; disease.

Monsel's Salt, Món-sel'z Sɵlt; dried subsulphate of iron.

Monsel's Solution, — Sɷ-lų́-ʃon; solution of subsulphate of iron; a styptic. [sickness."

Morbus Caducas, — Ka-dų́-kas; epilepsy, or "falling

Morbus Coxarius, Koks-ɑ́-ri-us; the hip disease.

Morgagni (Sinuses of,) Mɵr-gɑ́g-nį; three slight enlargements near the head of the aorta.

Moribundus, Mor-i-bún-dus; dying, or ready to die.

Morphia, Mɵ́r-fi-ɑ; an alkaloid from opium, a powerful narcotic.

Morphine, Mɵ́r-fin. Same as *Morphia*.

Morphosis, Mor-fɷ́-sis; morbid growth or organization.

Morrhuæ Oleum, Mo-rų́-ē ɷ'lē-um; cod-liver oil.

Mors Mɵrz; death; entire absence of life.

Morus Rubra, Mó-rus Rú-bra; the mulberry tree; the ripe fruit of which is slightly laxative.
Morus Tinctoria, — Tiŋk-tó-ri-a; a tree of South America that yields fustic.
Mother Liquor, Múđ-er Lík-or; a term applied to the solution from which crystals have been separated after formation.
Mother's Mark, —Mqrk; any of the peculiar marks on the skin of a child caused by mental impressions on the pregnant mother.
Motherwort, Múđ-er-wurt; *Leonurus Cardiaca;* used in female diseases.
Motores Oculorum, Mo-tó-rīz Ok-ų-ló-rum; a pair of nerves that gives motion to the eyeball.
Moxa, Móks-a; a substance of cotton, wool, etc., applied to the skin and burned, with the aid of a blow-pipe, to cause an issue and draw off diseased action from another part.
Moxosphyra, Moks-o-sfí-ra; an iron hammer, or piece of smooth metal, heated in boiling water, and applied to the skin as a counter-irritant.
Mucilage, Mų́-si-lej; a solution of gum in water; usually applied to the solution of gum Arabic.
Mucin, Mų́-sin; the animal matter of mucus.
Muciparus, Mų-síp-a-rus; productive of mucus.
Mucocele, Mų́-ko-sēl; a tumor in the mucous membrane; also a distention of the lachrymal sac.
Muco-Purulent, Mų́-ko-Púr-ų-lent; having the natures of mucus and pus combined.
Mucous, Mų́-kus; relating to or like mucus.
Mucous Follicles, — Fól-i-klz; small glands of the mucous membranes whose function it is to secrete mucus.
Mucous Membranes, — Mém-branz; those which line the cavities and canals that communicate with the outer air.
Mucronata, Mų-kro-ná-ta; the pointed cartilage of [the sternum.
Mucuna Pruriens, Mų-kų́-na Prú-ri-ens; a climbing plant of South America, that yields pods from which cowhage is obtained.
Mucus, Mų́-kus; one of the principal fluids of the [body.

Mulberry, Múl-ber-i; the fruit of the *Morus rubra*.

Mulberry Calculus, — Kál-kų-lus; a kind of urinary calculus that resembles the rough surface of the mulberry.

Mullein, Múl-en; *Verbascum Thapsus*, a common plant, the leaves and flowers of which are used as a demulcent.

Multifid, Múl-ti-fid; many-cleft, or much divided; applied to a muscle of the spine.

Multiparous, Mul-típ-a-rus; relating to animals that bring forth more than one at a birth.

Mumps, Mumps; parotitis, a disease of the parotid gland.

Muriates, Mų́-ri-ats; once applied to all salts of muriatic acid; now restricted to the salts with alkaloids.

Muriatic Acid, Mų-ri-át-ik As'id; a combination of equal volumes of chlorine and hydrogen; called also hydrochloric acid and spirit of salt.

Muscæ Volitantes, Mús-sē Vol-i-tán-tēz; an affection of the eyes, in which motes seem dancing before them.

Muscle, Mús-l; (*Musculus;*) a bundle of animal fibers.

Muscular, Mús-kų-lar; relating to or possessing muscle.

Musculi-Pectinati, Mús-kų-lį-Pek-ti-ná-tį; fibers within the auricles of the heart, resembling the teeth of a comb.

Musculo-Cutaneous, Mús-kų-lo Kų-tá-nē-us; apertaining to muscle and the contiguous skin.

Musculus, Mús-kų-lus; muscle, a portion of flesh capable of contraction and extension, causing motion, voluntary and involuntary.

Mushroom, Múʃ-rum; *Agaricus campestris*, a fungus vegetable production.

Musk, Musk; an odoriferous substance, secreted in a special sac by the male musk deer, (*Moschus moschiferus;*) used in medicine as a stimulant.

Musk-Root, — Rut; sumbul root; the root of a plant of Russia, used as a nervine.

Mustard, Mús-tard; the pungent seed of *Sinapis nigra*, mostly used in poultices as a rubefacient.

Mustard Oil, (essential,) —Oil; a pungent oil obtained by distilling black mustard seed with water.

Mutitas Atonica, Mų́-ti-tas A-tón-i-ka; dumbness resulting from imperfect action of the nerves of the tongue.
Mutitas Sudorum, — Sų-dṓ-rum; dumbness resulting from sympathy with deafness.
Myalgia, Mį-ál-ji-a; cramp; muscular pain.
Myasthenia, Mį-as-thḗ-ni-a; debility of the muscles.
Mycoderma, Mį-kō-dér-ma; a mucous membrane.
Mycodermitis, Mį-kō-der-mį́-tis; inflammation of a mucous membrane.
Mycophthalmia, Mį-kof-thál-mi-a; fungous inflammation of the eye.
Mycosis, Mį-kṓ-sis; a fungus tumor.
Mydriasis, Mi-drį́-a-sis; weakness of vision, resulting from an excessive humor of the eye.
Myelarius, Mį-ē-lá-ri-us; having vertebra and spinal marrow.
Myelitis, Mį-ē-lį́-tis; inflammation of the spinal marrow.
Myeloma, Mį-ē-lṓ-ma; a medullary tumor, of a brain-like consistency.
Myelosis, Mį-ē-lṓ-sis; the formation of a medullary tumor.
Myentasis, Mį-én-ta-sis; muscular extension, or stretching of the muscles.
Myitis, Mi-į́-tis; inflammation of a muscle.
Mylodus, Míl-ō-dus; a molar tooth.
Mylo-Hyoideus, Mį́-lō-Hį-ō-į-dē-us; muscle of the lower jaw and tongue.
Mylo-Pharyngeus, — Far-ín-jē-us; the *Constrictor superior* muscle of the pharynx.
Myo-Carditis, Mį́-ō-Kar-dį́-tis; inflammation of the muscles of the heart.
Myodes, Mį-ṓ-dēz; resembling a muscle.
Myoline, Mį́-ō-lin; the elementary substance of muscle.
Myology, Mį-ól-ō-ji; description of the nature and uses of muscles.
Myopathia, Mį-ō-pá-thi-a; pains in the muscles of the womb.
Myopia, Mį-ṓ-pi-a; near-sightedness.
Myosis, Mį-ṓ-sis; unusual contraction of the pupil of the eye.
Myotomy, Mį-ót-ō-mi; anatomy or dissection of a muscle.
Myrcia Acris, Mér-ʃi-a Ak'ris; a tree of the West Indies, from the leaves of which bay-rum is distilled.

Myrica Cerifera, Mír-i-ka Ser-íf-er-a; bayberry, a native shrub, the bark of which is used as a tonic and expectorant.
Myristica Moschata, Mir-ís-ti-ka Mos-ká-ta; a tree of the East Indies that yields nutmegs and mace.
Myrospermum, Mir-ω-spér-mum; a genus of South American leguminous trees, the source of the balsams of Peru and Tolu.
Myrrh, Mεr; a hard resinous exudation from the *Balsamodendron Myrrha*, used as a tonic and as a wash.
Myrtus Pimenta, Mér-tus Pi-mén-ta; synonym for *Eugenia pimenta*.
Mystachial, Mis-tá-ki-al; relating to the upper lip.
Mystax, Mís-taks; the upper lip; the moustache.

N

Naboth's Glands, Ná-boθ's Glandz; certain mucous follicles within the neck of the uterus.
Nævus Maternus, Né-vus Ma-tér-nus; maternal mark; a mark on the neck of a child at birth, and ever after, caused by the mother's longing for, or dislike of certain objects.
Nail, Nal; a horny appendage to the fingers and toes.
Nanocephalus, Nan-ω-séf-a-lus; a dwarfed head.
Nape of the Neck; *Nucha;* the back part, and including the spinal projection just above the shoulders.
Napiform, Náp-i-fərm; descriptive of one of the textures of cancer.
Narcodes, Nqr-kώ-dēz; affected with stupor.
Narcoma, Nqr-kώ-ma; stupor from the effect of narcotic medicine.
Narcosis, Nqr-kώ-sis; the action of narcotic drugs.
Narcotic, Nqr-kót-ik; stupefying; deadening.
Narcotin, Nq́r-kω-tin; an alkaloid of opium.
Narcotism, Nq́r-kω-tizm; the effect produced by narcotic drugs.
Naris, Ná-ris; (pl. Nares;) the nostril.

Narthex Assafœtida, Nạr-theks As-a-fét-i-da; an umbelliferous plant of Asia, from the fresh roots of which assafœtida exudes.

Nasal, Ná-zal; pertaining to the nose.

Nasal Fossæ, — Fós-ē; the cavities constituting the internal portions of the nose.

Nasturtium Armoracia, Nas-túr-ʃi-um Ar-mo-ré-ʃi-a; a synonym for *Cochlearia armoracia;* horse-radish.

Nasus, Ná-sus; the nose, including all its parts.

Nates, Ná-tēz; the buttocks, or posterior part of the body, on which we sit.

Natrium, Ná-tri-um; a name for sodium.

Natrum, (or Natron,) Ná-trum; a saline compound, mostly subcarbonate of soda. (Homœopathic)

Natrum Arsenicatum, — Ar-sen-i-ka-tum; a compound of arsenic, acid and sodium.

Naturalia, Nat-ų-rá-li-a; natural; applied to the parts of generation.

Nausea, Nó-ʃē-a; sickness of the stomach.

Nausea Marina, — Ma-rį-na; sea-sickness.

Nauseous, Nó-ʃē-us; causing nausea: disgusting.

Navel, Ná-vel; the cicatrix left from the umbilical cord, about the middle of the abdomen.

Navel-String, — Striŋ; the umbilical cord of the fœtus.

Navel-wort, Ná-vel-wurt. See *Cotyledon umbilicus.*

Naviculare, Nav-ik-ų-lá-rē; applied to a bone of the wrist, and also to one of the ankle.

Near-Sightedness. See *Myopy.*

Nebula, Néb-ų-la; a cloud or speck on the cornea of [the eye.

Neck, Nek; the part between the head and thorax.

Necrology, Nē-król-o-ji; a record of the number and causes of deaths.

Necroscopy, Nē-krós-ko-pi; a post mortem examination of a lifeless body.

Nectandra Rodiei, Nek-tán-dra Ro-di-é-į; a South American tree which yields bebeeru bark.

Neonatus, Nē-o-ná-tus; newly born.

Nephralgia, Nē-frál-ji-a; pain in the kidneys.

Nephria, Né-fri-a; "proposed as a synonym for Bright's Disease, or granulated kidney." (Thomas' Medical Dictionary.)

Nephritic, Nē-frit-ik; pertaining to the kidneys.
Nephritis, Nē-frị-tis; inflammation of the kidneys.
Nephritis, Albuminous, — Al-bɥ́-min-us; Bright's disease of the kidneys, characterized by albuminous urine.
Nephrotomy, Nē-frót-ɷ-mi; the operation of cutting into the kidney for the extraction of calculus.
Neroli, (Oil of) Nē-rɷ́-lị; an essential oil, distilled from orange flowers, and used as a perfume.
Nerves, Nɛrvz; long white cords, of delicate substance, that ramify through the body, arising in the brain and spinal cord, and whose office it is to convey sensation and volition to and from the brain.
Nervine, Nɛ́r-vin; relating to the nerves; also, a common name for *Cypripedium pubescens.*
Nervous, Nɛ́r-vus; affected by the nerves.
Neuralgia, Nɥ-rál-ji-ɑ; pain in a nerve.
Neurine, Nɥ́-rin; substance of the nerves.
Neuritis, Nɥ-rị-tis; inflammation of a nerve.
Neurology, Nɥ-ról-ɷ-ji; the science of the functions of the nerves.
Neuroma, Nɥ-rɷ́-mɑ; knotty tumors upon nerves.
Neuropathy, Nɥ-róp-a-ŧi; disease of a nerve.
Neurophthisis, Nɥ-róf-ŧi-sis; the weakening and wasting of nerves.
Neurosis, Nɥ-rɷ́-sis; nervous affections. [a nerve.
Neurotomy, Nɥ-rót-ɷ-mi; the dissection or division of
Neutralizing Cordial, Nɥ́-tral-ịz-iŋ Kɵ́rd-yal; cordial containing rhubarb, hydrastis, bi-carbonate of potassium, much used in bowel affections.
Nicotiana Tabacum, Ni-kɷ-ti-á-nɑ Ta-bá-kum; the tobacco plant, the leaves used as a sedative, and which yield an alkaloid (nicotin,) which is a powerful narcotic poison.
Nicotin, Ník-ɷ-tin; a volatile alkaloid obtained from tobacco. [eye-lids.
Nictitation, Nik-ti-tá-ʃon; a morbid quivering of the
Night-blooming Cereus, Nịt-blúm-iŋ Sí-rē-us; *Cereus grandiflorus,* a cactus plant, used in heart diseases.
Nightmare, Nịt-mɑr; *Ephialtes;* a horrible or oppressive dream.

Nightshade, (Deadly) Nįt-ʃad; the common name for *Atropa Belladonna.*

Nigrities Ossium, Nį-grí-ʃi-ēz Os'i-um; caries; blackness of bones.

Nisus, Nį-sus; the action of the diaphragm and abdominal muscles in expelling any matter from the body.

Nisus Formativus, — Fər-ma-tį-vus; plastic force, or the vital power in each organ of the body to perform its function.

Nitrates, Nį-trats; salts of nitric acid. The radical is hypothetical (NO^3.)

Nitre, Nį-ter; a term applied to nitrate of potassium; [saltpeter.

Nitre, sweet spirit of; a solution in alcohol of the peculiar ether obtained when nitric acid is distilled with ordinary alcohol.

Nitric Acid, Nį-trik As'id; a combination of the hypothetical radical (NO^3) with hydrogen, forming a salt of hydrogen, (HNO^3.)

Nitrite of Amyl, Nį-trįt of Am'il; an etherial liquid used extensively in sea-sickness.

Nitrite of Ethyl, — Eŧ'il; the chief therapeutical ingredient of spirit of nitrous ether.

Nitrites, Nį-trįts; salts of nitrous acid; characterized by the radical NO^2.

Nitrogen, Nį-trɷ-jen; an element of the atmosphere, and constituting a large portion of all organic bodies.

Nitro-Muriatic Acid, Nį-trɷ-Mų-ri-át-ik As'id; a mixture of muriatic and nitric acid; once known as *Aqua Regia.*

Nitrous Acid, Nį-trus As'id; a combination of NO^2 with hydrogen, forming HNO^2.

Nitrous Ether, — Ŀ'ŧer; the peculiar ether produced by the action of nitrous acid upon alcohol.

Nitrous Oxide, — Oks'įd; protoxide of nitrogen, or laughing gas.

Noctambulation, Nok-tam-bų-lá-ʃon, walking in one's [sleep.

Nocturnal Emission, Nok-túr-nal Ŀ-miʃ-on; spermatorrhœa; the involuntary emission of semen, at night, when asleep.

Node, Nɷd; a morbid excrescence of bones.

Nodose, Nɷ-dɷ́s; having nodes or knots; swollen in [places.

Nodular, Nód-ų-lar; relating to small nodes or knots
Nodule, Nód-ųl; a diminutive node or knot.
Nodus Cerebri, Nṓ-dus Sér-ē-brī; "knot of the brain;" a medullary substance uniting the cerebrum and cerebellum.
Noli me Tangere, Nṓ-li mē Tán-jer-ē; an ulcerous disease affecting the skin and sometimes the cartilages of the nose.
Noma, Nṓ-ma; "to eat away;" a corroding disease, often attacking the mouth and also the *pudenda* of female children.
Non Compos Mentis; "not sound of mind."
Non-metallic Elements. See Elements Non-metallic.
Nordhausen Sulphuric Acid, Nord-hȣ-sen Sul-fų́-rik As'id. See Fuming Sulphuric Acid.
Nosography, Nō-sóg-ra-fi; description of diseases.
Nosology, Nō-sól-ō-ji; classification of diseases.
Normal, Nór-mal; natural; in a healthy condition.
Nostalgia, Nos-tál-ji-a; home-sickness.
Nostomania, Nos-tō-má-ni-a; homesick madness.
Nostril, Nós-tril; the cavity on each side of the nose.
Nostrum, Nós-trum; "ours;" applied to private or patent medicines; a quack medicine.
Notalgia, Nō-tál-ji-a; pain in the back.
Nubecula, Nų-bék-ų-la; cloudy appearances in the urine, when in a morbid condition.
Nucha, Nų́-ka; the nape or back of the neck.
Nucleolus, Nų-klḗ-ō-lus; a small nucleus.
Nucleus, Nų́-klē-us; the kernel, or central point.
Numbness, Núm-nes; torpor; want of sensation.
Nutgalls, Nút-golz. See Galls.
Nutmegs, Nút-megz; the aromatic dried kernels of *Myristica moschata*, mostly used as a condiment.
Nux Vomica, Nuks Vóm-i-ka; the poisonous seed of *Strychnos Nux Vomica;* used in small doses as a general tonic; the source of the poisonous alkaloids, *strychnia* and *brucia*.
Nymphæ, Nim-fē; the internal membranous folds, or lips, of the vulva.
Nymphæa Odorata, Nim-fḗ-a Ō-dō-rá-ta; water lily, a native aquatic flower, the root of which is astringent and demulcent.

Nymphitis, Nim-fí-tis; inflammation of the nymphæ.
Nymphomania, Nim-fo-má-ni-a; excessive desire in females for coition.
Nymphoncus, Nim-fón-kus; a tumor or swelling of the nymphæ.
Nymphotomy, Nim-fót-o-mi; the removal of diseased nymphæ by the knife.

O

Oak, Ok; a common name for trees of the genus *Quercus*, the bark of several species is used as an astringent.
Oaricus, O-ár-i-kus; relating to the ovary.
Oarium, O-á-ri-um; the ovarium; an ovary.
Oat-Meal, Ot-mēl; a nutritious substance, the ground seed of the oat, (*Avena sativa.*)
Obesity, O-bés-i-ti; fatness; corpulence of body.
Obliquus Externus, Ob-lík-u-us Eks-tér-nus; a muscle of the abdomen that arises from the lower ribs.
Obliquus Inferior, — In-fé-ri-or; the shortest muscle of the eye.
Obliquus Internus, — In-tér-nus; a minor muscle of the abdomen, arising from the spine of the ilium.
Obliquus Superior, — Su-pé-ri-or; the longest muscle of the eye, arising from the optic foramen.
Oblongatis, Ob-long-gá-tis; extended; somewhat long.
Obovoid, Ob-ó-void; nearly egg-shaped, but with the small end downward.
Obstetrics, Ob-stét-riks; the art of assisting at child-birth, and treating the diseases connected therewith.
Obstetrix, Ob-stét-riks; a midwife.
Obstipation, Ob-sti-pá-shon; persistent costiveness, from which no relief can be obtained by evacuation.
Obstruent, Ob-strú-ent; shut up; astringent.
Obturator, Ob-tu-rá-tor; applied to muscles, foramina, etc., that close up.
Obturator Externus, — Eks-tér-nus; a muscle connected with the *trochanter major*, which rotates the thigh.

Obturator Internus, Ob-tų-rá-tor In-tér-nus; a muscle whose location is nearly the same as the last.
Obvolute, Ob'vǫ-lųt; wrapped, or rolled together.
Occipital, Ok-síp-i-tal; connected with the occiput, or back part of the head.
Occipito-Frontalis, — Fron-tá-lis; a muscle that extends from the occiput to the forehead.
Occiput, Ok'si-put; the back part of the head.
Occlusion, Ok-lų́-ʒon; imperforation; shut up.
Occult, Ok-últ; hidden; latent: not developed.
Ocellate, Ǫ-sél-at; having small spots like the pupil of the eye.
Ocellus, Ǫ-sél-us; small round spots, the center of which has a different color from the rest.
Octana, Ok-tá-nɑ; an intermittent fever that returns every eighth day.
Ocular, Ok'ų-lɑr; relating to the eye.
Oculate, Ok'ų-lat; spotted with figures resembling an eye.
Oculist, Ok'ų-list; one who gives special attention to diseases of the eye.
Oculus; Ok'ų-lus; the eye; the organ of sight.
Od, Od; the force or influence supposed to cause the phenomena of animal magnetism.
Odic, Ǫ'dik; relating to the force termed od.
Odontagra, Ǫ-dón-ta-grɑ; rheumatic toothache; also, an instrument for extracting teeth.
Odontalgia, Ǫ-don-tál-ji-ɑ; a violent toothache, resulting from caries and exposure of the nerve.
Odontia, Ǫ-dón-ʃi-ɑ; applied to all morbid conditions of the teeth.
Odontitis, Ǫ-don-tį́-tis; inflammation of a tooth.
Odontoid, Ǫ-dón-tǫd; tooth-like; resembling teeth.
Odontology, Ǫ-don-tól-ǫ-ji; science of the teeth.
Odorate, Ǫ'dǫ-ret; having a strong odor or scent.
Œdema, Ȩ-dḗ-mɑ; a swelling, caused by the effusion of a serous fluid into the cellular membrane.
Œdematus, Ȩ-dém-a-tus; relating to œdema.
Œnomania, Ȩ-nǫ-má-ni-ɑ; urine madness; *mania a potu.*
Œnothera Biennis; Ȩ-nót-er-ɑ Bį-én-is; evening primrose, a common native plant.
Œsophagitis, Ȩ-sof-a-jį́-tis; inflammation of the œsophagus.

Œsophagotomy, Ē-sof-a-gót-o-mi; the operation of opening the œsophagus for the removal of a foreign body.

Œsophagus, Ē-sóf-a-gus. See Esophagus.

Œstrum, Es'trum; the impulse of passion or desire, that can scarcely be controlled; especially applied to the sexual passions.

Officinal, Of-ís-i-nal; (gen. *officinalis*, from *officina*, "a shop";) applied to medicines that are authorized by the proper medical authorities to be prepared and kept on sale, as distinguished from those to be compounded from the prescription of a physician. The word *official*, "with authority," similar in meaning, is sometimes used, improperly, for *officinal*.

Oil, Oil; unctious or fatty matter, obtained from vegetable or animal bodies, not soluble in water.

Oils, Fixed; non-volatile oils.

Oils, Volatile, — Vól-a-til; essential oils; oils that may be distilled, and are usually obtained by distillation of plants, seeds, etc., with water.

Ointments, Oint'ments; medicated mixtures, for external application, softer than cerates.

Oleander, O-lē-án-der; *Rhododendron chrysanthum;* an acro-narcotic, recommended in rheumatism, gout, and syphilis.

Oleates, O'lē-ats; combinations of oleic acids.

Oleic Acid, O-lē-ik As'id; the acid of fluid oils.

Olecranon, O-lék-ra-non; end of the ulna at the elbow; the joint of the elbow.

Olein, O'lē-in; the pure oils, as olive oil, oleate of glyceryl.

Oleo-Resins, O'lē-o-Réz-inz; mixtures of resins and volatile oils.

Oleum, O'lē-um; latin name for oil.

Olfactory Nerves, Ol-fák-to-ri Nervz; a pair of nerves connected with the pituitary membrane of the nose, that carries to the brain the sense of smell.

Olibanum, O-líb-a-num; frankincense; a gum resin, obtained from several species of *Boswellia.*

Oligæmia, Ol-i-gē-mi-a; paucity or thinness of the blood.

Oligospermia, Ol-i-go-spér-mi-a; deficiency of semen.

Olive Oil, Ol'iv Ōl; a mild, bland oil, expressed from the fruit of *Olea Europœa*; used mostly as an external application in ointments, liniments, etc.

Omagra, Om'a-grɑ; pain or gout in the shoulder. [der.

Omarthritis, Om-ɑr-ŧrị-tis; inflammation of a shoul-

Omentitis, Ω-men-tị-tis; inflammation of the omentum.

Omentum, Ω-mén-tum; (*majus* and *minus;*) the folds of the peritoneum that cover the bowels.

Omo-Hyoideus, Om'ω-Hị-ω-ị-dē-us; applied to a muscle of the neck, that depresses the *os hyoides* and lower jaw.

Omphalic, Om-fál-ik; relating to the navel. [cus.

Omphalitis, Om-fa-lị-tis; inflammation of the umbili-

Omphalocele, Om'fal-ω-sēl; umbilicus hernia.

Omphaloncus, Om-fa-lón-kus; a hard swelling of the navel.

Onanism, Ω'nan-izm; the vice of masturbation.

Ontology, On-tól-ω-ji; the doctrine or theory of existence.

Onychia, Ω-ník-i-ɑ; a whitlow or abscess near the nail.

Onyx, Ω'niks; a purulent speck in the anterior chamber of the eye. [of the finger.

Onyxis, Ω-níks-is; an ingrowing of a nail into the flesh

Opercular, Ω-pér-kụ-lɑr; applied to that which closes or covers a cavity.

Ophthalmia, Of-ŧál-mi-ɑ; inflammation of the eye, whether internal, external, catarrhal, purulent or rheumatic.

Ophthalmic, Of-ŧál-mik; belonging to the eye, or relating to ophthalmia.

Ophthalmitis, Of-ŧal-mị-tis; inflammation of the ball of the eye and its membranes.

Ophthalmoblennorrhœa, Of-ŧal-mω-blen-ω-ré-ɑ; a discharge of mucus from the eye.

Ophthalmocarcinoma, Of-ŧal-mω-kɑr-si-nố-mɑ; cancer of the eye. [eye.

Ophthalmocele, Of-ŧál-mω-sēl; abscess or tumor of the

Opthalmoplegia, Of-ŧal-mω-plé-ji-ɑ; a paralysis of the muscle of the eye.

Ophthalmorrhœa, Of-ŧál-mω-rē-ɑ; extravasation of blood in the eye.

Opiate, Ѡ'pi-at; an anodyne; that which causes sleep.
Opisthotonos, Ѡ-pis-ŧót-ѡ-nos; a kind of tetanus that bends the body backwards.
Opium, Ѡ'pi-um; the dried juice obtained from the capsules of *Papaver somniferum;* a very powerful narcotic, and the source of morphine.
Opodeldoc, Ѡ-pѡ-dél-dok; a name applied to camphorated soap-liniment, in which an animal soap is substituted for the castile of the officinal process.
Opodeldoc Liquid,— Lík-wid; officinal camphorated soap-liniment.
Opponens Pollicis, Op'ѡ-nens Pól-i-sis; a muscle of the thumb and wrist.
Optic, Op'tik; relating to the organ of sight.
Optic Nerve, — Nɛrv; the medium of communication between the eye and brain.
Optic Thalamus, — Ŧál-a-mus; two eminences in the lateral ventricles of the brain, seat of the optic nerve.
Optics, Op'tiks; the science of light and vision.
Ora, Ѡ'ra; plural of *os*, a mouth.
Oral, Ѡ'ral; relating to a mouth; "by word of mouth."
Orange-Peel, Or'enj-Pēl; the dried fruit-rind of *Citrus Aurantium*, and *C. vulgaris*, used as an aromatic and tonic.
Orbicular, Ɵr-bík-ų-lar; having the shape of an orb.
Obiculare Os, Ɵr-bik-ų-lá-rē Os; a small bone of the ear, shaped like an orb.
Orbicularis Oculi, — Ok'ų-lį; a muscle connected with the nasal process and the superior maxillary bone.
Orbicularis Oris, — Ѡ'ris; the muscle constituting the body of the lips.
Orbicularis Palpebrarum, — Pal-pē-brá-rum; the muscle that shuts the eye.
Orbit, Ɵr'bit; the cavity in which the eye is set.
Orbital, Ɵr'bit-al; relating to the eye.
Orbito-Sphenoid, Ɵr'bi-tѡ-Sfē-nɵd; used to describe the orbital wing of the sphenoid bone.
Orcheitis, Ɵr-kē-į-tis; inflammation of the scrotum.
Orcheoplasty, Ɵr-kē-ѡ-plás-ti; the process of removing a diseased portion of the scrotum, and supplying its place with a healthy piece from an adjoining part.

Orchialgia, Θr-ki-ál-ji-ɑ; pain in the testicle.

Orchiocele, Θr'ki-ɷ-sɫl; hernia of the testicle.

Orchis, Θr'kis; the testicle.

Orchitis, Θr-kị-tis; inflammation of the testicle.

Organ, Θr'gan; any specific part of a vegetable or animal having an office to perform.

Organic, Θr-gán-ik; having organs; applied to diseases of the organic structure, as distinct from functional disease.

Organic Chemistry, — Kém-is-tri; that which treats of the properties of animal and vegetable matter.

Organic Life — Lịf; existence dependent upon organization, vegetable as well as animal.

Organic Molecules, — Mól-e-kɥlz; used by certain scientists to designate floating particles thought to exist in the male semen, as the primordial elements of existence.

Organism, Θr'gan-izm; vital economy; active life.

Organology, Θr-gan-ól-ɷ-ji; the branch of physiology which considers the organs of animal existence.

Orgasm, Θr'gazm; state of excitement, especially of the sexual organs.

Orifice, Or'i-fis: an aperture, or mouth.

Origanum Majorana, ɷ-ríg-a-num Ma-jɷ-ré-nɑ; sweet marjoram, a labiate plant, native of Europe; used as an aromatic.

Origanum, Oil of; a volatile oil distilled from *Origanum vulgare*, and mostly used in liniments. That which is sold as commercial oil of origanum is the oil of thyme.

Orobanche Virginiana, Or-ɷ-bán-kɫ Vɛr-jin-i-é-nɑ; beech-drops; synonym for *Epiphegus Virginiana*.

Orpiment, Θr'pi-ment; a native sulphide of arsenic, poisonous, but used associated with other substances, as a depilatory.

Orrhorrhœa, Or-ɷ-rɫ-ɑ; a discharge of serum.

Orrhymen, O-rị-men; a serous membrane.

Orris, Or'is: the root of *Iris Florentina*, chiefly used in tooth powders, and as a perfume for the breath.

Orthopædia, Θr-θɷ-pɫ-di-ɑ; the curing of deformities in children.

Orthophosphoric Acid, Θr-ŧω-fos-fŏr-ik As′id; the officinal phosphoric acid.
Orthopnœa, Θr-ŧop-nĕ-a; difficult respiration, requiring an erect position.
Os, Os; (gen. *oris;*) a mouth; an opening.
Os, Os; (gen. *ossis,* pl, *ossa;*) a bone.
Os Externus, — Eks-tĕr-nus; mouth of the vagina.
Os Femoris, — Fém-or-is; the long bone of the thigh.
Os Humeri, — Hų́-mer-ị; the bone of the arm, from the shoulder to the elbow.
Os Hyoides, — Hị-ω-ị́-dēz; a small bone at the base of the tongue, having the shape of the Greek letter *v.*
Os Iliacum, — I-lị́-a-kum; one of the two large bones of the pelvis.
Os Ilium — Il′i-um; the upper part of the *Os Innominatum.*
Os Internum, — In-tĕr-num; the mouth of the uterus.
Os Pubis, — Pų́-bis; a bone in the fœtal pelvis.
Os Tincæ, Os Tín-sē; orifice of the womb.
Os Ustum, Os Us-tum; bone-ash, which see.
Os Uteri, Yú-ter-ị; mouth, or opening of the uterus.
Oscheal, Os′kē-al; relating to the scrotum.
Oscheitis, Os-kē-ị́-tis; inflammation of the scrotum.
Oschelephantiasis, Os-kel-ē-fan-tị́-a-sis; a great enlargement of the scrotum.
Oscheocele, Os′kē-ω-sēl; hernia of the scrotum.
Oscitation, Os-i-tá-ʃon; the act of gnawing.
Osculator, Os-kų-lá-tor; the muscle of the lips.
Osculum, Os′kų-lum; a small mouth or opening.
Osmazome, Os′ma-zωm; the principle in muscular fiber which gives to it taste and flavor when cooked.
Osmunda Regalis, Os-mún-da Rē-gá-lis; buckhorn brake, a tonic.
Osphyarthritis, Os-fi-ạr-ŧrị́-tis; (*Osphyitis,*) inflammation of the loins; gout of the hip.
Ossa Convoluta, Os′a Kon-vω-lų́-ta; two turbinated bones of the nostrils.
Ossa Innominata, — In-nom-i-ná-ta; two large bones of the pelvis.
Osseous, Os′ē-us; bony; having the nature of bone.
Os Sepiæ, Os Sē-pi-ē; cuttle-fish bone.
Ossicula, Os-ík-ų-la; small bones.

Ossicula Auditus, Os-ík-ų-la Θ'di-tus; a small bone in the tympanum.
Ossiferous, Os-íf-er-us; containing bones.
Ostæmia, Os-tḗ-mi-a; excess of blood in a bone.
Ostalgia, Os-tál-ji-a; pain or soreness in the bones.
Osteanaphysis, Os-tē-a-náf-i-sis; the reproduction of a bone.
Ostein, Os'tē-in; the animal matter composing a bone.
Osteitis, Os-tē-ị-tis; inflammation of a bone.
Ostembryon, Os-tém-bri-on; a hardened embryo.
Osteocele, Os'tē-ω-sēl; hardening of the sac of a hernia; also, ossification of the testicles.
Osteodentine, Os-tē-ω-dén-tin; a change in the tissue of teeth, causing it to resemble both bone and dentine.
Osteodynia, Os-tē-ω-dín-i-a; chronic pain in a bone.
Osteology, Os-tē-ól-ω-ji; the science of bones.
Osteoma, Os-tē-ώ-ma; tumor of a bone.
Osteonecrosis, Os-tē-ω-nē-krώ-sis; death of a bone.
Osteosarcoma, Os-tē-ω-sąr-kώ-ma; growth of a cartilaginous mass within a bone, causing it to enlarge and sometimes fracture.
Osteotomy, Os-tē-ót-ω-mi; the dissection of bones.
Ostium, Os'ti-um; an opening; as that between the auricle and ventricle of the heart.
Ostium Abdominale, — Ab-dom-i-ná-lē; orifice of the Fallopian tube.
Otalgia, Ω-tál-ji-a; pain in the ear, or ear-ache. [ear.
Othelcosis, Ot-el-kώ-sis; discharge of matter from the
Oticus, Ot'i-kus; auricular; relating to the ear.
Otitis, Ω-tị-tis; inflammation of the ear. [from the ear.
Otoblenorrhœa, Ot-ω-blen-ω-rḗ-a; discharge of mucus
Otodynia, Ot-ω-dín-i-a; chronic pain in the ear.
Otology, Ω-tól-ω-ji; science of the ear. [ear.
Otoneuralgia, Ot-ω-nų-rál-ji-a; a nervous pain in the
Otoplasty, Ot'ω-plas-ti; the reparation of an injury to the external ear by transferring to it a sound portion of the integument.
Otorrhœa, Ot-ω-rḗ-a; a running from the ear.
Otoscope, Ot'ω-skop; an instrument by which the sound of air may be heard, in passing through the tympanic cavity.

Ounce Troy. Ȣns Trơ; 480 grains; used in compounding medicines.

Ovarialgia, Ɯ-va-ri-ál-ji-ɑ; pain in the ovary.

Ovarian Dropsy, Ɯ-vá-ri-an Dróp-si; the growth of encysted tumors in the ovaries, often acquiring great size.

Ovaritis, Ɯ va-rị-tis; inflammation of the ovary.

Ovary, Ɯ'va-ri; (*Ovarium;*) two oval bodies connected with the uterus by a broad ligament, and containing several small vesicles or ova.

Ovarian Pregnancy, Ɯ-vá-ri-an Prég-nan-si; extra-uterine pregnancy, the fœtus being found in the ovarium.

Oviduct, Ɯ'vi-dukt; the Fallopian tube, that carries the ovum from the ovary to the uterus.

Oviparous, Ɯ-víp-a-rus; applied to animals that bring forth their young by means of eggs.

Ovisac, Ɯ-vi-sak; the coating that encloses the ovum.

Ovula, Ov'ṷ-lɑ; a small unimpregnated egg; an ovule.

Ovulate, Ov'ṷ-lat; bearing or having ovules.

Ovulation, Ov-ṷ-lá-ʃon; a process of generation by placing in a membranous sac the nutritious matter from a female, and adding thereto the semen from a male.

Ovule, Ɯ'vṷl; a little egg, or unimpregnated ovum; also the seed of a plant.

Ovum, Ɯ'vum; an egg; applied also to the Graafian vesicle of mammalia.

Oxalates, Oks-ál-ats; salts of oxalic acid, found native in certain plants, such as rhubarb, wood sorrel, etc. Oxalate of cerium is used as a remedy for vomiting during pregnancy.

Oxalic Acid, Oks-ál-ik As'id; an organic acid, poisonous, and capable of being produced artificially from sugar, woody fiber etc.

Oxaluria, Oks-a-lṷ́-ri-ɑ; a condition of the urine indicating the presence of the oxalate of lime.

Ox-Gall, Oks-Gɑl; *fel bovinum;* the bile of the ox, dried to the consistency of a solid extract.

Oxide, Oks'ịd; combinations of oxygen with another element.

Oxyacid Salts, Oks-i-ás-id Səlts; an obsolete term, formerly used for salts that were supposed to be formed of the oxide of a metal and an anhydride.
Oxygen, Oks'i-jen; an elementary substance, which supports all animal life; it is a constituent of the atmosphere, of water, and most organic and many inorganic bodies.
Oxyopia, Oks-i-ṓ-pi-ɑ; acute sense of vision.
Oxyphonia, Oks-i-fṓ-ni-ɑ; a morbid condition of the larynx that causes a shrill voice.
Oxysalts, Oks'i-səlts. See Oxyacid Salts.
Oxyuris Vermicularis, Oks-i-ú-ris Vɛr-mik-ų-lá-ris; the tape-worm.
Oyster-Shell, Ӫs'ter-Σel; (*Ostrea Edulis,*) when burned the shell is used in medicine.
Ozæna, Ꙍ-zé-nɑ; a fetid ulcer in the nostril, that discharges purulent matter, and is sometimes attended with caries of the bones.
Ozone, Ꙍ'zɷn; allotropic form of oxygen, a powerful oxydizing and disinfecting agent.

P

P.; an abbreviation for *part*, *powder*, etc.
Pabulum; Páb-ų-lum; food; sustenance.
Pacchioni's Glands, Pak-i-ṓ-nį'z Glandz; small oval-shaped eminences on the membranes of the brain.
Pachyæma, Pak-i-é-mɑ; a thick state of the blood.
Pachyblepharum, Pak-i-bléf-a-rum; a morbid thickening of the eyelids.
Pacini, Pɑ-çé-nē; small whitish bodies, united with the cutaneous fibers of the palm of the hand and sole of the foot.
Pædatrophia, Ped-a-trṓ-fi-ɑ; want of nutrition; emaciation of children.
Pædiaphtha, Ped-i-áf-ϑɑ; the thrush of infants.
Painter's Colic, Pánt-er'z Kól-ik; *Colica Pictorum;* a form of colic attributed to working with lead.

Palatal, Pál-a-tal; relating to the palate.
Palate, Pál-et; the roof of the mouth.
Palatum Durum, Pál-a-tum Dú-rum; the hard palate, in the front of the mouth.
Palatum Molle, — Mól-ĕ; the soft palate, in the back part of the mouth.
Pale Bark, Pel Bɑrk; a variety of cinchona bark.
Paleontology, Pe-lĕ-on-tól-ɷ-ji; the science of fossil organic remains.
Paleozoology, Pe-lĕ-ɷ-zɷ-ól-ɷ-ji; the science of the fossil remains of animals.
Palma, Pál-mɑ; the hand, or the palm of the hand; also, the name of a tree.
Palma Christi, — Krís-tį; the *Ricinus communis*, or castor-oil plant.
Palmar Arch, Pál-mɑr Ārç; the name of the two arches formed by the blood-vessels in the palm of the hand.
Palmaris Brevis, Pal-mé-ris Bré-vis; a muscle of the wrist and the palm of the hand.
Palmaris Longus, — Lóŋ-gus; a muscle of the arm that moves the wrist, and is attached to all the fingers.
Palmaris Magnus, — Mág-nus; a muscle of the arm that bends the hand.
Palmula, Pal-mú-lɑ; "a little palm;" applied to the flat end of a rib.
Palpation, Pal-pé-ʃon; examination with the hand.
Palpebra, Pál-pĕ-brɑ; the eyelid.
Palpitation, Pal-pi-té-ʃon; a fluttering, morbid movement of the heart.
Palsy, Pél-zi; paralysis of any part of the body.
Panacea, Pan-a-sé-ɑ; a remedy said to be good for almost any disease.
Panado, Pa-né-dɷ; dry bread, boiled in water to the consistency of pap, and sweetened.
Panax Quinquefolium, Pé-naks Kwin-kwĕ-fɷ́-li-um; ginseng, synonym for *Aralia quinquefolia*.
Pancreas, Pán-krĕ-as; a long, flat gland, seated behind the stomach, that secretes the pancreatic juice.
Pancreatalgia, Pan-krĕ-a-tál-ji-ɑ; pain in the pancreas.
Pancreatic Duct, Pan-krĕ-át-ik Dukt; the canal leading from the pancreas to the duodenum.

Pancreatic Juice, Pan-krē-át-ik; Jṳs; the fluid which the pancreas secretes.
Pancreatoncus, Pan-krē-a-tón-kus; a tumor in the pancreas.
Pandemia, Pan-dḗ-mi-a; an epidemic.
Pandiculation, Pan-dik-ṳ-lā́-ʃon; yawning; gaping.
Panniculus, Pan-ík-ṳ-lus; a membranous covering.
Pantamorphia, Pan-ta-mór-fi-a; general deformity.
Pantatrophia, Pan-ta-trṓ-fi-a; entire want of nutrition.
Papaver Somniferum, Pa-pā́-ver Som-níf-er-um; the opium plant, native of Asia, extensively cultivated in India and Turkey for its yield of opium.
Papilla, Pa-píl-a; a pimple; applied to the small points on the skin that mark the terminations of nerves, and to red eminences on the tongue in scarlatina, etc.
Pappoose Root, Pa-pṓs Rōt; a name sometimes applied to blue cohosh, (*Caulophyllum thalictroides.*)
Pappus, Páp-us; the first soft beard on the chin.
Papula, Páp-ṳ-la; a soft, watery pimple.
Parablebsis, Par-a-bléb-sis; false or deceptive vision.
Parabisma, Par-a-bís-ma; excess of humors.
Paracentesis, Par-a-sen-tḗ-sis; a tapping of the abdomen, thorax, etc., for the discharge of fluid.
Paracusis, Par-a-kṳ́-sis; defective hearing.
Paraffin, Pár-a-fin; a white inodorous substance derived from coal tar or petroleum.
Paraguay Tea, Pár-a-gwe Tē; the leaves of *Ilex Paraguaiensis*, used as a nervous stimulant.
Paralysis, Par-ál-i-sis; loss of the power of motion, in any part of the body.
Paralysis Agitans, — Aj'i-tans; the shaking palsy.
Paralytic, Par-a-lít-ik; relating to paralysis.
Paramenia, Par-a-mḗ-ni-a; disordered menstruation.
Paraphimosis, Par-a-fi-mṓ-sis; constriction of the prepuce behind the *glans penis*.
Paraphonia, Par-a-fṓ-ni-a; a morbid change in the [voice.
Paraplegia, Par-a-plḗ-ji-a; paralysis, partial or complete, of either the upper or lower half of the body.
Parapsis, Par-áp-sis; defective sense of touch.
Parasite, Pár-a-sīt; an animal or plant that draws its sustenance from another.

Parasystocele, Par-a-sís-tō-sēl; disordered pulsations of the heart and arteries.

Paregoric Par-ē-gór-ik; camphorated tincture of opium, each ounce contains a small fraction less than two grains of opium.

Pareira Brava, Pą-rá-rą Brą́-vą; the root of *Cissampelos Pareira*; a diuretic.

Parenchyma, Par-én-ki-ma; the spongy tissue connecting the viscera, that is distinct from the ducts, nerves, etc.

Paries, Pá-ri-ēz; (pl. *Parietis;*) the walls or sides of a cavity, as the thorax, etc.

Parietal, Par-į-ē-tal; relating to the walls of a cavity.

Parietal Bones, — Bōnz; two quadrangular bones of the cranium.

Parilla, Yellow, Pa-ríl-a, Yél-ō; *Menispermum Canadense*, a native twining vine.

Parodynia, Par-ō-dín-i-a; false, or premature labor.

Paronychia, Par-ō-ník-i-a; a whitlow, or abscess on the finger.

Parotid, Par-ót-id; applied to the salivary glands, situated beneath each ear.

Parotid Duct, — Dukt; the channel through which the saliva is carried from the parotid gland to the mouth.

Parotitis, Par-ō-tį-tis; inflammation of the parotid gland, usually known as the mumps.

Paroxysm, Pár-oks-izm; periodical symptoms, or spasms of disease.

Parsley, Pą́rs-li; a common garden plant, *Petroselinum sativum*, the root used as a diuretic.

Partridge-berry, Pą́r-trij-ber-i; *Mitchella repens*, a pretty little plant, used as a diuretic and tonic.

Parturient, Pąr-tų́-ri-ent; child-bearing.

Parturition, Pąr-tų-rí-ʃon; the act of bringing forth a child.

Parulis, Pa-rú-lis; a gum-boil; inflammation of the gums.

Paruria, Pa-rú-ri-a; difficulty in urinating.

Par Vagum, Pąr Vá-gum; the eighth pair of nerves.

Pastinaca Sativa, Pas-ti-ná-ka Sa-tį-va; the parsnip; diuretic and demulcent.

Patella, Pa-tél-a; the knee-pan, or cap.
Pathema, Pa-thē-ma; instinctive passion or feeling.
Pathetic, Pa-thét-ik; applied to a muscle of the eye, and also to the fourth pair of nerves.
Pathogenesis, Path-o-jén-ē-sis; origin or generation of disease. [produce disease.
Pathogenic, Path-o-jén-ik; applied to such things as
Pathogeny, Path-ój-en-i; the branch of pathology that treats of the origin and progress of disease.
Pathology, Path-ól-o-ji; the doctrine of diseases; their nature and results.
Paullinia Sorbilis, Pa-lín-i-a Sór-bil-is; a climbing shrub of Brazil, the source of *guarana*.
Paunch, Panch; the stomach.
Peach, Pēch; *Amygdalus Persica*, a common cultivated fruit-tree, the leaves and kernels of which contain a small portion of hydrocyanic acid; and are used as a sedative.
Pectin, Pék-tin; the *os pubis;* a bone in the fœtal pelvis.
Pectinalis, Pek-ti-ná-lis; relating to the *os pubis;* a muscle of the thigh. [chest.
Pectoral, Pék-to-ral; appertaining to the breast or
Pectoralis Major, Pek-to-rá-lis Má-jor; a muscle that rises in the clavicle, and moves the arm forward.
Pectoralis Minor, — Mī-nor; a muscle of the third, fourth and fifth ribs, and connects with the shoulder bone. [the chest.
Pectorals, Pék-to-ralz; medicines used for diseases of
Pectoriloquy, Pek-to-ríl-o-kwi; a condition of the chest in which the voice seems to issue from the breast.
Pectus, Pék-tus; (pl. *Pectora;*) that part of the body between the neck and abdomen.
Pedes, Pē-dēz; (pl. of *pes*, a foot;) feet.
Pedialgia, Pē-di-ál-ji-a; pain or neuralgia in the feet.
Pediculation, Pē-dik-u-lá-shon; a morbid condition favoring the breeding of lice on the skin.
Pediculus, Pē-dík-u-lus; a louse, one of the parasites of the body.
Pediculus Pubis, — Pú-bis; the "crab louse," that infests the pubes, causing almost intolerable itching.
Pediluvium, Ped-i-lú-vi-um; any bath for the feet.

Pellicle, Pél-i-kl: a thin skin; a delicate membrane.
Pellis, Pél-is; the *cutis*, or entire skin.
Pelvic, Pél-vik; appertaining to the pelvis.
Pelvimeter, Pel-vím-ē-ter; an instrument for measuring the cavity of the pelvis. [of the body.
Pelvis, Pél-vis; a basin; the osseous cavity at the base
Pemphigus, Pém-fi-gus; a vesicular eruption, accompanied by fever, the vesicles from the size of a pea to a walnut.
Penis, Pḗ-nis; the male organ of generation.
Pennyroyal, Pen-i-rő-al; *Hedeoma Pulegioides*, a native herb, abounding in a highly aromatic and stimulant oil.
Penthorum Sedoides, Pen-ᵺώ-rum Sē-dω-į-dēz; a native plant, lately introdueed as a remedy for catarrh.
Peotomia, Pē-ω-tώ-mi-ɑ: amputation of the penis.
Pepo, Pḗ-pω. See *Cucurbita pepo*.
Pepper, Black, Pép-er, Blak; the dried berries of *Piper nigrum*, used as a stimulant.
Pepper, Cayenne, or Red, — Ka-én; the ripe pods of *Capsicum annuum*.
Peppermint, Pép-er-mint; *Mentha piperita*, a well known aromatic herb, the oil of which is used as a stimulant.
Pepsin, Pép-sin; a substance existing in gastric juice and the peptic glands, that is a powerful promoter of digestion.
Peptic, Pép-tik; promotive of digestion.
Per-; a prefix denoting the highest of several.
Peracute, Pér-a-kųt; very severe; acute.
Perchlorides, Pɛr-klώ-rįdz; the higher chlorides; ferric chloride, tincture of muriate of iron, is a solution of this salt in alcohol.
Percussion, Pɛr-kú-ʃon; the examination of the chest or other cavity, by gently striking the surface and noting the kind of sound produced.
Perforans, Pɛ́r-fω-rans; perforating; applied to a muscle that bends the fingers.
Perforation, Pɛr-fω-rá-ʃon; the use of the trepan, or other instrument, in piercing the cranium or other organ.

Perhydrate of Iron, Pɛr-hį-drat of Ī'urn; ferric hydrate; an antidote for arsenic, made by decomposition of ferric sulphate by means of solution of caustic soda, potassæ or ammonia water.

Peri-; a prefix signifying about, on all sides; very.

Pericardiac, Per-i-kạ́r-di-ak; about, or relating to the heart. [containing the heart.

Pericardium, Per-i-kạ́r-di-um; the membranous sac

Perichondrium, Per-i-kón-dri-um; a membrane that envelops the cartilages.

Pericranium, Per-i-krá-ni-um; a membrane that envelops the bones of the skull.

Peridesmium, Per-i-dés-mi-um; a membrane that encloses the ligaments.

Perididymis, Per-i-díd-i-mis; a serous covering that encloses the testes.

Periglottis, Per-i-glót-is; the velvety membrane covering the tongue.

Perimysium, Per-i-mís-i-um; a thin membrane that envelops the muscles.

Perinæocele, Per-i-nḗ-ω-sēl; hernia of the perineum.

Perinæum, Per-i-nḗ-um; the part between the anus and genital organs.

Perinephritis, Per-i-nē-frį́-tis; inflammation of the perinephrium.

Perinephrium, Per-i-nḗ-fri-um; a membrane that encloses the kidneys.

Periodicity, Pē-ri-od-ís-i-ti; the return, at regular intervals, of any symptoms or effects of diseases.

Periodoscope, Pē-ri-ód-ω-skωp; an instrument for ascertaining the time of menstruation, etc.

Periosteum, Per-i-ós-tē-um; a delicate membrane that invests the bones. [teum.

Periostitis, Per-i-os-tį́-tis; inflammation of the perios-

Periostoma, Per-i-os-tώ-mɑ; a morbid development on the surface of a bone.

Periphacus, Per-íf-a-kus; the capsule or sac that encloses the lens of the eye.

Peripneumonia, Per-i-nụ-mώ-ni-ɑ; acute bronchitis.

Peristaltic, Per-i-stál-tik; a peculiar movement of the bowels described as vermicular or worm-like.

Peristaphylinus, Per-i-staf-i-lį-nus; applied to muscles of the palate, *externus* and *internus*.

Peristoma, Per-ís-tɷ-mɑ; the margin of a mouth or opening.

Peristroma, Per-is-trṓ-mɑ; the villous, mucous coating of the intestines.

Perisystole, Per-i-sis-tɷ-lē; the slight pause between the contraction and dilatation of the heart, as death approaches.

Peritonæum, Per-i-tɷ-nē-um; a serous membrane that lines the abdomen, covering all its organs.

Peritonitis, Per-i-tɷ-nį-tis; inflammation of the peritoneum.

Perizoma, Per-i-zṓ-mɑ; the diaphragm.

Permanganate of Potassium, Pɛr-mán-ga-nat of Pɷ-tás-i-um; a salt ($K^2 Mn^2O^8$) that readily yields its oxygen to organic matters, and is used as a disinfectant.

Pernio, Pɛ́r-ni-ɷ; a chilblain.

Pernitrate of Iron, Pɛr-nį-trat of Ī'urn; ferric nitrate. *Liquor Ferri Nitratis*, is officinal.

Peronæus, Per-ɷ-nē-us; relating to the fibula; applied to the long, short, and third muscles of the leg.

Peroxide, Per-óks-id; a combination in which there is the highest degree of oxidation.

Persimmon, Per-sím-on *Diospyros Virginiana*, a native tree, the bark of which is astringent.

Perspiration, Pɛr-spi-rá-ʃon; sweat; the moisture that passes from the pores of the skin.

Perspiration, Insensible; transpiration, or the emission of vapor by the skin.

Persulphate, Pɛr-súl-fat; ferric sulphate; used to prepare ferric hydrate, and other officinal preparations of iron.

Perturbation, Pɛr-tur-bá-ʃon; disquiet, or disturbance of mind or body.

Pertussis, Pɛr-tús-is; the whooping cough.

Peru, Balsam of, Pē-rú, Bél-sam ov; a resinous substance obtained from *Myrospermum Peruiferum*, and used as a tonic and expectorant.

Peruvian Bark, Pē-rú-vi-an Bɑrk; a common synonym for cinchona bark.

Pervigilium, Per-vi-jíl-i-um; inability to sleep.
Pes, Pes; the foot, including the tarsus or instep.
Pes Anserinus, — An-ser-ị-nus; a plexus of nerves in the face, distributed like the foot of a goose.
Pessary, Pés-a-ri; a ball, or other instrument for inserting in the vagina to prevent a return of prolapsus.
Pestis, Pés-tis; the plague, a contagious fever.
Petechia, Pe-tḗ-ki-a; a purplish spot on the skin.
Petit, Canal of, Pá-tē; a small channel between the layers of the hyaloid membrane of the eye.
Petrifaction, Pet-ri-fák-ſon; the conversion of wood, or animal fiber into stone; sometimes used in the sense of *calcification*, when a soft part hardens like stone, but should not be comfounded with *ossification*.
Petroleum, Pē-tró-lē-um; "rock oil," a bituminous fluid, obtained by boring into the earth in certain geological formations.
Petrosal Sinus, Pē-tró-sal Sị-nus; applied to the superior and inferior sinus of the *dura mater*.
Petroselinum Sativum, Pē-tro-sē-lị-num Sa-tị-vum; parsley, a garden plant.
Peyer's Glands, Pị-er'z Glandz; also called *Peyer's patches;* clusters of very small mucous glands on the inside of the small intestines.
Phacitis, Fa-sị-tis; inflammation of the lens of the eye.
Phagedæna, Fag-e-dḗ-na; a virulent ulcer, that corrodes and spreads rapidly.
Phalanges, Fa-lán-jēz; the small bones of the fingers and toes.
Phallocarcinoma, Fal-o-kar-si-nó-ma; cancer of the penis.
Phallorrhœa, Fal-o-rḗ-a; gonorrhœa; flow of semen.
Phantasma, Fan-táz-ma; an apparition, caused by the morbid condition of the eye or brain.
Pharmaceutics, Far-ma-sú-tiks; the science of manufacturing and compounding medicines.
Pharmacist, Fár-ma-sist; (or *Pharmaceutist;*) a person skilled in Pharmacy.
Pharmacon, Fár-ma-kon; a drug, or medicine.
Pharamcopœia, Far-ma-ko-pḗ-ya; a treatise on the science of Pharmacy.

Pharmacy, Fą̈r-ma-si; the art of preparing medicines for sale; the place where they are prepared and sold.
Pharyngalgia, Far-in-gál-ji-a; pain in the pharynx.
Pharyngeal, Far-in-jē-al; pertaining to the pharynx.
Pharyngitis, Far-in-jị-tis; inflammation of the pharynx. [pharynx.
Pharyngoplegia, Far-in-gō-plé-ji-a; paralysis of the
Pharyngotomy, Far-in-gót-ō-mi; the act of opening into the pharynx with the knife.
Pharynx, Fár-iŋks; the region of the throat behind the nose, mouth and larynx, and above the œsophagus.
Phenol, Fé-nol; carbolic acid.
Philadelphia Fleabane, Fil-a-dél-fi-a Flé-ban; *Erigeron Philadelphicum*, a common weed, used as a diuretic.
Phimosis, Fị-mó-sis; a congenital constriction of the prepuce that prevents the glans penis from being uncovered. [vein.
Phlebectasia, Flē-bek-tá-si-a; an extended or swollen
Phlebitis, Flē-bị-tis; inflammation of a vein.
Phleborrhagia, Fleb-ō-rá-ji-a; sudden flow of blood from a ruptured vein.
Phlebotomy, Flē-bót-ō-mi; the opening of a vein for blood-letting.
Phlegm, Flem; a thick mucus discharged from the throat and lungs.
Phlegmasia, Fleg-má-ʃi-a; inflammation, with fever.
Phlegmatia Dolens, Fleg-má-ʃi-a Dó-lens; white or milk-leg, afflicting some women after child-birth, the inguinal glands swelling and becoming painful.
Phlegmatic, Fleg-mát-ik; full of phlegm; sluggish.
Phlegmon, Flég-mon; a red boil; inflammation in the cellular tissue.
Phlogistic, Flō-jís-tik; combustible, inflammable.
Phlogiston, Flō-jís-ton; once supposed to be the principle of combustion or inflammability existing in matter.
Phlogosis, Flō-gó-sis; external inflammation, as in erysipelas.
Phlyctæna, Flik-té-na; a small vesicle under the epidermis, containing a serous fluid.
Phonica, Fón-i-ka; diseases affecting the vocal organs.

Phoradendron Flavescens, Fω-ra-dén-dron Fla-vés-ens; mistletoe, a native parasite, commonly described as *Viscum flavescens.*

Phosphates, Fós-fats; compounds of phosphoric acid.

Phosphide, (or **Phosphuret**,) Fós-fịd; a combination of phosphorous with another element.

Phosphoric Acid, Fos-fór-ik As'id; an acid of phosphorous, $H^3 PO^4$; (the ordinary medicinal acid is called ortho-phosphoric acid.)

Phosphorus, Fós-fω-rus; an elementary substance obtained from bones, very inflammable, poisonous, and must be preserved beneath water and handled carefully. [light.

Photalgia, Fω-tál-ji-α; pain resulting from excessive

Photonosos, Fω-tón-ω-sos; snow-blindness; sun-stroke.

Photopsia, Fω-tóp-si-α; lucid vision, or internal sight.

Photuria, Fω-tụ́-ri-α; urine that has a light and shiny appearance.

Phrenic, Frén-ik; relating to the diaphragm.

Phrenica, Frén-ik-α; diseases affecting the mind.

Phrenitis, Frē-nị-tis; inflammation of the brain.

Phrenology, Frē-nól-ω-ji; the science of the mind, in conjunction with the brain.

Phrenzy, Frén-zi; phrenitis; excitement of the brain.

Phthisical, Tíz-i-kal; pertaining to phthisis; consumptive. [sumption.

Phthisic, Tíz-ik; *Phthisis Pulmonalis;* pulmonary con-

Phthoe, Fώ-ē; ulcers in the lungs.

Phyma, Fị-mα; a tubercle, or inflamed boil.

Phymatoid, Fị-ma-tωd; resembling a tubercle.

Physconia, Fis-kώ-ni-α; abnormal enlargement of the abdomen.

Physeter Macrocephalus, Fị-sē-ter Mak-rω-séf-a-lus; the sperm-whale, that yields spermaceti.

Physiatrica, Fis-i-át-ri-kα; the science of the healing qualities in nature's products.

Physic, Fíz-ik; the science of medicine in the cure of disease.

Physician, Fi-zí-ſan; a person educated for the practice of medicine, and authorized to practice by a chartered college.

Physiognomy, Fiz-i-óg-nọ-mi; the act of determining to some extent, the dispositions of men by observing their countenances.

Physiology, Fiz-i-ól-ọ-ji; the science of life, both animal and vegetable.

Physostigma Venenosum, Fị-sọ-stíg-ma Ven-ē-nó-sum; a woody African vine, which yields calabar beans.

Phytolacca Decandra, Fị-tọ-lák-a Dē-kán-dra; pokeweed, a common American weed, the dried berries and root of which are used as an alterative.

Pia Mater, Pị-a Má-ter; the delicate membrane which forms an innermost covering of the brain and spinal cord.

Pica, Pị-ka; the unnatural appetite, during pregnancy.

Picric Acid, Pík-rik As'id; carbazotic acid, or tri-nitro-carbolic acid, is made by the action of nitric acid upon carbolic acid. Picrate of ammonium is used in medicine. (See Carbazotate of ammonium.)

Pigmentum Nigrum, Pig-mén-tum Nị-grum; a dark pigment in the choroid membrane of the eye.

Piles, Pịlz; hemorrhoids; an inflamed condition of the veins of the anus.

Piliferous, Pị-líf-er-us; hairy; covered with hair.

Piliform, Píl-i-form; resembling hair.

Piline, Pị-lin; a fabric made of wool and sponge, and covered with a coating of India-rubber, used for poultices and fomentations.

Pill, (or **Pilula**,) Píl-ụ-la; a pellet or small ball of medicine, for swallowing whole.

Pilocarpin, Pil-ọ-kạr-pin: an alkaloid of jaborandi.

Pilocarpus Pinnatus, Pil-ọ-kạ́r-pus Pin-á-tus; a tree of South America, the leaves of which are used to promote perspiration; jaborandi.

Pilorum Arrectores, Pị-lṓ-rum A-rek-tṓ-rēz; the very small muscles that produce the effect called *cutis anserina*, or "goose skin," and also cause the hair of the skin to rise when one is frightened.

Pilose, Pị-lṓs; hairy, with distinct hairs.

Pilular, Píl-ụ-lar; appertaining to a pill.

Pimeladen, Pi-mél-a-den; a fatty gland.

Pimelitis, Pim-ĕ-lī-tis; inflammation of the adipose membrane.

Pimelosis, Pim-ĕ-ló-sis; obesity; fatness.

Pimento Berries, Pi-mén-tō Bér-iz; allspice, the fruit of *Eugenia Pimenta*.

Pimpinella Anisum, Pim-pi-nél-a A-nī-sum; an umbelliferous plant that yields aniseed.

Pimple, Pím-pl; a small round protuberance of the skin, filled with a watery fluid.

Pine, Pīn; a common name for the evergreen trees of the genus *Pinus*.

Pineal Gland, Pín-ĕ-al Gland; a small soft conical body, the size of a pea, found above the *tubercula quadrigemina* of the brain, supposed by Descartes to be the seat of the soul, but whose office is not yet learned.

Pinguecula, Pin-gwék-ū-la; a small tumor in the edge of the cornea.

Pinguedo, Pin-gwé-dō; a term for fat.

Pink-Root, Píŋk-rūt; the root of *Spigelia Marilandica*, used as an anthelmintic.

Pinna, Pín-a; the expanded portion of the external ear; also the lower part of each side of the nose.

Pinta, Pín-ta; "the blue stain," a disease that is prevalent in Mexico.

Pinus, Pī-nus; a large genus of evergreen trees, the source of tar, turpentine and rosin.

Pinus Canadensis, — Kan-a-dén-sis; a synonym in common use for *Abies Canadensis;* hemlock spruce.

Piper Cubeba, Pī-per Kū-bé-ba; a climbing vine of the East Indies, which yields cubeb berries.

Piper Nigrum,— Nī-grum: a vine of the West Indies, the dried fruit of which is black pepper.

Piperin, Píp-er-in; a very weak alkaloid of pepper.

Pipsissewa, Pip-sís-ĕ-wa; a native plant, *Chimaphila umbellata;* used as a diuretic and tonic.

Pistacia Lentiscus, Pis-tá-ʃi-a Len-tís-kus; the tree that yields mastic.

Pistil, Pís-til; the female organ of a plant that contains [the ovule.

Pistillate, Pís-til-at; having pistils.

Pit, Pit; in the plural, the cavities left in the skin after small-pox.

Pit of the Stomach; the external cavity over the stomach.
Pitaya Bark, Pi-tá-ya Bark; a variety of non-officinal cinchona bark.
Pitch, Black, Pic, Blak; the residue left from coal tar after distillation.
Pitch, Burgundy, — Búr-gun-di; a resinous substance obtained from *Abies excelsa*, and used in plasters.
Pituita, Pit-u-í-ta; phlegm; a viscid mucus.
Pituitary, Pit-ú-i-ta-ri; appertaining to phlegm.
Pituitary Gland, — Gland; a small round body, occupying the Sella Turcica, or depression, of the sphenoid bone.
Pituitary Membrane, — Mém-bran; the mucous membrane in the interior of the nose.
Pix Liquida, Piks Lík-wi-da; officinal name for tar.
Placebo, Pla-sé-bo; a medicine given the patient more to satisfy his wish than with the expectation of benefiting him.
Placenta, Pla-sén-ta; a roundish flat substance that forms in the uterus in conjunction with the fœtus, and to which the umbilical cord is attached, constituting the medium of communication between mother and child.
Placentitis, Pla-sen-tí-tis; inflammation of the placenta.
Pladarosis, Plad-a-ró-sis; a soft tumor within the eyelid.
Plague, Pleg; a kind of typhus fever, attended with carbuncles, hæmorrhage, and great prostration.
Planta, Plán-ta; the sole of the foot.
Plantago Major, Plan-tá-go Má-jor; the common plantain; a weed used as an alterative.
Plantar, Plán-tar; applied to arteries, muscles, ligaments, etc., of the foot.
Plantaris, Plan-tá-ris; a muscle that extends the foot
Plantigrade, Plán-ti-gred; applied to man and other animals that walk on the sole of the foot.
Planuria, Plan-ú-ri-a; discharge of urine through an artificial passage.
Planus, Plá-nus; flat; applied to the flat part of the ethnoid bone.

Plasma, Pláz-ma; the liquid forming the thick portion of the blood.

Plastic, Plás-tik; that may be formed or moulded, as [plaster.

Platiasmus, Pla-ti-áz-mus; imperfection of speech, by reason of thick! broad lips.

Plasters, Plás-terz. See *Emplastra*.

Platinum, Pla-tį-num; an elemental substance, that is unaffected by the action of most acids, and consequently valuable for chemical apparatus.

Platysma, Pla-tís-ma; an expansion or broadening.

Platysma Myodes, — Mį-ṓ-dēz; a broad muscle on the side of the neck.

Pledget, Pléj-et; a piece of lint, or compress, rolled in- [to oval shape.

Pleonasm, Plḗ-ο-nazm; a faulty development, in an extra number of parts.

Pleonexia, Plē-ο-néks-i-a; abnormal greediness, to the extent of being a disease.

Plethora, Pléth-ο-ra; fullness to repletion; plumpness.

Pleura, Plų́-ra; a serous membrane that lines the cavities of the thorax.

Pleura Costalis, — Kos-tá-lis; the part of the pleura that lines the parietes of the chest.

Pleura Pulmonalis, — Pul-mο-ná-lis; that part of the pleura that covers the lungs.

Pleuralgia, Plų-rál-ji-a; pain in the side, or in the [pleura.

Pleurapostema, Plų-ra-pos-tḗ-ma; a tumor or abscess in the pleura.

Pleurisy, (or **Pleuritis**,) Plų́-ri-si; inflammation of [the pleura.

Pleurisy-Root, Plų́-ri-si-Rut; *Asclepias tuberosa*, a native plant, also known as butterfly-weed; reputed as a remedy for pleurisy.

Pleurodynia, Plų-rο-dín-i-a; spasmodic pain in the muscles of the chest.

Pleuropneumonia, Plų-rο-nų-mṓ-ni-a; inflammation of the pleura and of the lungs at the same time.

Pleurorrhœa, Plų-rο-rḗ-a; an excess of fluid in the pleura.

Pleurospasmus, Plų-rο-spáz-mus; cramp in the side, or in the pleura.

Pleurothotonos, Plų-rο-thót-ο-nos; tetanus in which the body is curved to one side.

Pleximeter, Pleks-ím-ĕ-ter; a flat circular piece of ivory, or metal, by which mediate percussion is performed.

Plexus, Pléks-us; a network of nerves or blood-vessels. See *Axillary*, *Cardiac*, and *Choroid* plexus.

Plexus Pampiniformis, — Pam-pin-i-fór-mis; blood-vessels twined about the spermatic cord.

Plexus Pulmonicus, — Pul-món-i-kus; a junction of the eighth pair of nerves with the great sympathetic nerve.

Plica, Plį-kɑ; a disease attended with the glutinus matting of the hair.

Plicidentine, Plis-i-dén-tin; a change in the tissue of a tooth.

Plumbago, Plum-bá-gɷ; a form of carbon, commonly termed black lead.

Plumbum, Plúm-bum; the Latin name for the element lead.

Pneumarthrosis, Nų-mɑr-ŧró-sis; the secretion of air in a joint.

Pneumatica, Pų-mát-i-kɑ; diseases of the functions of respiration.

Pneumatocele, Nų-mát-ɷ-sēl; any hernia filled with air.

Pneumatometer, Nų-ma-tóm-ĕ-ter; an instrument for measuring the amount of air inhaled at a breath.

Pneumatosis, Nų-ma-tó-sis; the distention of a cellular membrane with wind.

Pneumogastric, Nų-mɷ-gás-trik; appertaining to both the lungs and stomach; applied also to the eighth pair of nerves, (*par Vagum.*)

Pneumonæmia, Nų-mɷ-né-mi-ɑ; an engorgement of blood in the lungs.

Pneumonalgia, Nų-mɷ-nál-ji-ɑ; pain in the lungs.

Pneumonia, Nų-mó-ni-ɑ; (*Pneumonitis;*) inflammation of the lungs; fever, pain in the thorax, increased by coughing; quick, hard pulse, and difficulty in breathing.

Pneumonic, Nų-món-ik; relating to the respiratory organs.

Pneumothorax, Nų-mɷ-ŧó-raks; the sudden accumulation of air in the sac of the pleura; a dangerous condition.

Pock, Pok; applied to the pustules of small-pox.

Podagra, Pód-a-grɑ; gout in the joints of the foot.

Podalgia, Pō-dál-ji-a; chronic pain in the foot; gout, or rheumatism.

Podarthritis, Pod-ar-thrī-tis; inflammation of the joints of the feet.

Podœdema, Pod-ē-dē-ma; a swelling of the feet.

Podophyllin, Pod-ō-fil-in; the precipitate obtained when concentrated tincture of mayapple (*Podophyllum peltatum*) root is poured into cold water.

Podophyllum Peltatum, Pod-ō-fil-um Pel-tá-tum; a common plant in the United States, known as may-apple or mandrake; the root is extensively used as a cathartic.

Podophyllum, Resin of; Podophyllin.

Poison, Pó-zon; any animal, mineral or vegetable substance, which, when applied to the surface or taken into the body, causes such a derangement of the system as to induce disease or lead to death.

Poison-Vine, — Vīn ; a common name for *Rhus Toxicodendron*, a poisonous vine of the United States.

Poke, Pōk; *Phytolacca decandra*, a common weed.

Polemonium Cæruleum, Pol-ē-mṓ-ni-um Sē-rú-lē-um; Greek valerian; a nervine.

Polemonium Reptans, — Rép-tans; a native plant, sometimes used as an alterative.

Pollen, Pól-en; the powder of flowers, which is the fecundating principle of plants.

Pollex, Pól-eks; the thumb, or great toe.

Pollution, Po-lú-ʃon; the emission of semen in an unnatural way.

Polygala Senega, Pō-líg-a-la Sén-ē-ga; seneca snake-root; a native plant, the root of which is used as an expectorant.

Polygonatum Giganteum, Pō-lig-ō-ná-tum Jī-gán-tē-um ; Solomon's Seal, a native plant, the root used as a tonic.

Polygonum Bistorta, Pō-líg-ō-num Bis-tór-ta; a European plant, bistort, the root of which is an astringent.

Polygonum Hydropiper, — Hī-dróp-i-per; water-pepper, a common weed, used as a stimulant, often described as *Polygonum Punctatum*.

Polymnia Uvedalia, Pɷ-lím-ni-ɑ Yu-vē-dā-li-ɑ; an indigenous plant, lately recommended as a remedy for enlarged spleen.
Polyopia, Pol-i-ṓ-pi-ɑ; abnormal vision, in which objects are multiplied.
Polypodium Vulgare, Pol-i-pṓ-di-um Vul-gā́-rē; polipod, a native fern, used as a pectoral.
Polypus, Pól-i-pus; a tumor in the natural cavities of the body, as the nose, uterus, etc.
Polysarcia, Pol-i-sár-ʃi-ɑ; excessive flesh; corpulency.
Polytricum Juniperinum, Pɷ-lít-ri-kum Jų-nip-ē-rį-num; hair-cap moss, a diuretic.
Pomegranate, Púm-gran-et; *Punica granatum*, an ornamental tree of the Mediterranean.
Pompholyx, Póm-fɷ-liks; a watery pimple, or sac, on the skin, without inflammation.
Pomum Adami, Pṓ-mum A-dā́-mį; the cartilaginous projection on the front part of the neck.
Pons Hepatis, Pons Hép-a-tis; "bridge of the liver," the part connecting the lobes.
Pons Tarini,— Ta-rį́-nį; the ash-like substance forming the floor of the third ventricle of the brain.
Pons Varolii, — Va-rṓ-li-į; the *corpus annulare*, a part of the medullary substance uniting the cerebrum, cerebellum, and medullary oblongata.
Poples, Póp-lēz; the ham, or posterior part of the knee-joint.
Poplitæus, Pop-li-tḗ-us; a muscle of the thigh and leg, that articulates the knee-joint.
Popliteal, Pop-li-tḗ-al; applied to muscles, nerves, etc., of the ham.
Poppy, Póp-i; *Papaver somniferum*, the plant that yields opium; the ripe capsules, known as poppy-heads, are a feeble sedative.
Populus Balsamifera, Póp-ų-lus Bəl-sam-íf-er-ɑ; (*var candicans*, Gray;) a tree of the Northern United States, the buds of which are known as Balm of Gilead.
Pore, Pɷr; in the plural, minute openings or passages, that exist in all bodies; in the skin they are the extremities of internal exhalant vessels.
Poroma, Pɷ-rṓ-mɑ; a hard or callous part.
Porphyrisma, Pər-fi-ríz-mɑ; scarlitina, or scarlet fever.

Porrigo, Po-rị-gō; an eruptive disease known as scald-head, or ring-worm of the scalp.

Porta, Pór-tɑ; "a gate:" applied to the passage-ways of the liver.

Portal Circulation, Pór-tal Sɛr-kụ-lá-ʃon; that part of the venous circulation of the blood that makes an extra circuit before uniting with the rest of the blood.

Portal Vein, — Van; a vein that unites with most of the organs within the abdomen.

Portio Dura, Pór-ʃi-ō Dụ́-rɑ; the hard, or facial nerve.

Portio Mollis, — Mól-is; the soft, or auditory nerve.

Porus, Pó-rus; the hard skin, or callus; also, a pore or opening.

Porus Opticus, — Op'ti-kus; a point in the optic nerve, where the central artery passes through.

Posology, Pō-sól-ō-ji; the science of the quantity and frequency of doses.

Posterior Auris, Pōs-tḗ-ri-or Θ'ris; a fleshy fiber or muscle behind the ear.

Posthitis, Pos-ṫị-tis; inflammation of the prepuce.

Post-Mortem, Pōst-Mór-tem; the formal or official examination of a dead body.

Post Partum — Pɑ́r-tum; applied to hæmorrhage, etc., after parturition.

Potash, (or **Potassæ**,) Pót-aʃ; caustic potash.

Potassæ Caustic, Pō-tás-ē Kés-tik. See *Caustic Potash.*

Potassium, Pō-tás-i-um; an elementary substance, the base of the potassium salts.

Potassium Hydrate, — Hị-drat; caustic potash.

Potentilla Canadensis, Pō-ten-tíl-ɑ Kan-a-dén-sis; cinquefoil, five-finger; a native herb, used as a tonic and astringent.

Potentilla Tormentilla, — Tɵr-men-tíl-ɑ; tormentil, a European plant, the root of which is a powerful astringent.

Potion, Pó-ʃon; a medicine to be taken as a drink.

Potomania, Pō-tō-má-ni-ɑ; delirium tremens.

Pot-Pourri, Pot-Pú-rē; a mixture of fragrant plants, flowers and roots.

Poultice, Pól-tis; a soft preparation of bread and milk, flax-seed, or oat-meal, spread on a cloth, for applying to sprains, or sores.

Poupart's Ligament, Pú-pqrt's Líg-a-ment; a ligament that extends from the ilium to the *os pubis*.

Pox, Poks; the vulgar name for syphilis.

Præcordia, Prē-kór-di-a; the anterior part of the thorax.

Precipitant, Prē-síp-i-tant; the substance that produces a precipitate.

Precipitate, Prē-síp-i-tat; the substance left in the bottom of the vessel after the process of precipitation.

Precipitation, Prē-sip-i-tá-ʃon; the chemical action which results in a substance separating from a liquid in which it was dissolved.

Precipitated Chalk, Prē-síp-i-tat-ed Ȼok; carbonate of calcium, thrown from solution by a carbonated alkali.

Pregnancy, Prég-nan-si; the condition of being with child, or bearing young.

Prepensile, Prē-pén-sil; adapted to the catching hold of objects, as fingers, tails, etc.

Premature Labor, Pré-ma-tųr Lá-bor; that which comes on before the allotted period of gestation.

Premaxillary, Prē-máks-i-la-ri; applied to the incisor part of the superior maxillary.

Premolar, Prē-mṓ-lar; applied to the first pairs of molar, or bicuspid teeth, in each jaw.

Prepared Chalk, Prē-pąrd Ȼok; washed chalk.

Prepuce, Pré-pųs; the membrane covering the end of the glans penis, and also the clitoris.

Presbyopia, Pres-bi-ṓ-pi-a; defective vision, resulting in far-sightedness, attending old age.

Prescription, Prē-skríp-ʃon; a written, or partly printed and partly written, direction for the preparation of medicine for a patient.

Presentation, Prē-zen-tá-ʃon; the position in which a child presents itself in the uterus at birth.

Presphenoid, Prē-sfé-nơd; applied to the anterior part of the sphenoid bone in infancy.

Priapism, Prį-a-pizm; a morbid erection of the penis, without or with desire.

Prickly Ash, Prík-li Aʃ; *Xanthoxylum Americanum*, a native shrub, the bark and berries of which are used as a stimulant.

Pride of India, Prįd ov In'di-ɑ; *Melia Azedarach*, a tropical tree.

Primæ Viæ Prį-mē Vį-ē; the primary passages, as the stomach and intestines.

Primalia, Prį-má-li-ɑ; applied to growths which are the lowest in the scale of existence.

Primigenious, Prį-mi-jé-ni-us; primitive; first born.

Primipara, Prį-míp-a-rɑ; a mother who has been delivered of her first child.

Probang, Prɷ́-baŋ: a piece of whalebone with an ivory point, for pressing down into the stomach any substance that may have caught in the œsophagus.

Primrose, Evening, Prím-rɷz, Ɛv'niŋ; *Œnothera biennis*, a common native plant with yellow flowers.

Prince's Pine, Príns-ez Pįn; a common name for *Chimaphila umbellata*.

Prinos Verticillatus, Prį-nos Vɛr-tis-i-lá-tus; black alder. See *Ilex verticillata*.

Privet, Prív-et; *Ligustrum vulgare*, a shrub common in cultivation.

Probe, Prɷb; an instrument with which to examine wounds.

Process, Pró-ses; any outgrowth or projection of bone or other tissue; also the method of performing a chemical operation.

Procidentia, Pros-i-dén-ʃi-ɑ; a prolapsus; the falling or depression of an organ or part, as the eye, anus, etc.

Practalgia, Prak-tál-ji-ɑ; pain in the rectum.

Proctica, Prók-ti-kɑ; diseases of the anus.

Proctitis, Prok-tį-tis; inflammation of the anus and rectum.

Proctocele, Prók-tɷ-sēl; prolapsus ani, or hernia of the rectum.

Proctodynia, Prok-tɷ-dín-i-ɑ; spasms of pain in the rectum.

Proctotomy, Prok-tót-ɷ-mi; the making of an incision into the rectum, as for *fistula in ano*.

Prodrome, Prɷ́-drɷm; a precursor, as one disease is sometimes the forerunner of another.

Profluvia, Prɷ-flų́-vi-ɑ; profuse discharges, or flux, with fever.

Profundus, Prɷ-fún-dus; deep-seated; applied to arteries, etc., of the arm and thigh.

Profucio, Prω-fŭ-ʃi-ω; loss of blood or other fluid.
Prognosis, Prog-nώ-sis; the knowledge of the nature of a disease, obtained from early symptoms.
Prolabium, Prω-lá-bi-um; the front part of the lip.
Prolapsus, Prω-láp-sus; a falling and protrusion of any part, as the anus, uterus, etc.
Prolapsus Ani, — Ɛ́'nį; a falling of the extremity of the anus.
Prolapsus Iridis, — Ir'i-dis; the protrusion of the iris through an injury of the cornea.
Prolapsus Uteri, — Yú-ter-į; the falling of the womb, and its protrusion from the vulva.
Promontory, Próm-on-tω-ri; a projection from the cavity of the tympanum.
Promontory of the Sacrum, — Sá-krum; the projecting part of the sacrum.
Pronation, Prω-ná-ʃon; the act of turning the hand with the palm downwards.
Pronator Quadratus, Prω-ná-tor Kwod-rá-tus; a muscle which passes from the ulna to the radius, and that turns the hand inwards.
Pronator Teres, — Tḗ-rḗz; a muscle which passes from the inner condyle of the humerus to the radius.
Proof Spirit, Prωf Spír-it; alcohol, diluted with water until of the Sp. Gr. 0.920, is officinal in the British Pharmacopœia.
Prophylactic, Prof-i-lák-tik; applied to means used to prevent disease, and preserve health.
Prophylaxis, Prof-i-láks-is; the use of means necessary for the preservation of health.
Prosector, Prω-sék-tor; one who prepares a subject for dissection, or dissects for another. [face.
Prosopalgia, Pros-ω-pál-ji-a; neuralgia; pain in the
Prostatalgia, Pros-ta-tál-ji-a; pain in the prostate gland.
Prostate, Prós-tat; applied to a gland situated in front of the orifice of the male urinary bladder.
Prostatitis, Pros-ta-tį-tis; inflammation of the prostate gland.
Prosthesis, Prós-θḗ-sis; the substitution of an artificial part for one destroyed.

Protein, Prō-tē-in; a nitrogenous substance analogous to fibrin, erroneously supposed to form the substance from which all albuminoids were derived.

Protoplasm, Prō-tō-plazm; a nitrogenous substance, possessing vital principles, essential in the organization of all living beings, even the lowest.

Protuberance, Prō-tū-ber-ans; an eminence, or process, or swelling.

Proud Flesh, Prsd Fleʃ; a fungus; an unhealthy growth of flesh in a sore.

Proximate Cause, Próks-i-met Kez; that which comes next to the disease itself.

Prunus Lauro-cerasus, Prú-nus Le-rō-sē-rá-sus; cherry-laurel, an Asiatic evergreen tree, the leaves of which contain a small portion of prussic acid, and when distilled with water yield cherry-laurel water.

Prunus Serotina, — Sē-rót-i-na; the wild cherry, a native forest tree, the bark of which is extensively used as a tonic. (This tree is often described as *Prunus Virginiana*, which see.)

Prunus Virginiana, — Vɛr-jin-i-á-na; the choke-cherry, a native shrub, the bark not used medicinally. See *Prunus serotina*.

Prurigo, Prū-rį-gō; a papulous eruption on the skin, attended with itching.

Pruritus, Prū-rį-tus; excessive itching; prurigo.

Prussian Blue, Prúʃ-an Blū; ferrocyanide of iron, used generally in connection with quinia.

Prussiate of Potash, Prúʃ-i-et ov Pót-aʃ; ferrocyanide of potassium, or yellow prussiate of potash.

Prussic Acid, Prús-ik As'id; hydrocyanic acid, a powerful poison; used in a diluted form for whooping cough.

Psellismus, Sel-ís-mus; stammering; hesitation in speech.

Pseudæsthesia, Sū-des-thé-si-a; false sensation; as pain in a limb that has long been amputated.

Pseudarthrosis, Sū-dar-thró-sis; growth of a false joint.

Pseudoblepsia, Sū-dō-blép-si-a; false vision.

Pseudomembrane, Sū-dō-mém-bran; false membrane, the effect of inflammation.

Psoadicus, Sō-ád-i-kus; appertaining to the loins.

Psoæ, Sṓ-ē; applied to muscles of the loins.
Psoas Abscess, Sṓ-as Ab'ses; an abscess of the loins.
Psoas Magnus, — Mág-nus, a muscle extending from the last dorsal vertebra to the os femoris, and which moves the thigh forward.
Psoas Parvus, — Pą́r-vus; a muscle extending from the last dorsal vertebra to the pelvis, and which bends the spine upon the pelvis.
Psora, Sṓ-ra; the itch; scabies.
Psoriasis, Sō-rį́-a-sis; scaly tetter, a cutaneous disease.
Psoriasis Guttata, — Gu-tá-ta; small patches of scaly eruption, without inflammation.
Psoriasis Infantilis, — In-fan-tį́-lis; a dry tetter on the cheeks, breast, etc., affecting infants.
Psychical, Sį́-ki-kal; relating to the mind.
Psychology, Sį-kól-ō-ji; the science of the soul or mind; mental philosophy.
Psychometry, Sį-kóm-ē-tri; the art professed by Dr. J. R. Buchanan, in 1842, and others since, of measuring or reading mind by sympathetic impressions derived from feeling one's head or his manuscript.
Psychosis, Sį-kṓ-sis; disease or affection of the mind.
Ptelia Trifoliata, Tḗ-li-a Trį-fō-li-á-ta; the wafer ash, a native shrub or small tree, the bark of which is used as a tonic.
Pteris Aquilina, Tér-is Ak-wi-lį́-na; the common brake, an astringent fern.
Pterocarpus Marsupium, Ter-ō-kąr-pus Mąr-sų́-pi-um; an Indian tree which yields the astringent gum kino.
Pterygium, Ter-íj-i-um; a membranous fiber on the internal canthus of the eye.
Pterygoid Tér-i-gœd; formed like a wing.
Pterygoideus Externus, Ter-i-gœ́d-ē-us Eks-tér-nus; a muscle extending from the pterygoid process to the anterior part of the lower jawbone.
Pterygoideus Internus, — In-tér-nus; a muscle extending from the pterygoid process of the sphenoid bone to the inner angle of the lower jaw.
Pterygo - Pharyngeus, Tér-i-gō-Far-in-jḗ-us. Same as the *Constrictor superior* muscle of the pharynx.

Ptosis, Tó-sis; a falling, applied to the eyelid.

Ptyalagogue, Tį-ál-a-gog; a syalagogue, or medicine to increase the flow of saliva.

Ptyalin, Tį́-a-lin; an albuminous principle in saliva.

Ptyalism, Tį́-a-lizm; salivation, an excessive flow of saliva.

Ptyalum, Tį́-a-lum; saliva, which see.

Puberty, Pų́-ber-ti; the period approaching maturity, when the young are capable of reproduction.

Pubes, Pų́-bēz; the external region of the organs of generation, which after puberty is covered with hair.

Pubic, Pų́-bik; appertaining to the pubes.

Puccoon, Red, Pu-kún; *Sanguinaria Canadensis*, the blood root.

Puccoon, Yellow; the common name for *Hydrastis Canadensis*, yellow root.

Pudenda, Pų-dén-da; (sing. *Pudendum*,) the parts of generation, taken as a whole.

Pudenda Virorum, — Vį-ró-rum; the male generative organs taken collectively.

Pudenda Muliebre, — Mų-li-é-br; the female generative organs, collectively.

Pudic, Pų́-dik; relating to the pudenda.

Puerpera, Pų-ér-pē-ra; one who has recently given birth to a child.

Puerperal, Pų-ér-pē-ral; relating to child-bearing.

Puerperal Fever, — Fé-ver; a febrile condition sometimes resulting from parturition.

Puerperium, Pų-er-pé-ri-um; state of women during confinement.

Pug, (*or* **Pugillus**,) Pų-jíl-us; a small quantity, that can be taken between the thumb and finger.

Pulmo, Púl-mo; the Latin for lung.

Pulmometer, Pul-móm-ē-ter; an instrument for ascertaining the capacity or strength of the lungs.

Pulmonaria Officinalis, Pul-mo-ná-ri-a Of-is-i-ná-lis; a European demulcent plant.

Pulmonary, Púl-mo-na-ri; relating to the lungs.

Pulmonary Artery, — Ar′-ter-i; it rises in the right ventricle of the heart, divides, and one branch passes into each lung, which carry the blood there for aeration.

Pulmonary Consumption, — Kon-súm-ʃon; a fatal disease of the lungs, accompanied with cough, exhaustive expectoration, hectic fever, etc.

Pulmonary Plexus, — Pléks-us; a network of nerves back of the bronchia.

Pulmonary Veins, — Vanz; arising in the lungs, they unite and form four trunks that issue from each lung, and open into the left auricle of the heart.

Pulmonitis, Pul-mo-nį-tis; pneumonia; inflammation of the lungs.

Pulp, Pulp; soft pith, applied to the core of the teeth.

Pulsatilla, Pul-sa-tíl-a; *Anemone Pulsatilla*, a little European flower; the entire plant is used in nervous diseases.

Pulsation, Pul-sá-ʃon; any throbbing sensation; the action of the heart, felt wherever the arteries reach.

Pulse, Puls; the beating of the radial artery, at the wrist, caused by the propulsion of blood from the heart. The number of beats per minute, in good health, is, in a child of one year, 120; two years 110; three years 90; puberty 80; adult 70; old age 60.

Pulse, Dicrotic, — Dį-krót-ik; a double or rebounding pulsation.

Pulse, Feeble; weak in force though full in measure.

Pulse, Full; firm and of the average frequency.

Pulse, Hard; unyielding to firm pressure.

Pulse, Intermittent, with an occasional omission of a beat, indicative of heart disease.

Pulse, Irregular; unequal in force and frequency.

Pulse, Quick; one in which the beat is sudden, though regular.

Pulse, Tense, or Wiry; as if stretched and small.

Pulsus Cordis, Púl-sus Kór-dis; the beat of the heart against the thorax.

Pulvis, Púl-vis; powder; any medicine reduced to powder.

Pumpkin Seed, Púmp-kin Sēd; the seed of *Cucurbita pepo;* diuretic and anthelmintic.

Puncta Lachrymalia, Púŋk-ta Lak-ri-má-li-a; two small outlets of the lachrymal ducts, in the eyelids, for the escape of the tears.

Punctum, (*pl.***Puncta**,) Púŋk-tum; a point, or spot.

Punctum Cæcum, Púŋk-tum Sē-kum; the point of the retina, from which the optic nerve-fibers radiate, which is insensible to light.

Punctum Saliens, — Sā-li-ens; the first point of motion after the fecundation of the germ, supposed by some to be the first pulsation of the heart of the embryo.

Punica Granatum, Pū-ni-ka Gran-ā-tum; the pomegranate tree; the bark of the root is used as a vermifuge, especially for the expulsion of the tape-worm.

Pupil, Pū-pil; the dark round opening in the iris, through which the light passes to impress the image of an object on the retina.

Pupillary Membrane, Pū-pil-a-ri Mém-bran; a very thin membrane that, in the fœtus, closes the opening in the iris.

Purgation, Pur-gā-ʃon; the evacuation of the bowels.

Purgative, Púr-ga-tiv; any medicine that promotes free action of the bowels, but less violent than a cathartic.

Purging Cassia, Púrj-iŋ Káʃ-i-a; *Cassia fistula*, the pods of which are a mild cathartic.

Puriform Pū-ri-form; resembling the nature of pus.

Purpura, Púr-pu-ra; a disease in which livid spots appear on the skin, with general debility and sometimes fever.

Purulent, Púr-u-lent; full of pus; having the nature of [pus.

Pus, Pus; matter produced from inflamed animal texture, of the consistency of cream.

Push, Puʃ; a pustule, or inflammatory swelling.

Pustule, Pús-tul; a small protuberance of the cuticle enclosing pus.

Putrefaction, Pu-trē-fák-ʃon; the decomposition, or rotting, of animal matter.

Putrescence, Pu-trés-ens; a condition of rottenness.

Putrid Fever, Pū-trid Fē-ver. See Typhus Fever.

Pyæmia, Pi-ē-mi-a; a purulent condition of the blood, resulting in abscesses in different parts.

Pyelitis, Pi-ē-li-tis; inflammation of the pelvis of the [kidney.

Pyesis, (or **Pyosis**,) Pi-ē-sis; the formation of pus.

Pyloric, Pi-lór-ik; appertaining to the pylorus.

Pylorus, Pi-lō-rus; the lower apperture of the stomach.

Pyogenic, Pį-ꞷ-jén-ik; producing pus.
Pyramid, Pír-a-mid; a bony projection in the tympanum, in shape like a pyramid.
Pyramidalis, Pir-am-i-dá-lis; a triangular muscle in the back part of the pelvis, that rotates the thigh outward, and the pelvis inward.
Pyramidalis Nasi, — Ná-sį; a muscle of the nose.
Pyrethrum Parthenium, Pir-ŧ-ŧrum Pɑr-ŧŧ-ni-um; feverfew, a European plant, often cultivated in gardens.
Pyretic, Pir-ét-ik; febrile; relating to fever.
Pyrexia, Pir-éks-i-ɑ; a condition of fever.
Pyriformis, Pír-i-fór-mis; a muscle that passes from the pelvis to the great trochanter of the femur.
Pyrogenesia, Pir-ꞷ-jen-ŧ-si-ɑ; the generation of fire.
Pyromania, Pir-ꞷ-má-ni-ɑ; a mania for setting houses on fire.
Pyrophosphoric Acid, Pir-ꞷ-fos-fór-ik As'id; an acid made by heating phosphoric acid to a temperature sufficient to remove the element of water.
Pyrophosphates, Pir-ꞷ-fós-fats; salts of pyrophosphoric acid. The pyrophosphate of iron is used in medicine.
Pyrosis, Pir-ꞷ́-sis; water-brash, or heart-burn.
Pyrosphyra, Pir-os-fį-rɑ; a metal instrument, to be heated and used for cauterizing.
Pyroxylon, Pir-óks-i-lon; gun cotton.
Pyrus Malus, Pį-rus Má-lus; the apple tree.

Q

Q. P.; abbreviation of *quantum placet*, "as much as you please."
Q. S.; *quantum sufficit*, "what will suffice."
Quackery, Kwák-er-i; the pretensions of uneducated practitioners of medicine; also, undignified acts of competent professionals.
Quadratus Femoris, Kwod-rá-tus Fém-ꞷ-ris; a muscle passing from the ischium to the femur.

Quadratus Genæ, Kwod-rá-tus, Jḗ-nē; a muscle that depresses the lower lip.

Quadratus Lumborum, — Lum-bṓ-rum; a muscle between the last rib and the crest of the ilium, that moves the loins to one side.

Quadriceps Extensor, Kwód-ri-seps Eks-tén-sor; the extensor muscle of the knee.

Quadrigemina Tubercula, Kwod-ri-jém-i-na Tų-bér-kų-la; four small oval muscles, located below the posterior commissure of the brain, called the *nates* and *testes*.

Quadrumana, Kwod-rú-ma-na; animals having four extremities terminating with hands.

Qualitative, Kwól-i-ta-tiv; relating to quality.

Quarantine, Kwór-an-tēn; the detention of passengers and goods coming in from a port where a contagious disease prevailed, until thoroughly disinfected.

Quartan, Kwór-tan; occurring once in four days, as fever and ague.

Quassia, Kwóʃ-i-a; a bitter tonic, the wood of *Simaruba excelsa*.

Queen of the Meadow, Kwēn ov ðe Méd-ō; *Eupatorium purpureum*, a native plant; the name is also applied to *Spiræa tomentosa*.

Queen's Root, Kwēn'z Rut; a common name for *Stillingia sylvatica*.

Quercus, Kwér-kus; the oak family of trees. The inner barks of *Q. alba* and *Q. tinctoria* are officinal, and used as astringents.

Quercus Infectoria, — In-fek-tṓ-ri-a; the dyer's oak of Asia, which produces galls.

Quevenne's Iron, Ka-ven'z Ī'urn; iron by hydrogen, which see.

Quick Lime, Kwik Līm; lime unslacked, which see.

Quicksilver, Kwik-sil-ver; a synonym for the element mercury.

Quillaia Saponaria, Kwi-lá-a Sap-ō-ná-ri-a; the soap tree, an evergreen of South America, the bark of which is used as an errhine.

Quince Seed, Kwins Sēd; the seed of *Cydonia vulgaris*, which are demulcent.

Quinia, or **Quinine,** Kwín-i-a or Kwi-nín; (Fr. Kinín;) the most valuable of the cinchona alkaloids, the sulphate of quinia being mostly used.

Quinidia, or **Quinidine,** Kwin-íd-i-a, or Kwín-i-din; an alkaloid from cinchona bark, in little demand.

Quinine Flower, Kwi-nín Flŏ-er. See *Sabbatia Elliotii.*

R

R.; in prescriptions, means Recipe, "take."

Rabies, Rá-bi-ēz; madness, caused by the bite or scatch of an animal, the saliva, it is supposed, being affected with a diseased virus.

Rabies Canina, — Ka-ní-na; hydrophobia, caused as above, and so named because the patient cannot endure the presence of water.

Race Ginger, Ras Jin-jer; common black ginger root.

Rachialgia, Rak-i-ál-ji-a; pain in the spine.

Rachitis, Ra-kí-tis; inflammation of the spine, strictly; but also applied to the rickets, which see.

Radicals, Rád-i-kalz; a term given to elements and compounds which form roots for series of salts.

Ragweed, Rág-wēd; *Ambrosia artemisiæfolia,* a native troublesome weed.

Rale, Rel; (Fr., "a rattle;")applied to certain sounds, termed "moist," "dry," or "sonorous," that indicate a morbid condition of the bronchia or vesicles of the lungs.

Ramentum, Ra-mén-tum; any substance reduced to scales by filing; sometimes applied to a hair-like growth.

Ramollissement, Ra-mol-is-mañ; French for "softening."

Ramose, Ra-mós; divided into branches.

Ramulus, Rám-u-lus; a ramule, or small branch.

Rancid, Rán-sid; stale, or rank; applied to fat or oil.

Ranula, Rán-u-la; a tumor under the tongue, resulting from obstructions in the salivary or mucous glands.

Ranunculus Bulbosus, Ra-nún-ku-lus Bul-bó-sus; crowfoot; buttercup; an acrid plant, the fresh bulb of which was formerly used as a vesicant.

Raphania, Ra-fá-ni-a; a disease of Germany, attended with spasms of pain in the joints.

Raphe, Rá-fē; a seam or cord, as between the hemispheres of the brain, in the scrotum, etc.

Rash, Raʃ; redness and eruption of the skin.

Rat's Bane, Rát's Ban; formerly the common name for arsenious acid.

Rattlesnake's Master, Rát-l-snak's Más-ter; a common name applied to *Eryngium yuccæfolium*, and in the Southern States to *Liatris squarrosa*.

Rattle Weed, Rát-l Wēd; a common name for *Cimicifuga racemosa*, applied to it on account of its dry rattle-like fruit.

Raucedo, Re-sé-dω; hoarseness, resulting from inflammation of the mucous membrane.

Reaction, Rē-ák-ʃon; the revival of the vital powers after great or prolonged depression, sometimes effected by irritants or stimulants.

Reagent, Rē-á-jent; a test, employed by chemists in ascertaining the quality or quantity of different substances.

Receptaculum Chyli, Rē-sep-ták-ų-lum Kį-lį; the lower part of the thoracic duct.

Reclination, Rek-lin-á-ʃon; the operation for cataract, in which the lens of the eye is turned in a horizontal position.

Recrementitious Humor, Rek-rē-men-tí-ʃus Yú-mor; a secretion that is returned whence it came, as the saliva, which being first separated from the blood is returned to it.

Recrudescence, Rek-rω-dés-ens; increased violence of a disease, after temporary indications of a favorable termination.

Rectalgia, Rek-tál-ji-a; pain in the rectum.

Rectitis, Rek-tį-tis; inflammation of the rectum.

Rectum, Rék-tum; the lower section of the intestines, terminating in the anus.

Recti Abdominis, Rék-tį Ab-dóm-i-nis; a long flat muscle in the front of the abdomen, reaching from the pubes to the three lower ribs, and bending the chest in respiration.

Recti Capitis, Rék-tį Káp-i-tis; five muscles, reaching from the cervical vertebra to the occipital bone.

Recti Femoris, — Fém-ǫ-ris; muscles extending from the pelvis to the patella.

Recti Laterales, — Lat-er-á-lēz; straight muscles of the side of the trunk.

Recurrent, Rē-kúr-ent; applied to branches of arteries and nerves which turn back in their course.

Red Bark, Red Bąrk; that variety of cinchona bark yielded by the *Cinchona succirubra.*

Red Cedar, Red Sé-dar; *Juniperus Virginiana*, a native evergreen.

Red Clover, — Klǿ-ver; *Trifolium pratense*, a common cultivated plant, the dried flower-heads are the portion used.

Red Lead, — Led; red oxide of lead, used in preparing certain ointments and plasters.

Red Phosphorous, — Fós-fǫ-rus; amorphous phosphorous, made by exposing ordinary phosphorous to about 450° Fah., in a closed vessel, from which air is excluded.

Red Precipitate, — Prē-sip-i-tat; red oxide of mercury; murcuric oxide.

Red Puccoon. See Bloodroot.

Redintegration, Rē-din-tē-grá-ʃon; the reproduction of a part that has been destroyed.

Reduced Iron, Rē-dųst Ī'urn; iron by hydrogen, [which see.

Reduction, Rē-dúk-ʃon; replacing a dislocated bone, or joint; replacing a hernia.

Reflect, Rē-flékt; to turn back on itself.

Reflection, Rē-flék-ʃon; the retroversion of the uterus; the doubling back of a membrane.

Reflex Action, Ré-fleks Ak'ʃon; a term much used of late to signify "the reflection by an efferent nerve of an impression conveyed to a nervous center by an afferent nerve." (Dunglison.)

Reflux, Ré-fluks; the return of the blood to the heart.

Refrigerant, Rē-frij-er-ant; medicines that reduce the heat of the blood or body.

Regeneration, Rē-jen-er-á-ʃon; the reproduction or growth of matter lost by disease.

Regimen, Réj-i-men; habits in regard to food; methods of eating and drinking, for the preservation of health.

Regurgitation, Rē-gur-ji-tá-ʃon; the return of food or drink, after swallowing.

Remittent Fever, Rē-mit-ent Fé-ver; any fever that subsides at regular intervals, but does not wholly cease.

Ren, Ren; the kidney, whose function is to secrete the urine.

Renal, Ré-nal; appertaining to the kidneys.

Repellent, Rē-pél-ent; a medicine, or agency, that causes a disease to recede from the surface.

Repriments, Rép-ri-ments; remedies for the repression of fluxes, as astringents, acids, etc.

Reproduction, Rē-prɷ-dúk-ʃon; the procreation of organized beings or bodies.

Reptant, Rép-tant; creeping, as a reptile.

Resection, Rē-sék-ʃon; amputation, by trimming off broken parts.

Resinoid, Réz-i-nɵd; a substance that is obtained from plants, and does not admit of classification with resins, oils, etc. Sometimes the so-called resinoids of the market are simply dried solid extracts.

Resins, Réz-inz; substances obtained from plants, insoluble in water, not volatile, resemble somewhat camphors, usually soluble in alcohol.

Resolution, Rez-ɷ-lų́-ʃon; the gradual termination of inflammation, without suppuration.

Resolvent, Rē-zól-vent; a substance that dissolves or terminates inflammatory tumors.

Resonance, Réz-ɷ-nans; a reverberation of the voice, as if sounding in an unusual place, indicating a morbid condition of the lungs.

Resorption, Rē-sérp-ʃon; the absorption of a fluid after it has once been regularly deposited.

Respirable, Rē-spír-a-bl; air or gas that may safely be inhaled.

Respiration, Res-pi-rá-ʃon; the act of breathing, consisting of both inspiration and expiration; in health, the respiration of infants is 35 to the minute; at two years old 25; at puberty 20; in the adult 18.

Retching, Réç-iŋ; involuntary and ineffectual efforts to vomit.

Rete, Ré-tē; a net; applied to interlacings of fibers, nerves, etc.
Rete Mucosum, — Mų-kó-sum; the tissue underlying the cuticle that gives color to the skin.
Rete Testis, — Tés-tis; the network of tubes into which the vascular system of the testicles is gathered.
Reticular, Rē-tík-ų-lar; resembling a net.
Reticulum, Rē-tík-ų-lum; a little net.
Retiferus, Rē-tíf-er-us; marked with lines like a net.
Retiform, Rét-i-fərm; shaped in the form of a net.
Retina, Rét-i-na; the expansion of the optic nerve, which forms the inner coat of the eye, being the organ of visual perception.
Retinacula, Ret-i-nák-ų-la; bands which serve to hold the tendons close to the bones, in the wrist, ankle, etc.; also the ridge around the ileo-cæcal valve.
Retinitis, Ret-i-nį-tis; inflammation of the retina.
Retort, Rē-tórt; an earthen, glass, or metal vessel, used in distillation.
Retraction Rē-trák-ʃon; shortening, or drawing back.
Retractor, Rē-trák-tor; applied to muscles that withdraw the parts to which they are attached; also, a piece of linen used in amputation.
Retrahens Auriculum, Rét-ra-hens Ɵ-rík-ų-lum; one of the muscles of the auricle of the ear.
Retrocedent, Ret-rɷ-sé-dent; passing from the outer part of the body to an internal part, as rheumatism.
Retroflexed, Ré-trɷ-flekst; bent backward.
Retroflexio Uteri. Same as *Retroversio Uteri*.
Retroversion, Rē-trɷ-vér-ʃon; turning backward, as in the case of the bladder, uterus, etc.
Retroversio Uteri, Ré-trɷ-vér-ʃi-ɷ Yú-ter-į; a displacement of the uterus so that the bottom is turned toward the concavity of the sacrum, and the mouth and neck are pressed over against the *ossa pubis*.
Rhachiæus, Ra-ki-é-us; relating to the spine.
Rhachiasmus, Ra-ki-ás-mus; incipient epilepsy, manifested by spasms in the muscles of the neck.
Rhachioparalysis, Rak-i-ɷ-par-ál-i-sis; paraplegia, or paralysis of the spine.
Rachis, Rá-kis; the spine; the vertebral column.

Rhamnus Catharticus, Rám-nus Ka-ŧɋr-ti-kus; buckthorn, the berries of which are a violent purgative.

Rhamnus Frangula, — Fráŋ-gɥ-lɑ; a European tree, the bark of which is used as a cathartic.

Rhamnus Purshiana, — Pur-ʃi-á-nɑ; a Western tree, the bark of which is recommended as a laxative.

Rhatany, Rát-a-ni; the root of a South American shrub, *Krameria triandra*, which is a powerful astringent.

Rhegma, Rég-mɑ; a rupture, as the bursting of an abscess.

Rheum, Rɯm; a thin watery discharge from the mucous membranes.

Rheumatism, Rɯ́-ma-tizm; a neuralgic disease; sometimes confined to the joints; and at others to the muscles; sometimes with great inflammation, and at others little; always painful, and difficult to cure.

Rheumatic, Rɯ-mát-ik; relating to rheumatism.

Rheumatism Root, Rɯ́-ma-tizm Rɯt; *Jeffersonia diphylla.*

Rheum Palmatum, Rɯm Pal-má-tum; the rhubarb plant, a native of Asia, the root of which is a valuable cathartic.

Rhinalgia, Ri-nál-ji-ɑ: pain in the nose.

Rhinitis, Ri-nị-tis; inflammation of the nose.

Rhinoplasty, Rị-nɷ-plas-ti; the formation of a new nose from the skin of the forehead.

Rhinopolypus, Rị-nɷ-pól-i-pus; polypus or tumor in the nose.

Rhinorrhagia, Rị-nɷ-rá-ji-ɑ; excessive bleeding from the nose.

Rhododendron Maximum, Rɷ-dɷ-dén-dron Máks-i-mum; a native showy shrub, known as rosebay, stimulant and astringent.

Rhomboideus, Rom-bɷ-ị-dĭ-us; a muscle in the back of the neck that moves the scapula.

Rhoncus, Rón-kus: a rattling sound in the throat. See Rale.

Rhubarb, Rɯ́-bɑrb; the root of *Rheum palmatum*, a cathartic, possessing also astringent properties.

Rhus Glabra, Rus Glá-brɑ; sumach, a native shrub, the berries of which contain malic acid, and are used as a refrigerant; the bark is astringent.

Rhus Toxicodendron, Rus Toks-i-kō-dén-dron; a poisonous vine of the United States, the leaves of which are used in nervous diseases; the poisonous principle of the vine is volatile, and produces inflammation and painful eruptions of the skin.

Rhyas, Rī-as; a disease of the eye, in which the caruncula lachrymalis is affected, causing a constant flow of tears.

Ricinus Communis, Rís-i-nus Kom-ū-nis; the castor-oil plant, the seeds of which abound in a fixed viscid oil, which is extensively used as a carthartic.

Rickets, Rik-ets; rachitis: a disease of children, in which a crooked spine, distorted limbs, and general debility are the result.

Rigor, Rig-or; sudden chilliness and shivering.

Rima Glottidis, Rī-ma Glót-i-dis; the opening between the vocal cords of the larynx.

Rimose, Rī-mṓs; full of openings or cracks.

Ringworm, Riŋ-wurm; a vesicular disease, in which the pustules arise on an inflamed base, and unite in circles or rings.

Risus, Rī-sus; laughter, an involuntary movement of the lips and muscles of the face.

Risus Sardonicus — Sar-dón-i-kus; a convulsive laugh, or spasm of the face, resulting from tetanus.

Rochelle Salt, Rō-ʃél Selt; tartrate of sodium and potassium, used as a laxative and a component of Seidlitz Powders.

Rock Rose, Rok Rōz; a common name for frostwort; *Helianthemum Canadense*.

Roll Sulphur, Rōl Súl-fur; brimstone; sulphur melted and run into moulds.

Roman Chamomile, Rṓ-man Kám-ō-mīl; *Anthemis nobilus*, designated *Roman* in contradistinction to the German chamomile, *Matricaria Chamomilla*.

Rosa Centifolia, Rṓ-sa Sen-ti-fṓ-li-a; a cultivated double rose, the petals of which are distilled in water to make rose-water.

Rosemary, Rṓz-me-ri; *Rosmarinus officinalis*, a labiate plant, cultivated in gardens, and mostly used in domestic practice.

Rose Oil, Rœz Œl; otto of rose, a sweet scented oil, obtained from roses.

Rose Water, — Wé-ter; a sweet scented water, made by distillation of water from roses.

Roseola, Rœ-sḗ-œ-la; a rash, or eruption of pimples.

Rosin, Róz-in; the residuum after distillation of turpentine from the oleo-resin of the pine.

Rotator, Rœ-tá-tor; applied to muscles employed in producing circular movements.

Rottlera Tinctoria, Rot-lḗ-ra Tiŋk-tœ́-ri-a; a Euphorbiaceous tree of India, from the fruit of which Kameela is obtained.

Rottlerin, Rot-lḗ-rin; a crystalline resin of Kameela.

Round Ligament, Rȣnd Líg-a-ment; a short ligament that connects the head of the femur with the cotyloid cavity.

Round Ligaments; two cords that extend from the sides of the uterus, through the abdominal rings, to the groins.

Rubefacient, Rɯ-bē-fá-ʃent; any application that excites redness of the skin.

Rubeola, Rɯ-bḗ-œ-la; the measles, a kind of inflammatory fever, with sneezing, cough, and eruption of the skin.

Rubeoloid, Rɯ-bḗ-œ-lœd; resembling measles.

Rubia Tinctorum, Rɯ́-bi-a Tiŋk-tœ́-rum; a plant of Europe that yields madder.

Rubus Villosus, Rɯ́-bus Vi-lœ́-sus; the common blackberry, the root of which is astringent.

Ructus, Rúk-tus; eructation, or belching.

Rue, Rɯ; *Ruta graveolens*, a garden plant, used as a stimulant.

Rugose, Rɯ-gœ́s; wrinkled and rough.

Rumex Acetosella, Rɯ́-meks As-ē-tœ-sél-a; sheep-sorrel, a common weed, with a sour juice; used as a refrigerant.

Rumex Crispus, — Krís-pus; yellow dock, a weed, the root of which is astringent and tonic.

Rupia, Rɯ́-pi-a; a pustular eruption, the discharge from which thickens into scabs.

Rupture, Rúp-tɥr. Same as *Hernia*, which see.

Ruta Graveolens, Rú-ta Gráv-ĕ-ō-lens, rue, a European plant, used as a stimulant.
Rutidosis, Ru-ti-dó-sis; (or *Rhytidosis*,) a shrinking and puckering of the cornea, considered a sign of approaching death.
Ruyschiana, Rœs-ki-á-na; the internal membrane of the choroid coat of the eye.
Rye, Rī; *Secale cereale*, a common cultivated grain, the diseased seed, enlarged by a fungus growth, are known as ergot, or blasted rye.

S

S.; *Semissis*, "half;" sometimes written *ss*.
Sabadilla, Sa-ba-díl-a. See *Veratrum Sabadilla*.
Sabbatia Angularis, Sa-bá-ʃi-a Aŋ-gū-lá-ris; American centaury, a native herb, used as a bitter tonic.
Sabbatia Elliottii, — El-i-ót-i-ī; a southern plant; lately introduced as an antiperiodic under the name quinine flower.
Saccharated Carbonate of Iron, Sák-a-ra-ted, —; Vallet's iron mass, carbonate of iron freshly precipitated, mixed with sugar and dried.
Saccharum, Sák-a-rum; cane sugar.
Saccharum Lactis, — Lák-tis; sugar of milk.
Sacculated, Sák-ū-la-ted; made like a sac; encysted.
Saccule, Sák-ūl; a little sac or bag.
Sacculus Cordis, Sák-ū-lus Kór-dis; the pericardium.
Sacculus Lachrymalis, Lak-ri-má-lis; the beginning of the lachrymal duct.
Sacculus Laryngis, — Lar-ín-jis; a small pouch connecting with the ventricle of the larynx.
Sacculus Proprius, — Pró-pri-us; the smaller sac of the vestibulum of the ear.
Sacer Ignis, Sá-ser Ig'nis; "sacred fire;" the erysipelas.
Sacer Morbis, — Mór-bis; a term for epilepsy.
Sacrolumbalis, Sak-rō-lum-bá-lis; a muscle of the sacrum, connecting with the six lower ribs.

Sacrum, Sá-krum; the posterior bone of the pelvis.

Safflower, Sáf-flɤ-er; American saffron; the florets of *Carthamus tinctorius*.

Saffron, Sáf-ron; the dried central organs, or stigmas, of the flowers of *Crocus sativus*.

Sage, Sej; *Salvia officinalis*, a common garden plant, used as an aromatic tonic.

Sagittal Suture, Sáj-i-tal Sų́-tųr; that which unites the parietal bones.

Sago, Sá-gɷ; the nutritious starch obtained from the pith of an East Indian palm tree, *Sagus Rumphii*.

Saint Anthony's Fire, Sant An'tɷ-ni'z Fįr. See *Erysipelas*.

Saint John's Wort, — Jonz-wurt; *Hypericum perforatum*, a troublesome naturalized weed.

Saint Vitus' Dance, — Vį-tus Dɑns. See *Chorea*.

Sal, Sal. See Salt. [nium.

Sal Ammoniac, Sal A-mɷ́-ni-ak; chloride of ammo-

Salicin, Sál-i-sin; a neutral crystalline body obtained from willow bark.

Salicylic Acid, Sal-i-síl-ik As'id; an organic acid first obtained from a species of spiræa; now made from carbolic acid. It is used in acute rheumatism, and as an antiseptic. [glands; spittle.

Saliva, Sa-lį-vɑ; the fluid secreted by the salivary

Salivary Glands, Sál-i-va-ri Glandz; the glands underneath and back of the lower jaw.

Salivation, Sal-i-vá-ʃon; an excessive secretion of saliva; sometimes caused by the improper use of murcury.

Salix, Sá-liks; the generic name for the numerous species of willows; the bark of *S. alba* is officinal, and used as a tonic.

Salpingitis, Sa.-pin-jį-tis; inflammation of the Fallopian tube.

Sal Prunelle, Sal Prɯ-nél; nitrate of potassium, melted and cast into bullets; almost out of use.

Salt, (**Common**,) Sɵlt; chloride of sodium. A term once used to note the substance formed by the union of an acid and an alkali. [potassium.

Saltpeter, Sɵlt-pé-ter; the common name for nitrate of

Salt of Sorrel, Selt of Sór-el; a crystalline substance obtained by combining acid oxalate of potassium with oxalic acid. Sometimes oxalic acid is sold for it.

Salvatella, Sal-va-tél-a; a vein on the back of the hand, tributary to the basillic vein.

Salvia Officinalis, Sál-vi-a Of-i-si-ná-lis, the sage plant, tonic, stimulant and carminative.

Sambucus Canadensis, Sam-bú-kus Kan-a-dén-sis; the common elder, a native shrub, the dried flowers of which are sudorific.

Sanation, San-á-ʃon; a cure; the act of healing.

Sanative, Sán-a-tiv; having the power to cure.

Sandal Wood Oil, Sán-dal Wud Ōl; an essential oil of the yellow sandal wood, used in gonorrhœa.

Sanguinaria Canadensis, San-gwin-á-ri-a Kan-a-dén-sis; blood-root, a native plant, the root of which is expectorant and stimulant.

Sanguinarin, (or **Sanguinarina,**) San-gwín-er-in; an acrid pungent white alkaloid of *Sanguinaria Canadensis*. It forms salts that are red.

Sanguineous, San-gwín-ē-us; appertaining to blood, abounding in blood.

Sanies, Sá-ni-ēz; a thin fetid discharge from ulcers, rarely tinged with blood.

Sanitary, Sán-i-ta-ri; relating to health.

Santonin, Sán-to-nin; a very weak organic base, usually classed as a glucoside; the active principle of Levant wormseed, used as an anthelmintic.

Santorini, (**Tubercles of,**) San-to-rí-ni; small projections at the top of the arytenoid cartilages, for the support of the ligaments of the glottis.

Saphena, Sa-fē-na; applied to a vein and nerve near the surface of the skin, and passing from the knee to the ankle.

Sapid, Sáp-id; possessing or imparting taste.

Sapo, Sá-po; soap. Castile soap is used in soap liniment and pills.

Saponaria Officinalis, Sap-o-ná-ri-a Of-is-i-ná-lis; soapwort, bouncing-bet; an introduced weed, used as an alterative.

Sarcitis, Sar-sí-tis; inflammation of the muscles; rheumatism.

Sarcocele, Sq́r-sō-sēl; a kind of cancer, or a fleshy growth about the testicle.

Sarcodes, Sqr-kṓ-dēz; fleshy; resembling flesh.

Sarcolemma, Sqr-kō-lém-a; a sheath that surrounds the particles of muscle forming a fiber.

Sarcology, Sqr-kól-ō-ji; that branch of anatomy which treats of the soft parts of the body.

Sarcoma, Sqr-kṓ-ma; a fleshy tumor, of many varieties.

Sarcomatous, Sqr-kóm-a-tus; relating to sarcoma.

Sarcophagus, Sqr-kóf-a-gus; flesh-eating.

Sarcoptes, Sqr-kóp-tēz; a small insect that stings the flesh; the *Acarus Scabies*, or itch insect.

Sarcosis, Sqr-kṓ-sis; a morbid growth of flesh.

Sardonic Laugh, Sqr-dón-ik Lqf. See *Risus Sardonicus*.

Sarothamæ Scoparius, Sar-óth-a-mē Skō-pá-ri-us; the broom, diuretic and cathartic.

Sarracenia Purpurea, Sar-a-sé-ni-a Pur-pų-ré-a; a native swamp plant, the root of which is used in dyspepsia.

Sarsaparilla, Sqr-sa-pa-ríl-a; the roots of a South American vine, *Smilax Officinalis*, used as an alterative in syphilitic diseases.

Sartorius, Sqr-tṓ-ri-us; the longest muscle of the body extending from the spinous process of the ilium to the inner part of the head of the tibia.

Sassafras, Sás-a-fras; an indigenous small tree, the bark from the root of which is an aromatic stimulant, and the pith of the stems forms with water a mucilaginous wash.

Sativus, Sa-tį́-vus; a specific name applied to plants that grow in fields, or are cultivated.

Saturation, Sat-ų-rá-ʃon; the act of filling water or other liquid with as much of a soluble body, salt, for instance, as it will dissolve.

Satyriasis, Sat-i-rį́-a-sis; morbid sexual desire in men.

Satureia Hortensis, Sat-ų-rį́-a Hor-tén-sis; summer savory, an aromatic garden herb.

Savine, Sá-vin. See *Juniperus Sabina*.

Saxifraga, Saks-íf-ra-ga; a genus of herbs, several species of which possess alterative properties.

Scabies, Ská-bi-ēz; the itch, a cutaneous disease, developing into irritable scaly patches in different parts of the body.

Scald Head, Skeld Hed; an eruption, like ringworm, of the scalp.

Scale, Skel; small whitish lamina, or crusts of diseased cuticle, that fall off and are reproduced.

Scalenus, Ska-lé-nus; two muscles, the *anticus* and *posticus*, that arise in the vertebræ of the neck and connect with the first and second ribs, and are used in moving the neck.

Scalp, Skalp; the integument that covers the skull.

Scalpel, Skál-pel; a small straight bladed knife used in dissecting operations.

Scammony, Skám-ω-ni; a gum resin exuded from the roots of the *Convolvulus Scammonia;* a very active cathartic.

Scapula, Skáp-ų-la; the shoulder-blade.

Scapulalgia, Skap-ų-lál-ji-a; pain in the shoulder-blade.

Scarf-Skin, Skqrf-Skin; the epidermis or cuticle.

Scarification, Skar-i-fi-ká-ʃon; the making of small incisions into the surface of the skin, to draw blood or cause local depletion.

Scarlatina, Skqr-la-tį-na; scarlet fever, contagious, and attended with a scarlet eruption on the skin; it is *simple*, *anginose*, or *malignant*, according to the violence of the attack.

Scarlet Fever, Skq́r-let Fé-ver. Same as *Scarlatina.*

Scheroma, Skē-rώ-ma; insufficient lachrymal secretion.

Schneiderian Membrane, Snį-dé-ri-an Mém-bran; the pituitary membrane that lines the cavities of the nose.

Sciatic, Sį-át-ik; relating to nerves and vessels of the ischium.

Sciatica, Sį-át-i-ka; rheumatism in the hip-joint.

Scilla Maritima, Síl-a Mar-i-tį-ma; squill, a European plant, the dried bulbs of which are much used as an expectorant.

Scirrhogastria, Skir-ω-gás-tri-a; incipient cancer of the stomach.

Scirrhus, Skír-us; a hard tumor affecting the glands, often ending in cancer.

Scleremus, Sklē-ré-mus; a hardening of the cellular tissue.

Scleriasis, Sklē-rī-a-sis; a hardening, sometimes of the eye-lids, female genital organs, etc.
Sclerosis, Sklē-rṓ-sis; tkickening by condensation.
Sclerotica, Sklē-rót-i-ka; the hard membrane of the eye called the "white of the eye."
Scorbutic, Skor-bū́-tik; having the nature of or affected [by scurvy.
Scorbutus, Skor-bū́-tus; the scurvy, a disease causing a bloated countenance, livid spots on the skin, foul breath, loose teeth, and spongy gums.
Scotoma, Skō-tṓ-ma; darkness; obscure vision.
Scouring Rush, Skōr-iŋ Ruʃ; *Equisetum hyemale*, which see.
Scrobiculate, Skrō-bík-ū-lat; having small furrows or [cavities.
Scrobiculus, Skrō-bík-ū-lus; a pit, or small hollow.
Scrobiculus Cordis, — Kór-dis; the cavity of the heart, the pit of the stomach.
Scrofula, Skróf-ū-la; the king's evil: a swelling of the glands of the neck, causing imperfect suppuration.
Scrophularia Nodosa, Skrof-ū-lā́-ri-a Nō-dṓ-sa; figwort, carpenter's square, a common plant in the United States and Europe.
Scrotal, Skrṓ-tal; appertaining to the scrotum.
Scrotal Hernia, — Hér-ni-a; hernia in which part of the vicera protrudes into the scrotum.
Scrotocele, Skrṓ-tō-sēl. Same as *Scrotal Hernia*.
Scrotum, Skrṓ-tum; the sac or pouch that encloses the testicles.
Scullcap, Skúl-kap: *Scutellaria lateriflora*, a valuable [nervine.
Scurf, Skurf; dandriff; small scaly particles that rub loose from the skalp, when in an unhealthy condition.
Scurvy, Skúr-vi . See *Scorbutus*.
Scurvy-grass,. Skúr-vi-gras ; *Cochlearia officinalis*, a diuretic.
Scybala, Síb-a-la; dry and hard lumps in the excrement.
Scytoblastema, Sī-tō-blas-tḗ-ma; growth of the skin.
Sea-Sickness, Sē-Sík-nes; nausea, vomiting and gastric distress, caused by the undulating motions of a vessel at sea.
Sebaceous, Sē-bā́-ʃus; fatty; applied to glands that accumulate fat.
Sebiferous, Sē-bíf-er-us; oily, or fat-producing.

Secale Cereale, Sē-ká-lē Sē-rē-á-lē; the rye plant.
Secale Cornutum, — Kor-nú-tum; the former official name for ergot, which see.
Secernent, Sē-sér-nent; secretory; applied to vessels that separate different materials from the blood, for various purposes.
Second Intention, Sék-ond In-tén-ʃon; the healing of a wound by the several stages of suppuration, granulation and sicatrization.
Secretion, Sē-kré-ʃon; the process by which various organs separate different fluids or substances from the blood; the thing secreted.
Sectio Cæsarea, Sék-ʃi-ō Ses-a-ré-a. See *Cæsarean operation.*
Sectio Nympharum, — Nim-fá-rum. See *Nymphotomy.*
Secundine, Sék-un-din; in the plural applied to the afterbirth.
Sedation, Sē-dá-ʃon; the effect of a sedative.
Sedative, Séd-a-tiv; that which allays irritability.
Sediment, Séd-i-ment; particles in a fluid that settle to the bottom of a vessel.
Seidlitz Powders, Séd-lits Pọ́-derz; powders composed of Rochelle salts and bicarbonate of sodium mixed, to be added in solution to tartaric acid, thus making an effervescing drink.
Sella Turcica, Sél-a Túr-si-ka; the slight cavity in the clinoid process of the sphenoid bone in which lodges the pituitary gland.
Semeiology, Sem-i-ól-o-ji; the science of the symptoms of disease.
Semeiotic, Sem-i-ót-ik; relating to the symptoms of disease.
Semen, Sé-men; the seed of plants; the male sperm of animals.
Semi-, Sém-i-; a prefix meaning half.
Semilunar Ganglia, Semi-lú-nar Gáŋ-gli-a; the abdominal ganglia on the sympathetic nerve.
Semilunar Valves, — Valvz; a triplet of valves at the head of the aorta, and three others where the pulmonary artery begins.
Semimembranosus, Sem-i-mem-bran-ó-sus; a muscle extending from the head of the tibia to the lower end of the femur.

Seminal, Sém-i-nal; relating to seed or semen.
Semination, Sem-i-ná-ʃon; the distribution of seeds, or the depositing of semen in the uterus.
Seminiferous, Sem-i-níf-er-us; relating to vessels that carry the seminal fluid.
Semi-Spinales, Sém-i-Spi-ná-lēz; (*s. colli* and *s. dorsi,*) muscles connecting the transverse and spinous processes of the vertebræ.
Semi-Tendinosus, Sémi-Ten-din-ó-sus; a muscle extending from the ischium to the tibia.
Seneca Oil, Sén-ē-ka Oil; crude petroleum.
Senecio Aureus, Sen-é-ʃi-o Θ-ré-us; life-root; a native plant, used as a diuretic.
Senega, or **Seneka**, Sén-ē-ga, *or* Sén-ē-ka; *Polygala Senega*, an indigenous herb, the root of which is used as an expectorant. [tieth year.
Senectus, Sē-nék-tus; old age, beginning with the six-
Senile, Sé-nil; appertaining to old age.
Senna, Sén-a; the leaflets of *Cassia acutifolia* and *C. elongata*, an efficient purgative.
Sensorium, Sen-só-ri-um; the seat of sensation; the brain, or ganglia at the base of the brain.
Sensorium Commune, — Kóm-u-nē; also applied to the brain, where the nerves of sensation concentrate.
Sepia Officinalis, Sé-pi-a Of-is-i-ná-lis; a shell fish of the Mediterranean, the source of cuttle-fish bone.
Septæmia, Sep-té-mi-a; a morbid condition of the blood.
Septic, Sép-tik; putrefying; causing putrefaction.
Septum, Sép-tum; a division, or partition.
Septum Auricularum, — Θ-rik-u-lá-rum; the partition separating the right ventricle of the heart from the left.
Septum Cerebelli, — Ser-ē-bél-i; divides the cerebellum perpendicularly. [the heart.
Septum Cordis, — Kór-dis; divides the ventricles of
Septum Lucidum, — Lú-si-dum; separates the lateral ventricles of the brain.
Septum Nasi, — Ná-si; the division between the nostrils.
Septum Pectiniforme, Pek-tin-i-fór-mē; a partial tendinous division between the *corpora cavernosa* of the penis.

Septum Scroti, Sép-tum Skrṓ-tī; the partition separating the testicles.

Septum Transversum, — Trans-vér-sum; that which separates the thorax from the abdomen; also applied to a division between the semicircular canals of the ear.

Sequela, Sē-kwḗ-la; a secondary manifestation of disease, succeeding the original attack.

Sequestrum, Sē-kwés-trum; a dead part of bone cast out from a wound or ulcer.

Serolin, Sér-ō-lin; an oily substance in the blood.

Serous, Sḗ-rus; thin, watery; resembling serum.

Serpentaria, Ser-pen-tā́-ri-a; *Aristolochia Serpentaria*; Virginia snakeroot, a native herb, the root of which is used as a stimulant.

Serpigo, Ser-pī́-gō; ring-worm or tetter.

Serratus Magnus, Ser-á-tus Mág-nus; a large muscle of the thorax, stretching from the lateral surface of the ribs to the scapula.

Serratus Posticus, — Pos-tī́-kus; a muscle passing from the lumbar region to the ribs.

Serum, Sḗ-rum; the fluid part of the blood, *i. e.* blood without its corpuscles and fibrin.

Sesamoid, Sés-a-moid; applied to the small bones formed in tendons, as at the roots of the thumb and great toe.

Sesamum Indicum, Sés-a-mum In'di-kum; benne, the leaves of which form a demulcent drink, used in dysentery and diarrhœa; the seeds furnish oil of benne.

Sesqui-, Sés-kwi-; a prefix meaning one and a half; applied to compounds formed with three molecules of one element and two of another.

Seton, Sḗ-ton; a minute channel made under the skin with a seton needle, carrying one or more threads, which are kept there and daily moved back and forth, to cause suppuration and discharge of matter.

Seven Barks, Sév-en Barks; *Hydrangea arborescens*, a common indigenous shrub.

Shaking Palsy, Σák-iŋ Pól-zi; an affection of the muscles, causing them to alternately contract and relax.

Shampooing, Σam-pú-iŋ; a vapor bath, accompanied with rubbing, kneading, etc., by an attendent.

Sheep Laurel, Σīp Lé-rel; *Kalmia latifolia*, the leaves of which are reputed poisonous to sheep.

Sheep Sorrel, Σīp Sór-el; *Rumex Acetosella;* a native common plant, containing oxalic acid and having an agreeable sour taste.

Sherbet Σér-bet; a mildly stimulating drink, made of the juice of any fruit, water, sweetened and flavored.

Sherry Wine, Σér-i Wįn; *Vinum Xericum.*

Shin, Σin; the fore part of the leg, between the ankle and knee.

Shingles, Σiŋ-glz; herpes, or tetter, a skin disease, in which the vesicles spread across or around the waist.

Shoulder, Σώl-der; the humerus; the arm from the shoulder-joint to the elbow.

Shoulder-Blade, — Blɑd; the scapula, a broad flat bone, extending from the shoulder joint to the vertebræ.

Shower-Bath, Σŏ-er Bɑθ; the application of water to the whole body, by falling some distance from a sprinkler.

Sialadenitis, Sį-al-a-den-į-tis; inflammation of a salivary gland.

Sialagogue, Sį-ál-a-gog; a medicine that increases the flow of saliva.

Sialine, Sį́-a-lįn; relating to saliva.

Sialoid, Sį́-a-lɵd; resembling saliva.

Sialoncus, Sį-a-lón-kus; a tumor under the tongue, caused by an interrupted flow of saliva.

Siccant, Sík-ant; drying; possessing the quality of drying.

Sigmoid Flexure, Síg-mɵd Fléks-ųr; a portion of the colon in shape something like the Greek letter sigma.

Sigmoid Valves, — Valvz; the semi-lunar valves of the aorta and pulmonary artery.

Silk-Weed, (**Common**,) Sílk-wīd; *Asclepias Cornuti*, a native plant with a milky juice.

Silphium Laciniatum, Síl-fi-um La-sin-i-é-tum; rosin-weed or compass plant, a native resinous plant, used as a stimulant.

Silver, Síl-ver; *Argentum*, a metallic element, white, malleable, and soluble in nitric acid.

Silver, Fused Nitrate; lunar caustic, made by fusing nitrate of sllver and pouring into molds.

Simaba Cedron, Sím-a-ba Sí-dron; a tree of Central America. See Cedron Seed.

Simaruba Excelsa, Sim-a-rú-ba Ek-sél-sa; a tree of the West Indies, the wood of which is the well known tonic Quassia.

Simple Cerate, Sím-pl Sí-rat; a mild dressing for wounds, made of two parts of lard and one of white wax.

Simple Syrup, Sím-pl Sír-up; a saturated solution of white sugar in water.

Sinapis Nigra, Si-ná-pis Nį-gra; black mustard, a common European plant, naturalized in many parts of the United States; a synonym for *Brassica nigra*.

Sinapism, Sín-a-pizm; a rubefacient poultice made of mustard, ground linseed, and vinegar.

Sinciput, Sín-si-put; the fore part of the head.

Sinew, Sín-ų; a tendinous cord, that connects muscle with bone.

Singultus, Sin-gúl-tus; hiccup, a convulsive action of the diaphragm. [membrane.

Sinus, Sį́-nus; a long depression or cavity, in a bone or

Sinus Pocularis, — Pok-ų-lá-ris; a depression in the male urethra, which leads into the prostatic vessel.

Sinus Urogenitalis, — Yu-ro-jen-i-tá-lis; a sinus existing in the embryo, in connection with the generative apparatus.

Sinus Venosus, — Vē-nó-sus; applied to the main portion of the auricles of the heart, to distinguish them from the auricular appendages.

Siphonia, Sį-fó-ni-a; a tropical genus of trees, the source of most of the commercial caoutchouc.

Siriasis, Sir-į́-a-sis; synonymous with sunstroke.

Skeleton, Skél-ē-ton; the bones of an animal; it is termed *natural* when the bones are connected by their own ligaments; *artificial*, when held together by wires.

Skin, Skin; the covering of animal organization, composed of three membranes, viz: the outside *cuticle* or epidermis, the *rete mucosum*, and the *cutis vera*, the innermost or true skin.

Skin Bound, — Bound; a hardening of the tissue in infancy, that causes the skin to seem too tight for the body.

Skull, Skul; the cranium, or bones of the top of the head.

Slavering, Sláv-er-iŋ; drivelling; involuntary flow of saliva.

Sleeplessness, Slīp-les-nes; insomnia; inability to sleep.

Slippery-Elm, Slíp-er-i-Elm; *Ulmus fulva*, the inner bark of which is extensively used as a demulcent.

Slough, Sluf; any decayed part of the body separating from the rest, and dropping off.

Small-Pox, Smel-Poks; variola, a contagious fever.

Smart-Weed, Smqrt-Wīd; *Polygonum Hydropiper;* water pepper.

Smegma, Smég-ma; soap, or grease; also applied to the secretion from the sebaceous follicles of the skin and prepuce.

Smilacina Racemosa, Smį-la-sį-na Ra-sī-mó-sa; false Solomon's Seal, a native plant, the root of which is sometimes used as a tonic.

Smilax Officinalis, Smį-laks Of-is-i-ná-lis; a woody vine of South America, which yields sarsaparilla root.

Snakeroot, Black, Snák-rut; *Cimicifuga racemosa;* **S. Button**, *Liatris spicata;* **S. Canada**, *Asarum Canadensis;* **S. Seneke**, *Polygala Senega;* **S. Virginia—**, *Aristolochia Serpentaria;* all of which see.

Sneezing, Snīz-iŋ; a convulsive effort of the respiratory muscles, resulting from irritation of the nasal membrane.

Sneezewort, Snīz-wurt; *Helenium autumnale*, the dried flowers of which are used as an errhine.

Soap, Sop; the officinal soap is made of olive oil and soda; it is used in liniments and laxative pills.

Soap-Liniment, (Camphorated,) — Lín-i-ment; liquid opodeldoc.

Soapwort, Sóp-wurt. See *Saponaria officinalis*.

Socotrine Aloes, Sók-o-trin Al'oz; aloes yielded by the *Aloe Socotrina;* it is the best variety of aloes.

Soda, Só-da; bicarbonate of sodium, or baking soda, is generally known as simply soda.

Soda Caustic, — Kós-tik; hydrate of sodium.

Sodium, Só-di-um: an elemental (metallic) substance, the base of the salts of sodium.

Softening of the Brain; a degeneration of the substance of the brain, sometimes to a soft fatty consistency, and sometimes to a semi-liquid condition, the causes of which are but little known. [the mouth.

Soft Palate, Soft Pál-et; the back part of the roof of

Solanum Dulcamara, Sɷ-lá-num Dul-ka-má-ra; bittersweet, used as an alterative.

Solar Plexus, Sɷ́-lar Pléks-us; nervous ganglia surrounding the semi-lunar ganglia of the abdomen.

Soleus, Sɷ́-lĕ-us; a muscle that extends from the knee to the ankle, and moves the foot.

Solidago Odora Sol-i-dá-gɷ ɷ-dɷ́-ra; golden-rod, a native plant, stimulant and carminative.

Solidists, Sól-id-ists; those who accept the theory that all diseases are the result of morbid changes in the solid parts of the animal organization.

Solitary Glands; Bruner's Glands, mucous follicles in the membrane of the intestines.

Solomon's Seal, Sól-ɷ-mon'z Sĕl; *Polygonatum giganteum*, a common native plant. [*mosa.*

Solomon's Seal, False, — — Fels; *Smilacina race-*

Soluble Glass, Sól-ų-bl Glas; solution silicate of sodium.

Solution, Sɷ-lų́-ʃon; the dissolving of a solid substance in a liquid, so that it becomes invisible.

Solution Acetate of Ammonium,— As'ĕ-tat ov A-mɷ́-ni-um; spirits of Mindererus.

Solution Chlorinated Soda, — Klɷ-ri-nát-ed Sɷ́-da; Labarraque's disinfecting solution.

Solution Citrate Magnesium, — Sį-trat Mag-nĕ-ʒi-um; a mild cathartic solution, containing also free carbonic acid.

Solution Perchloride of Iron, — Pɛr-klɷ́-rįd ov Ɨ'urn; solution ferric chloride, used for making tincture chloride of iron, and known as solution of muriate of iron.

Solution Subacetate of Lead, — Sub-ás-ĕ-tat ov Led; Goulard's Extract, made by boiling litharge with acetate of lead and water.

Solution Subsulphate of Iron, — Sub-súl-fat ov Ɨ'urn; Monsel's Solution, used as a styptic.

Solution of Continuity; the breaking of connection, or separation of parts, as by a cut or blow.

Solvent, Sól-vent; any liquid, or other agent, capable of dissolving a substance.

Somatology, Sω-ma-tól-ω-ji; anatomy; the science of the human body.

Somnambulism, Som-nám-bų-lizm, sleep-walking, during which the body seems to respond to the dreams of the mind.

Somnifera, Som-níf-er-a; agents that have the power of causing sleep.

Somnolent, Sóm-nω-lent; disposed to sleep.

Somnolism, Sóm-nω-lizm; a kind of sleep caused by animal magnetism.

Sonitus, Són-i-tus; a buzzing or humming sound in the [ears.

Sophistication, Sof-is-ti-ká-ʃon; the adulteration of food or medicine.

Sopiens, Sώ-pi-ens; that which induces sleep.

Sopor, Sώ-por; deep, heavy sleep.

Soporific, Sω-por-íf-ik; causing deep sleep.

Sordes, Sér-dēz; matter cast out of ulcers, or that collects on the teeth during some fevers.

Sore Throat, Sωr Ħrωt. See *Cynanche.*

Sorrel, Sór-el; *Rumex Acetosella.* See Sheep Sorrel.

Sound, Sɜnd; an instrument with which to search the bladder for calculus.

Southernwood, Súđ-ern-wụd; *Artemisia Abrotanum*, a fragrant herb.

Spanish Flies, Spán-iʃ Flįz; cantharides, a European beetle that is used to produce blisters.

Spanish Needles. See *Bidens bipinnata.*

Spanæmia, Spa-nē-mi-a; poverty of the blood.

Spasm, Spazm; an involuntary contraction of the muscles, as in cramp, lockjaw, etc.

Spasmodes, Spas-mώ-dēz; affected with spasms.

Spasmus Caninus, Spás-mus Ka-nį-nus; a convulsive laugh in tetanus.

Spastic, Spás-tik; applied to muscles that draw to or [from.

Spatula, Spát-ų-la; a knife for mixing medicines.

Spearmint, Spér-mint, *Mentha viridis*, an aromatic labiate plant.

Specific, Spĕ-sif-ik; applied to medicines prepared for any special form of disease.

Specific Gravity, — Gráv-i-ti; the weight of a substance compared with water as unity, or the comparative weight of equal bulks or volumes at sixty degrees (60° F.)

Spectrum, Spék-trum; a figure, real or imaginary.

Speculum, Spék-ų-lum; an instrument for expanding natural openings, so as to facilitate their examination.

Sperm, Spεrm; the seminal fluid of animals.

Sperm-Cell, — Sel; small cellular bodies found in sperm.

Spermatic, Spεr-mát-ik; appertaining to semen or seed.

Spermatic Canal, — Ka-nál; an opening in the abdominal parietes through which the spermatic cord passes.

Spermatocele, Spεr-mát-ω-sĕl; a swelling of the testicles, from morbific causes.

Spermatorrhœa, Spεr-mat-ω-rĕ-ɑ; gonorrhœa; the involuntary emission of semen, resulting from prostration of the generative system.

Spermatochesis, Spεr-mat-ω-kĕ-sis; suppression or retention of the seminal secretion.

Spermatozoa, Spεr-mat-ω-zώ-ɑ; (or *Spermatozoon;*) various minute bodies, discoverable by the microscope, in the semen, supposed to constitute its fecundating power.

Sphacelation, Sfas-ĕ-lá-ʃon; complete mortification.

Sphacelismus, Sfas-ĕ-lis-mus; phrenitis; inflammation of the brain.

Sphenoid Bone, Sfĕ-nød Bωn: a wedge-shaped bone at the base of the skull.

Sphenopalatine, Sfĕ-nω-pál-a-tin; relating to the sphenoid and palatine bones; applied to an artery, foramen, and ganglia of nerves.

Sphenostaphylinus, Sfĕ-nω-staf-i-lį-nus; levator muscles of the soft palate.

Sphincter, Sfiŋk-ter; applied to muscles that surround natural openings, and close by contraction.

Sphincter Ani, — Ɐ'nį; (*Externus* and *Internus*,) muscles that close the anus.

Sphincter Oris, Sfiŋk-ter Ω'ris; a muscle that closes the mouth.
Sphygmodes, Sfig-mώ-dēz; throbbing; having pulse.
Sphygmometer, Sfig-móm-ē-ter; an instrument for ascertaining the rapidity of the pulse.
Spice Bush, Spįs Buʃ; *Lindera Benzoin*, a native shrub.
Spigelia Marilandica, Spį-jé-li-a Ma-ri-lán-di-ka; a southern plant, the root of which (pink root,) is an excellent anthelmintic.
Spika, Spį-ka; a bandage shaped like a spike of wheat [or barley.
Spicula, Spik-ų-la; a splinter of bone.
Spiloma, Spį-ló-ma; a stain; the mother's mark.
Spina Ventosa, Spį-na Ven-tó-sa; a disease of the bones, in which the texture expands with matter formed within, and the whole becomes spongy.
Spinal, Spį-nal; appertaining to the spine.
Spinal Cord, — Kerd. Same as Spinal Marrow.
Spinal Column, — Kól-um. See Vertebral Column.
Spinal Marrow, — Már-ω; the spinal cord, or medullary substance in the vertebral column.
Spinal Meningitis, — Men-in-jį-tis; inflammation of the membrane of the spinal cord.
Spinal Nerves, — Nɛrvz; a system of nerves that are a prolongation of the *medulla spinalis*.
Spinalis Dorsi, Spį-ná-lis Dór-sį; short, flat, fleshy fibers, located on either side of the interspinal ligament.
Spine, Spįn; the vertebral column, or back-bone.
Spintherismus, Spin-ter-ís-mus; scintillation; the apparant dropping of sparks from the eyes.
Spiracula, Spir-ák-ų-la; "breathing holes;" respiratory pores of the skin.
Spiræa Tomentosa, Spį-ré-a Tω-men-tó-sa; hardhack, a native shrub, the root of which is used as an astringent.
Spirit, Spír-it; any distilled or alcoholic liquor.
Spirit of Nitrous Ether; solution of nitrous ether in alcohol.
Spirit Proof, — Prωf; of B. P. is made by mixing five pints of rectified spirit with three pints of distilled water; corresponding nearly with diluted alcohol of the U. S. P.

Spirit Rectified, Spír-it Rék-ti-fīd; alcohol of Sp. gr. 0.838, containing sixteen per cent. of water, corresponding nearly with alcohol of the U. S. P. Sp. gr. 0.835.

Spirit of Wine, — Wīn; an old name for alcohol.

Spiritus, Spír-it-us; the soul, or spirit; also, the officinal name for spirits.

Spirometer, Spir-óm-ē ter; an instrument for ascertaining the amount of air breathed into or from the lungs at one time.

Spitting Blood, Spít-iŋ Blud. See *Hæmoptysis*.

Splanchnic, Spláŋk-nik; pertaining to the viscera, and applied to cavities of the cranium, chest and abdomen; also to nerves of the stomach.

Splanchnology, Splaŋk-nól-ω-ji; the science which treats of the nature of the viscera.

Spleen, Splēn; a viscus body in the left hypochondrium, supposed to have something to do in the development of blood.

Splenalgia, Splē-nál-ji-α; pain in the spleen.

Splenetic, Splē-nét-ik; pertaining to, or affected by disease of the spleen; fretful.

Splenious, Splé-ni-us; resembling the spleen.

Splenitis, Splē-nī-tis; inflammation of the spleen.

Splenius, Splé-ni-us; a muscle located in the back of the neck, that divides into the *splenius capitis* and the *splenius colli;* they rotate the head.

Splenization, Splen-i-zá-ʃon; descriptive of the lungs in the first stage of pneumonia, when their tissue resembles the spleen.

Splenohæmia, Splen-ω-hé-mi-α; congestion of the spleen.

Splint, Splint; a thin strip of wood, pasteboard, or tin, for use in holding fractured bones in position.

Splint-Bone, Splint-Bωn; the fibula.

Spondylitis, Spon-di-lī-tis; inflammation of any part of the vertebræ.

Spondylus, Spón-di-lus; a vertebra; also the vortex.

Sponge, Spunj; a porous substance, of animal origin, used in surgery; also by Homœopathists, as a medicine.

Spongiose, Spún-ji-ωs; spongy; porous, like sponge.

Sporadic, Spω-rád-ik; limited to a locality; not epidemic.

Sprain, Spran; (originally *strain;*) a sudden twist of a joint, causing laceration of ligaments without dislocation.

Spumescent, Spɥ-més-ent; frothy, foam-like.

Spurge, Spurj; a name applied to several plants of the genus *Euphorbia*.

Spurred Rye, Spurd Rį; common name for ergot.

Sputum, Spɥ́-tum; saliva; also phlegm.

Squama, Skwá-mɑ; skin diseases in which the cuticle scales off.

Squamate, Skwá-mat; having, or resembling scales.

Squamous Suture, Skwá-mus Sɥ́-tɥr; that which unites the squamous part of the temporal bone to the parietal.

Squamula, Skwám-ɥ-lɑ; a small scale from the skin.

Squill, Skwil; *Scilla maritima*, a bulbous plant that grows in the Mediterranean countries, the dried roots of which are used in cough-syrups.

Squinting, Skwínt-iŋ. See *Strabismus*.

Squirting Cucumber, Skwért-iŋ Kɥ́-kum-ber; *Momordica Elaterium*, the source of elaterium.

Stadium, Stá-di-um; a stage, or period, applied to the course of a disease.

Staff, Stɑf; a grooved steel instrument for entering the urethra and guiding the knife in lithotomy.

Stalactic, Sta-lák-tik; oozing, or dripping out.

Stamen, Stá-men; the male organ of flowers.

Stamina, Stám-i-nɑ; strength; vigor of constitution.

Stammering, Stám-er-iŋ; broken and halting articulation.

Stapedius, Sta-pḗ-di-us; a muscle of the ear.

Stapes, Stá-pēz; one of the bones of the internal ear.

Staphisagria, Staf-i-sá-gri-ɑ. See Stavesacre.

Staphyle, Stáf-i-lē; the uvula.

Staphylitis, Staf-i-lį́-tis; inflammation of the uvula.

Staphyloma, Staf-i-lṓ-mɑ; a dropsical disease of the cornea of the eye.

Staphylotomy, Staf-i-lót-ɷ-mi; excision of part of the uvula.

Star-Anise, Stɑr-An'is; the fruit of *Illicium Anisatum*, used as an aromatic.

Starch, Stɑrç: amylum, a white vegetable substance, found in many plants.

Star Grass, Stąr Gras; *Aletris farinosa*, a native plant, the root of which is used as a tonic.

Statice Limonium, Stát-i-sē Li-mṓ-ni-um; marsh rosemary, a plant found in salt marshes, the root of which is astringent.

Stavesacre, Stávz-ak-er; the seed of the *Delphinium Staphisagria*, used as a stimulant to the urinary organs.

Steatocele, Stē-át-ω-sēl; a sebaceous enlargement of the scrotum.

Steatodes, Stē-a-tṓ-dēz; sebaceous; full of fat. [stance.

Steatoma, Stē-a-tṓ-ma; a tumor filled with a fatty sub-

Stegnosis, Steg-nṓ-sis; constriction of the pores; also stoppage of the evacuations.

Steno's Duct, Stḗ-nω'z Dukt; the parotid duct.

Stenosis, Stē-nṓ-sis. Same as Stegnosis.

Stercoraceous, Stεr-kω-rá-ʃus; vomiting when fecal matter is thrown up; the peristaltic or inverse action of the intestines.

Sterelmintha, Ster-el-mín-ϑa; intestinal worms, termed solid because they have no abdominal cavity.

Sterility, Ster-íl-i-ti; inability to procreate offspring.

Sternalgia, Stεr-nál-ji-a; pain in the sternum.

Sterno-Cleido-Mastoideus, Stέr-nω-Klį́-dω-Mas-tω-į́-dē-us; a muscle in the anterior part of the neck, extending to the upper part of the sternum; it carries the head forward, and inclines it to one side.

Sterno-Hyoideus, — Hį-ω-į́-dē-us; a muscle arising from the hyoid bone, and extending to the posterior surface of the sternum.

Sterno-Thyroideus, — Ϧį-rω-į́-dē-us; a muscle extending from the outer surface of the thyroid cartilage to the second rib.

Sternum, Stέr-num; the *os pectoris*, or breast-bone.

Sternutation, Stεr-nų-tá-ʃon; frequent sneezing.

Stertor, Stέr-tor; loud and harsh respiration; snoring in natural sleep. [lungs.

Stethæmia, Steϑ-ḗ-mi-a: a conjestion of blood in the

Stethometer, Steϑ-óm-ē-ter; an instrument for ascertaining the condition of the action of the heart during disease.

Sthenic, Sϑén-ik; having strength, vigor, activity.

Stigma, Stíg-ma; a speck on the skin; a mark.
Still-Born, Stil-Born; born lifeless.
Stillicidium, Stil-i-sid-i-um; a flowing, drop by drop, as urine in stricture.
Stillingia Sylvatica, Stil-ín-ji-a Sil-vát-i-ka; queen's root, a native southern plant, the root of which is an alterative.
Stimulant, Stím-u-lant; a medicine capable of increasing the organic activity of the animal functions.
Stimulus, Stím-u-lus; "a whip," a stimulant.
Stitch, Stiç; a sharp pain, like that caused by a needle.
Stomach, Stúm-ak; a membranous sac, one of the principal organs of digestion.
Stomach-Ache, — Ek; colic; cardialgia.
Stomach Pump, — Pump; a kind of syringe for extracting the contents of the stomach in case of poison, or of conveying fluids thereto.
Stomachic, Stω-mák-ik, relating to the stomach.
Stomatic, Stω-mát-ik applied to medicines for the mouth.
Stomatitis, Stω-ma-tí-tis; inflammation of the mouth.
Stone, Stωn; calculus, a stone-like concretion, found in the bladder, kidney, etc.
Stone-Crop, (**Virginia**,) — Krop; *Penthorum sedoides.*
Stone-Root, — Rut; the root of *Collinsonia Canadensis*, which is a native labiate plant.
Stool, Stul; evacuation; the fæces discharged.
Storax, Stó-raks; an aromatic balsam obtained from the inner bark of *Liquidambar orientale*, used as an expectorant.
Strabismus, Stra-bís-mus; squinting; a distortion of one or both eyes.
Strabotomy, Stra-bót-ω-mi; a surgical operation for the cure of strabismus.
Stramonium, Stra-mó-ni-um; *Datura Stramonium*, a very common weed.
Strangulated, Stráŋ-gu-la-ted; choked; applied to hernia that cannot be reduced.
Strangury, Stráŋ-gu-ri; difficulty in passing urine.
Stremma, Strém-a; a sprain, or luxation.
Stria, Strí-a; a line, or mark under the skin, that appears in some fever.

Striated, Strį-at-ed; marked with long lines.
Stricture, Strík-tųr; the contraction of a canal, duct, or intestine.
Stridor Dentium, Strį-dor Dén-ʃi-um; gritting or grating of the teeth, in gastric affections. [body.
Stroma, Strṓ-ma; the base or bed of any organ of the
Stronger Alcohol, Stróŋ-ger Al'kō-hol; Alcohol Fortius U. S. P.; specific gravity 0.817.
Stronger Ether, — Ē'ter; ether purified by distillation from chloride of calcium. [human kidneys.
Strongylus, Strón-ji-lus; a worm rarely found in the
Strophulus, Stróf-ų-lus; an eruption of different kinds peculiar to infants.
Struma, Strú-ma; scrofula; follicular bronchocele.
Strumous, Strú-mus; of a scrofulous nature.
Strychnia, or **Strychnine**, Strík-ni-a, or Strík-nin; an organic base, derived from nux vomica, very poisonous.
Strychnia Solution, — Sō-lų́-ʃon; officinal in B. P., in which two fluid drachms contain one grain of strychnia.
Strychnos Ignatia, Strík-nos Ig-ná-ʃi-a; a tree of the Phillipine Islands, the source of Ignatia beans.
Strychnos Nux Vomica, — Nuks Vóm-i-ka; a tree of the East Indies, the seeds of which are the well known poisonous nux vomica.
Stupor, Stų́-por; drowsiness; loss of sensibility.
Sty, or **Stye**, Stį; a kind of tumor on the eyelids.
Stylo-Glossus, Stį-lō-Glós-us; a muscle extending from the styloid process to the root of the tongue, which it raises.
Stylo-Hyoideus, — Hį-ō-į-dē-us; a muscle in the side of the neck, connected with the styloid process and the *os hyoides*.
Stylo-Mastoid, — Más-tǝd; applied to the foramen through which passes the *portio dura* of the seventh pair of nerves.
Stylo-Pharyngeous; — Far-in-jḗ-us; a muscle of the neck, connected with the pharynx, which it raises.
Stymatosis, Stį-ma-tṓ-sis; violent erection of the penis, with sanguineous discharge.

Styptic, Stíp-tik; an agent having the power to check or stop bleeding.

Styrax Benzoin, Stį-raks Ben-zώ-in; a tree of the East Indies that yields the fragrant benzoin resin.

Sub.; a prefix meaning "under;" thus: subchloride of mercury is the lower chloride, or calomel.

Subclavian, Sub-klá-vi-an; applied to an artery, muscles, vessels, etc., situated under the clavicle. [skin.

Subcutaneous, Sub-kų-tá-nĭ-us; located beneath the

Sublimated, Súb-li-me-ted: vaporized by heat, and condensed; as sublimated or sublimed sulphur, etc.

Sublimis, Sub-lį-mis; applied to muscles situated more superficially than others of the same locality, as the *flexor digitorum communis* muscle.

Subluxation, Sub-luks-á-ʃon; partial dislocation.

Submaxillary, Sub-máks-il-a-ri; applied to a gland under the lower jaw.

Suborbitar, Sub-ór-bit-ar; applied to an artery, canal, fissure, and nerves, located beneath the orbitar cavity of the eye.

Subplacenta, Sub-pla-sén-ta; the *deciduary vera*, or that part of the placenta that lines the uterus.

Subscapular, Sub-skáp-ų-lar; applied to the fossa, muscles, and nerves, situated mainly beneath the shoulder blade.

Substantia Nigra, Sub-stán-ʃi-a Nį-gra; a dark colored matter found in the peduncles of the brain.

Subsultus, Sub-súl-tus; twitching, as the spasmodic contraction of the tendons.

Succedaneum, Suk-sĭ-dá-ni-um; a substitute, as one medicine for another. [amber.

Succinic Acid, Suk-sin-ik As'id; an acid obtained from

Succus, Súk-us; the juice of plants; also applied to certain animal fluids.

Succussion, Su-kúʃ-on; sudden agitation of the body, in examining the chest for the presence of a liquid in the thorax.

Sudamen, Sų-dá-men; milliary eruption, attending diseases in which there is much sweating.

Sudation, Sų-dá-ʃon; perspiration; much sweating.

Sudorific, Sų-dω-ríf-ik; producing sweat.

Suffocation, Suf-ɷ-ká-ʃon; suspended respiration, caused by smothering or the inhalation of noxious gas.
Suffusion, Su-fų́-ʒon; the diffusion of blood or some humor under the skin.
Sugar, Σúg-ɑr; a sweet substance obtained from cane and other plants, composed of carbon, oxygen, and hydrogen.
Sugar of Lead, — ov Led; the common name for acetate of lead.
Sugar of Milk; the sweet principle of milk.
Suggillation, Suj-i-lá-ʃon; ecchymosis; livid spots on dead bodies, caused by decay.
Sulcus, Súl-kus; a groove or furrow in the bones and other organs.
Sulphates, Súl-fats; salts of sulphuric acid.
Sulphides or **Sulphurets**, Súl-fi̧dz or Súl-fų-rets; the union of sulphur and another element.
Sulphites, Súl-fi̧ts; salts of sulphurous acid.
Sulphocarbolic Acid, Sul-fɷ-kɑr-ból-ik As'id; an acid made by heating sulphuric acid and carbolic acid.
Sulphur, Súl-fur; an element, of volcanic origin and inflammable, hence commonly called brimstone; used extensively in the arts and in medicine, and the origin of all sulphur compounds.
Sulphuric Acid, Sul-fų́-rik As'id; the higher acid $H^2 SO^4$, made from sulphurous acid gas, steam and nitric acid vapor.
Sulphurous Acid, Súl-fur-us As'id; the product of the combustion of sulphur in the atmosphere dissolved in water, H^2SO^3.
Sumach, Sú-mak; *Rhus glabra*, a native shrub, with bright scarlet berries, which are refrigerant.
Sumbul, Súm-bul; musk-root, a nervous stimulant obtained from an unknown plant of Russia.
Summer Complaint, Súm-er Kom-plánt; diarrhœa, or cholera infantum.
Summer Savory, — Sá-vɷ-ri; *Satureja hortensis*, a garden plant, used as a stimulant.
Sunflower Seed, Sún-flɤ-er Sēd; the seed of *Helianthus annuus;* used as an expectorant and diuretic.
Sun-Stroke, Sun-Strɷk. See *Coup de Soleil*.
Superfetation, Sų-per-fē-tá-ʃon; a second impregnation of a female before maturity and delivery of the first.

Superior Arch, Sų-pḗ-ri-or Arç. See Vértebral Arch.

Superior Auris, — Θ'ris; a muscle of the ear that lifts it upwards.

Supinator, Sų-pi-ná-tor; a muscle of the hand that turns [the palm upwards.

Suppositories, Su-póz-i-tɷ-riz; medicated concrete oils, used for introducing medicines into the rectum or vagina.

Suppuration, Sup-ų-rá-ʃon; the formation of matter under the skin, or within an organ.

Suppuratives, Súp-ų-ra-tivz; medicines that cause local inflammation and suppuration.

Supra-, Sų́-pra-; a prefix meaning *above*, as *supra-scapula*, above the shoulder.

Supracostales, Sų-pra-kos-tá-lēz; applied to the *levatores costarum* muscles, that lie upon the ribs.

Surdity, Súr-di-ti; difficulty of hearing.

Surgery, Súr-jer-i; the art of treating disease by manual operations, and with instruments.

Suspensorium Hepatis, Sus-pen-sɷ́-ri-um Hép-a-tis; the ligament which suspends the liver.

Suspensorius Testis, — Tés-tis; the cremaster muscle that supports the testicle.

Suspirium, Sus-pír-i-um; a short, but deep and audible breathing; a kind of sighing.

Sutura, Sų-tų́-ra; a suture, something like a seam. See Coronal, Sagittal, and Squamous Sutures.

Suture, Sų́-tųr; a seam, as in the junction of bones; also, in surgery, the joining of the lips of a wound by needle and thread.

Swamp Dogwood, Swomp Dóg-wud; *Cornus sericea.*

Sweet Fern, Swēt Fern; *Comptonia Asplenifolia*, a native plant, but *not* a fern.

Sweet Flag, — Flag. See *Acorus Calamus.*

Sweet Marjoram, — Mar-jɷ́-ram; *Origanum Majorana*, a garden plant.

Sweet Spirit of Nitre, Swēt Spír-it ov Nị-ter; nitrous ether, dissolved in alcohol.

Swine-Pox, Swịn-Poks; varicella, in which the vesicles are generally pointed, and the fluid they contain clear.

Swooning, Swún-iŋ; syncope, or suspension of consciousness.

Syaladenitis, Sį-al-a-den-į-tis. See *Sialadenitis*.
Sycoma, Sį-kṓ-ma; a kind of wart, like a fig.
Sycosis, Sį-kṓ-sis; an eruptive disease, on hairy portions of the face and scalp.
Sydenham's Laudanum, Sį́-den-ham'z Ló-da-num; an old preparation, nearly identical with officinal wine of opium.
Symblepharon, Sim-bléf-a-ron; a diseased adhesion of the eyelid to the globe of the eye.
Symbol. See Chemical Symbol.
Sympathetic, Sim-pa-thét-ik; similar to, or associated in function and action.
Sympathetic Nerve, — Nerv; also called the Great Sympathetic, and the Splanchnic Nerve; the organic nervous system, consisting of a series of ganglia, extending along the spine, and communicating with the thirty pairs of spinal nerves, etc.
Symphoresis, Sim-fo-rē-sis. Same as Congestion.
Symphysis, Sím-fi-sis; the natural joining of bones, by cartilages, etc.
Symphysotomy, Sim-fi-sót-o-mi; the operation of enlarging the diameter of the pelvis, to facilitate parturition.
Symphytum Officinale, Sím-fi-tum Of-is-i-ná-lē; comfrey, a well known domèstic remedy for coughs.
Symplocarpus Fœtidus, Sim-plo-kár-pus Fét-i-dus; skunk cabbage, a native marsh plant, the root of which is used as an antispasmodic. (This plant is described as *Ictodes fœtidus* and also as *Dracontium fœtidum*.
Symptom, Sím-tom; a sign or indication of the character of a disease.
Symptomatic, Sim-tom-át-ik; relating to symptoms; defining a disease that is only a symptom of another.
Syn-, Sin-; a prefix meaning *with*, or *union with*.
Synarthosis, Sin-ar-thrṓ-sis: a joint that does not admit of perceptible movement.
Synchondrosis, Sin-kon-drṓ-sis; a junction of bones united by intervening cartilages.
Synchondrotomy, Sin-kon-drót-o-mi; the operation of separating the union of bones, as the *ossa pubis*, in child-birth.

Synchronous, Sín-krω-nus; occurring at the same, or in corresponding time. [the eye.

Synchysis, Sín-ki-sis; the mingling of the humors of

Synclonus, Sín-klω-nus; applied to diseases in which there is a tremulous action of the muscles. [sy.

Synclonus Bolismus, — Bω-lís-mus; the shaking pal-

Syncope, Sin-kω-pē; fainting, or swooning, in which there is a partial suspension of respiration and of the heart's action.

Syndesmitis, Sin-des-mī-tis; inflammation of the articular ligaments.

Syndesmosis, Sin-des-mώ-sis; the joining of bones by means of ligaments.

Syndesmus, Sin-dés-mus; a ligament or bandage.

Synechia, Sin-ē-kī-ɑ; an adhesion of the iris to the cornea, or to the crystalline lens.

Synergy, Sín-er-ji; the united action of different organs in the production of the same result, as in digestion.

Synezisis, Sin-ē-zī-sis; the contraction, or entire closing of the pupil of the eye.

Syneurosis, Sin-ų-rώ-sis; the joining of bones by intermediate membranes.

Synocha, Sín-ω-kɑ; an inflammatory fever. [joints.

Synosteology, Sin-os-tē-ól-ω-ji; the philosophy of the

Synosteosis, Sin-os-tē-ώ-sis; the organic union of bones by osseous deposits. [joints.

Synosteotomy, Sin-os-tē-ót-ω-mi; dissection of the

Synovia, Sín-ώ-vi-ɑ; an oily secretion that lubricates the joints.

Syntenosis, Sin-ten-ώ-sis; a joint in which the bones are held together by tendons.

Synthesis, Sin-θē-sis; in surgery, the reuniting of parts.

Syphilelcos, Sif-i-lél-kos; chancre, a syphilitic ulcer.

Syphilides, Sif-il-i-dēz; skin eruptions arising from syphilis.

Syphilis, Síf-i-lis; the venereal disease; pox.

Syphiloid, Síf-i-lθd; resembling syphilis.

Syphilolepis, Sif-i-lól-ē-pis; a syphilitic scale, or scaly eruption.

Syringe, Sir-ínj; an instrument for injecting water, or medicated liquids into any opening or cavity.

Syringotomy, Sir-in-gót-ɷ-mi; the operation of cutting open a fistula.

Syrups, Medicated, Sír-ups, Méd-i-ka-ted; solution of medicinal substances with water and sugar.

Syrupus, Sír-up-us; officinal name for syrup, or sirup.

Syspasia, Sis-pá-si-ɑ; a convulsion or spasm.

Systatica, Sis-tát-i-kɑ; diseases which simultaneously affect the powers of sensation.

Systemic Circulation, Sis-tém-ik Sɛr-kɥ-lá-ʃon: the general circulation, in contradistinction to the pulmonary circulation.

Systole, Sís-tɷ-lē; the contraction of the heart, preceding its dilatation, (*diastole*,) in causing the circulation of the blood.

T

T-Bandage; a bandage made in the form of a letter T, for applying dressings to the groins, perinæum, etc.

Tabes, Tá-bēz; wasting, or consumption of the body; applied also to parts of the body.

Tabes Scrofulosa, — Skrof-ɥ-lṓ-sɑ; a disease of the mesenteric glands.

Tabula Vitrea, Táb-ɥ-lɑ Vít-rē-ɑ; the internal plate of the back of the cranium.

Tag Alder, Tag Al'der; *Alnus serrulata*, the bark of which is used as an alterative.

Tænia, Tē-ni-ɑ; the tape-worm; long, flat, and jointed.

Tænia Hippocampi, — Hip-ɷ-kám-pị; a white band at the angles of the lateral ventricles of the brain.

Tænia Lata, — Lá-tɑ; a tape-worm that sometimes grows to the enormous length of sixty yards.

Tænia Solium, — Sṓ-li-um; similar to the last named.

Taliacotian, Tal-i-a-kṓ-ʃan; the construction of a new external nose, by turning down a flap of the skin, from the forehead, or other part of the face.

Talipes, Tál-i-pēz; the deformity called club-foot.
Talpa, Tál-pa; "a mole"; applied to a tumor on the head, supposed to burrow.
Tamarinds, Tám-a-rindz; the agreeably tart fruit of *Tamarindus Indica*, used as a refrigerant.
Tampon, Tam-pon, or Tom-pon; a plug; a rag or sponge used for plugging.
Tanacetum Vulgare, Tan-a-sē-tum Vul-gá-rē; tansy, a garden plant, native of Europe.
Tannic Acid, or **Tannin**, Tán-ik As'id, or Tán-in; an astringent principle of certain plants; obtained, in its purity from galls.
Tansy, Tán-zi; *Tanacetum vulgare*, a garden plant, used as a tonic.
Tapeworm, Táp-wurm. See *Tænia*.
Tapioca, Tap-i-ó-ka; the peculiar starch obtained from the roots of *Janipha Manihot*, a very nutritious substance.
Tapping, Táp-iŋ; paracentesis; puncturing the abdomen or thorax for the escape of fluids.
Tar, Tar; a black semi-fluid substance, obtained from the wood of several species of pine trees.
Taraxacum Dens-Leonis, Tar-áks-a-kum Dens-Lē-ó-nis; dandelion, the root of which is used as a tonic and aperient; synonym for *Leontodon Taraxacum*.
Taraxis, Ta-ráks-is; a slight inflammation of the eye.
Tarsal, Tár-sal; relating to the instep; also the thin cartilaginous plates in the eyelids.
Tarsus, Tár-sus; the instep: also the cartilage in the eyelids.
Tartar, Cream of. See Cream of Tartar.
Tartar, Crude, Tár-tar, Krud. See *Argol*.
Tartar Emetic, — Ē-mét-ik; tartrate of antimony and potassium.
Tartaric Acid, Tar-tár-ik As'id; an acid obtained from cream of tartar, and found in the juices of many fruits.
Tartrates, Tár-trats; salts of tartaric acid.
Taxis, Táks-is; the operation by which any organ or part is replaced in its natural position by the hand.
Tear, Tēr; the fluid secreted by the lachrymal gland.
Teething, Tēd-iŋ; the cutting of teeth in children.
Tela, Tē-la; a web; the texture of a membrane.
Tela Araneæ, Tē-la A-ré-nē-ē. See Cobwebs.

Tela Choroidea, Tē-la Kō-rō-ị-dē-a; the membranous extension of the *pia mater.*

Temperament, Tém-per-a-ment; the peculiar powers, susceptibilities, and predilections of different organizations.

Temple, Tém-pl; the depression on each side of the forehead.

Temporal, Tém-pō-ral; relating to the temples, and applied to arteries, veins, muscles and nerves of that locality.

Tenaculum, Ten-ák-ų-lum; a small hook, used in dissecting, and by surgeons, in taking up arteries, etc.

Tendinous, Tén-din-us; relating to or like tendons.

Tendo Achillis, Tén-dō A-kíl-is; the large tendon above the heel.

Tendon, Tén-don; a white strong cord, that connects a muscle with a bone.

Tenesmus, Tē-nés-mus; painful inclination to evacuate but without any discharge.

Tenotomy, Ten-ót-ō-mi; the operation of dividing a tendon, to remedy a distortion or accident.

Tensor, Tén-sor; applied to muscles that extend parts to which they are attached.

Tensor Vaginæ Femoris, — Va-jí-nē Fém-ō-ris; a muscle extending from the spine of the ilium to the *fascia lata.*

Tent, Tent; a roll of lint, or piece of sponge, used for keeping open a sinus, wound, etc.

Tentaculum, Ten-ták-ų-lum; a feeler; applied to appendages used as instruments of exploration.

Tentorium, Ten-tṓ-ri-um; a horizontal partition of the brain, dividing the cerebrum and cerebellum.

Ter-; the prefix meaning *three.*

Terebinthina, Ter-ē-bín-ti-na; officinal name for turpentine.

Terebra, Ter-ḗ-bra; in surgery, a trepan.

Teres, Tḗ-rēz; the major and minor muscles extending from the scapula to the humerus.

Tertian, Tér-ʃan; an intermittent fever in which the paroxysm returns every third day.

Testa Præparata, Tés-ta Prep-a-rá-ta; oyster shell, calcined and powdered.

Testes, Tés-tēz; (sing. *Testis;*) the testicles, two glandular organs whose function it is to secrete the semen.

Testes Cerebri, — Sér-ē-brį; the inferior tubercles of the *corpora quadragemina*. [ticle.

Testitis, Tes-tį-tis; orchitis; inflammation of the tes-

Test Papers, Test Pá-perz; papers colored with solutions of vegetable substances, such as litmus and tumeric, used for testing acids and alkalies.

Tetanic, Tē-tán-ik; relating to tetanus.

Tetanus, Tét-a-nus; a morbid condition, in which there are violent spasmodic contraction of the muscles, closing of the jaws, and rigidity of the limbs.

Tetter, Tét-er; psoriasis; a herpetic eruption.

Thalami Nervorum Opticorum, Ħál-a-mį Nɛr-vώ-rum Op-ti-kώ-rum; posterior ganglion of the cerebrum.

Thalamus, Ħál-a-mus; a white substance constituting the base of the lateral ventricles of the brain; also the base of a nerve.

Thanatodes, Ħan-a-tώ-dēz; mortal; causing death.

Thanatology, Ħan-a-tól-ω-ji; a consideration of the causes of death.

Thapsia Garganica, Ħáp-si-ɑ Gɋr-gán-i-kɑ; a European plant that yields a resin, which is used as an irritant. [cord.

Theca, Ħé-kɑ; the membranous covering of the spinal

Theca Vertebralis, — Vɛr-tē-brá-lis; an extension of the *dura mater*.

Thelitis, Ħē-lį-tis; inflammation of the nipple.

Theine or **Theia**, Ħé-in or Ħē-į-ɑ; an alkaloid obtained from tea and coffee.

Theobroma Cacao, Ħē-ω-brώ-mɑ Ka-ká-ω; a tree of South America, from the fruit of which chocolate and cacoa butter are obtained.

Theomania, Ħē-ω-má-ni-ɑ; insanity resulting from religious excitement.

Therapeutics, Ħer-a-pų́-tiks; the science of the curative powers of medicines and their uses in treating diseases.

Therapeutist, Ħer-a-pų́-tist; one who is skilled in, and practices therapeutics.

Theriocatarrhus, Ħē-ri-ω-ka-tɋ́r-us. See Hay Fever.

Therioma, Ħē-ri-ṓ-ma; any very malignant ulcer.
Thermal, Ħḗr-mal; relating to warmth or heat.
Thigh, Ħị; the *femur*, that part of the lower limb between the hip and knee.
Third Pair of Nerves. See *Motores Oculorum.*
Thomsonianism, Tom-sṓ-ni-an-izm: the Botanic system, originated by a Dr. Thomson, of New England; it rejects all minerals and blood-letting.
Thoracic, Ħo-rás-ik; relating to the thorax.
Thoracic Duct, — Dukt; the trunk of the absorbent and lymphatic vessels.
Thorax, Ħṓ-raks; the chest, containing the lungs and heart.
Thornapple, Ħórn-ap-l; a common name for *Datura Stramonium.*
Threadworm, Ħréd-wurm; a worm an inch and a half or two inches long, found in the colon and cœcum.
Thoroughwort, Ħúr-o-wurt; *Eupatorium perfoliatum;* the name refers to the position of the leaves on the stem.
Throat, Ħrot; the pharynx, or fore part of the neck.
Thromboid, Ħróm-bed; similar to a thrombus.
Thrombus, Ħróm-bus; a small hard tumor, caused by the effusion of blood after a contusion or the bleeding of a patient in that locality.
Thrush, Ħruʃ; aphthæ, or white ulcers on the tongue and membranes of the mouth.
Thuja Occidentalis, Ħú-ja Ok-si-den-tá-lis; arbor vitæ, a native evergreen tree.
Thyme, Tịm; *Thymus vulgaris*, a labiate plant of Europe that yields an aromatic volatile oil.
Thymol, Tị́-mol; thymic acid, obtained by decomposition of oil of thyme; used as an antiseptic.
Thymus Gland, Ħị́-mus Gland; an oblong glandular body, behind the sternum.
Thyreocele, Ħị́-rē-o-sēl; bronchocele, or swelling of the thyroid gland.
Thyreo-Hyoideus, Ħị́-rē-o-Hị-o-ị́-dē-us; a muscle that draws the larynx and thyroid bone nearer each other.
Thyroid, Ħị́-red; shaped like a shield.
Thyroid Cartilage, — Ká̤r-til-ej; the large cartilage of the larynx, called Adam's apple.

Thyroid Gland, Ħį-rɵd Gland; a gland lying in front of the windpipe, on the horns of the thyroid cartilage, the seat of goitre. [leg.

Tibia, Tíb-i-a; the shin-bone, or largest bone of the

Tibialis, Tib-i-á-lis; applied to two muscles of the tibia, the *anticus* and *posticus*. [face.

Tic Douloureux, Tik Dúı-lɯ-rɯ; nervous pain in the

Tiglii Oleum, Tíg-li-į Ɯ'lē-um. See Oil of Croton.

Tinctures, Tíŋk-tųrz; solutions of soluble constituents of plants, or other medicinal substances, in alcohol, or mixtures of alcohol and water. [eruption.

Tinea, Tín-ē-a; the scaldhead, a species of cutaneous

Tinnevelly Senna, Tin-ē-vél-i Sén-a; a variety of senna obtained from India.

Tinnitus Aurium, Ti-nį-tus Θ'ri-um; ringing in the ears, a symptom of certain diseases.

Tissue, Tíʃ-ų; a distinct, organized structure.

Tissue, Mucous, — Mų́-kus; the tissue lining cavities that open to the external air. [which are closed.

Tissue, Serous, — Sē-rus; a tissue that lines cavities

Titubation, Tit-ų-bá-ʃon; an unsteady, staggering gait, resulting from spinal disease.

Tobacco, Tɷ-bák-ɷ; the dried leaves of *Nicotiana Tabacum*, used in medicine as a sedative.

Tobacco, Indian, — In'di-an; a common name for *Lobelia inflata*.

Tocology, Tɷ-kól-ɷ-ji; the science of parturition.

Tolu, (Balsam of,) Tɷ́-lų; an aromatic resin exuded from *Myrospermum Toluiferum*, and used as an expectorant. [*pia mater*.

Tomentum, Tɷ-mén-tum; small fibrous vessels in the

Tongue, Tuŋ; the organ of speech, and also one of the organs of taste.

Tongue-Tied, — Tįd; an adhesion of the edges of the tongue to the gums.

Tonic, Tón-ik; a tenacious contraction of the muscles; also applied to medicines that excite the vital functions.

Tonka Bean, Tóŋ-ka Bēn; the seed of *Dipterix odorata*, chiefly used for flavoring purposes.

Tonsil, Tón-sil; a small oval gland in the arches of the fauces.

Tonsillitis, Ton-sil-ị-tis; inflammation of the tonsils.
Toothache, Túθ-ak; pain in the nerve of a tooth.
Tooth-Rash, — Ráʃ; an eruption on different parts of the body of children during dentition.
Tophus, Tώ-fus; a calcareous substance in the joints of those afflicted with gout; also, a kind of tartar on the teeth.
Torcular Herophili, Tór-kų-lɑr Hē-róf-i-lị; a cavity where the sinuses of the *dura mater* unite.
Tormentil, Tór-men-til; the astringent root of *Potentilla Tormentilla.*
Tormina, Tór-mi-nɑ; dysentery, with griping pains in [the bowels.
Torpid, Tór-pid; benumbed; incapable of motion.
Torpor, Tór-por; numbness; want of sensation.
Torsion, Tór-ʃon; twisting; applied to a manipulation for the arrest of hemorrhage.
Torticollis, Tor-ti-kól-is; the affection termed wry- [neck.
Torus, Tώ-rus; the muscular part of the arm or leg.
Tourniquet, Túr-ni-ke; an instrument for compressing arteries in making amputations, to prevent hemorrhage.
Toxical, Tóks-i-kal; poisonous.
Toxicodendron, Toks-i-kω-dén-dron. See *Rhus Toxi-* [*codendron.*
Toxicodermitis, Toks-i-kω-der-mị-tis; inflammation of the skin, resulting from external poisoning.
Toxicohæmia, Toks-i-kω-hé-mi-ɑ; poisoning of the blood.
Toxicology, Toks-i-kól-ω-ji; the science of poisons.
Toxicosis, Toks-i-kώ-sis; applied to diseases which are caused by poisoning.
Trabecula, Tra-bék-ų-lɑ; applied to minute fibers, extending out from certain membranes.
Trachea, Tra-ké-ɑ; the wind-pipe, a cartilaginous canal for conveying air to the lungs.
Tracheal, Trák-ē-al; relating to the trachea; applied to the respiration heard through the stethoscope.
Tracheitis, Trak-ē-ị-tis; the croup, or inflammation of the trachea.
Trachelagra, Tra-kél-a-grɑ; rheumatism, or gout in [the neck.
Trachelismus, Trak-ē-lís-mus; a spasm of the muscles of the neck, causing it to be turned back; a symptom of epilepsy.

Trachelo-Mastoideus, Tra-kē-lω - Mas-tω-į-dē-us ; a muscle of the neck that draws the head back.

Tracheotomy, Trak-ē-ót-ω-mi; the making of an incision into the wind-pipe.

Trachoma, Tra-kώ-mα; ophthalmania, in which there is roughness on the internal coat of the eyelid, causing much pain.

Tractus Motorius, Trák-tus Mω-tώ-ri-us; an extension of the eminences of the *medulla oblongata*, from which the motor nerves arise.

Tractus Opticus, — Op′ti-kus; the course of the optic nerve, in its devious windings.

Tragacanth, Trág-a-kanθ; a white, flaky substance, obtained from *Astragalus verus*, and used as an excipient, in pills and troches.

Tragicus, Tráj-i-kus; a muscle of the ear.

Tragus, Tré-gus; the part of the ear opposite the lobe.

Trailing Arbutus, Trél-iŋ Ar-bų-tus; *Epigœa repens*, gravel plant; diuretic and astringent.

Transfusion, Trans-fų-ʒon; the transfer of blood from the veins of a healthy person to those of a patient; also the injection of any other fluid in the same way.

Transversalis Abdominis, Trans-ver-sá-lis Ab-dóm-in-is; a large flat muscle, having a transverse direction from the false ribs to the crest of the ilium, which supports the bowels.

Transversalis Colli, — Kól-į; a muscle of the posterior and lateral part of the neck and back.

Transversalis Dorsi, — Dér-sį; a muscle extending along the vertebral gutters, and whose use is to straighten the spinal column.

Transverse Suture, Trans-vẽrs Sú-tųr; a scarcely recognizable suture that joins the bones of the skull with those of the face.

Transversus Auris, Trans-vẽr-sus Θ′ris; a muscular ligament of the external ear.

Transversus Pedis, — Pē-dis; a muscle extending from the metatarsal bone of the large toe to that of the small one.

Transversus Perinæi, — Per-i-nē-į; a muscle of the posterior part of the perinæum, whose office is to compress the urethra and sustain the rectum.

Trapezium, Tra-pḗ-zi-um; the first bone of the second row of bones in the wrist.

Trapezius, Tra-pḗ-zi-us; a muscle in the back part of the neck and shoulder, having various attachments; it elevates and depresses the shoulder, head, etc.

Treacle, Trḗ-kl; *Syrupus Fuscus*, U. S. P., or molasses.

Trembles, Trém-blz; milk-sickness; also mercurial tremor.

Tremor Cordis, Trḗ-mor Kórdis; palpitation of the heart.

Tremor Mercurialis, — Mer-kū-ri-á-lis; a shaking palsy, superinduced by mercurial vapors.

Trepan, Trē-pán; an instrument for sawing away a portion of the skull-bone.

Trephine, Trē-fīn; the modern instrument for removing parts of the skull by a series of perforations.

Tresis, Trḗ-sis; a perforation or cut, in a soft part.

Triads, Trī́-adz; elements and radicals that are trivalent.

Triamines, Trī-ám-i-nēz; organic bases, considered as derived from three molecules of ammonia.

Triangularis Labiorum, Trī-aŋ-gū-lá-ris Lab-i-ṓ-rum; a muscle of the lips, of triangular form.

Triangularis Sterni, — Stér-nī; a muscle in the front but inner part of the chest, that depresses the ribs in respiration.

Triceps, Trī-seps: three-headed, as applied to muscles.

Triceps Extensor Cruris, — Eks-tén-sor Krú-ris; a muscle of the leg having three sources.

Triceps Extensor Cubiti, — — Kū́-bi-tī; a muscle extending from the shoulder-blade to the elbow, that extends the fore-arm.

Trichia, Trī́-ki-a; (or *Trichiasis;*) an inversion of the eyelashes.

Trichina, Tri-kī́-na; a species of entozoa, found in the muscle of swine especially; when such diseased pork is eaten, these parasites multiply in the intestines, and migrate to the muscles, causing death.

Trichocephalus, Trī-kō-séf-a-lus; the thread-worm, generally found in the cœcum and intestines.

Trichosis, Trī-kṓ-sis; a morbid condition, or deficiency, of hair.

Trichuris, Trī-kū́-ris; the long hair-worm.

Tricuspid, Trį-kús-pid; three-pointed; applied to a valve of the heart.

Trifacial, Trį-fá-ʃal. See *Trigemini*.

Trifolium Pratense, Trį-fó-li-um Pra-tén-sē; red clover.

Trigemini, Trį-jém-i-nį; the fifth pair of encephalic nerves, consisting of three branches.

Trigone, Tri-gón; the vesical triangle, a space between the orifice of the urethra and those of the ureters.

Trigonella Fœnumgræcum, Trig-o-nél-a Fē-num-grē-kum; a European plant that yields fenugreek seed.

Trilabe, Trį-lab; a three-armed instrument, for extracting substances from the bladder.

Trillium Erectum, Tril-i-um Ē-rék-tum; beth or birth root, an indigenous three-leaved plant, the root of which is astringent.

Trinitro-carbolic Acid, Trín-i-tro-kar-ból-ik As'id; picric acid.

Triosteum Perfoliatum, Trį-ós-tē-um Per-fo-li-á-tum, fever-root, an indigenous herb.

Triplopia, Trip-ló-pi-a; abnormal vision, in which an object appears tripled.

Tripod, Vital, Trį-pod Vį-tal; the heart, lungs and brain, so termed because essential to life.

Trismus, Trís-mus; tetanus, or locked-jaw.

Trismus Nascentium; — Na-sén-ʃi-um; locked-jaw of infants, within two weeks of birth.

Trisplanchnic Nerve, Trį-spláŋk-nik Nerv. See *Sympathetic Nerve*.

Triticum Repens, Trít-i-kum Rē-pens; couch-grass; dog-grass; a common weed in cultivated ground, used as a diuretic.

Triturate, Trít-u-rat; to rub down in a mortar.

Trivalence, Triv-a-lens; the property possessed by certain atoms and radicals of displacing three atoms of hydrogen or other univalent elements.

Trochanter, Tro-kán-ter; the major and minor processes on the femur.

Troches, Tró-kēz; small flattened pieces of confectionary, containing medicinal substances.

Trochlea, Trók-lē-a; a pulley; applied to certain tendons, as that at the upper part of the orbit of the eye.

Trochlearis, Trok-lē-á-ris; the *obliquus superior* muscle which passes through the trochlea.

Trochoid, Tró-kød; a movable connection, in which one bone rotates upon another, as the radius and ulna.
Trophical, Tróf-i-kal; relating to nourishment.
Trophoneurosis, Trof-ω-nų-rώ-sis; atrophy; a morbid condition of the powers of nutrition.
Truss, Trus; a bandage, or pads and straps, designed to support weak parts, as in hernia.
Tube, Tųb. See *Eustachian* and *Fallopian*.
Tuber, Tų́-ber; an enlargement, excrescent, or knob.
Tubercle, Tų́-bɛr-kl; a swelling or small tumor.
Tubercula, Tų-bɛ́r-kų-lɑ; small hard tumors.
Tubercula Quadrigemina, — Kwod-ri-jém-i-nɑ; four oval-shaped bodies in the brain, above the *pons varolii*.
Tubercular Phthisis, Tų-bɛ́r-kų-lɑr Tį-sis; consumption, attended with tubercles in the lungs.
Tuberculum, Annulare, Tų-bɛ́r-kų-lum An-ų-lá-rē; the *pons varolii*, which see.
Tubuli, Tų́-bų-lį; many minute vessels located in groups in different parts of the body.
Tubuli Recti, — Rék-tį; numerous small tubes appertaining to the testicle; termed also the *corpus highmorianum*.
Tubuli Seminiferi, — Sem-i-níf-er-į; the body of small tubular cords that compose the testicle.
Tubuli Uriniferi, — Yu-ri-níf-er-į; a series of eight or ten *fasciculi* in connection with the kidneys.
Tulpii Valva, Túl-pi-į Vál-vɑ; the ileo-cæcal valve.
Tumefaction, Tų-mē-fák-ʃon; tumescence; an enlargement or swelling.
Tumid, Tų́-mid; distended; enlarged.
Tumeric Paper, Tų-mér-ik Pá-per; paper colored yellow with tincture of tumeric; alkalies change the color to brown.
Tumor, Tų́-mor; a morbid local enlargement, without inflammation; of two kinds: sarcomatous, or fleshy and solid; or encysted and soft.
Tumor Ovarii, — Ω-vá-ri-į; tumor of the ovaries, which are either solid or encysted.
Tunica, Tų́-ni-kɑ; a coat; a membranous envolope.
Tunica Adnata, — Ad-ná-tɑ; the internal membrane of the eyelids.

Tunica Albuginea Oculi, Tú-ni-ka Al-bu-jín-ē-a Ok'u-li; the white sclerotic coat of the muscles that move the eye.

Tunica-Albuginea Testis, — — Tés-tis; the white fibrous envelope enclosing the testicle.

Tunica Arachnoides, — Ar-ak-no-i-dēz; the thin white membrane separating the *dura mater* and *pia mater*.

Tunica Choroides, — Ko-ro-í-dēz; the choroid membrane, or inner coat of the eyeball.

Tunica Communis, — Kom-ú-nis; the coating that encloses the spermatic cord and testicle.

Tunica Vaginalis Testis, — Vaj-i-ná-lis Tés-tis; the membranous coat that covers the testis.

Turbinated Bones, Túr-bin-a-ted Bonz; two top-shaped bones in the nostrils.

Turgescence, Tur-jés-ens; an excess of any of the humors of the body.

Turkey-Corn, Túr-ki-Kern; corydalis, the tubers of *Dicentra Canadensis.*

Turmeric, Túr-mer-ik; the powdered root of the *Curcuma longa*, mostly used as a coloring matter and as a test for acids.

Turpentine, Túr-pen-tin; an oleoresin obtained from several species of pines.

Turpentine, Spirits of; a volatile oil obtained by distillation from turpentine.

Turpeth Mineral, Túr-peth Mín-er-al; yellow oxysulphate of mercury.

Tussilago Farfara, Tus-i-lá-go Fár-fa-ra: colts-foot herb; used in coughs and pulmonary affections.

Tussis Convulsiva, Tús-is Kon-vul-sí-va; the hooping-cough.

Twin-Leaf, Twín-Lēf; *Jeffersonia diphylla;* the root is used as an expectorant.

Tylosis, Ti-ló-sis; an inflammation of the eyelids, in which they become knotty and hard.

Tympanites, Tim-pan-í-tēz; distention of the abdomen with air in the intestinal tubes.

Tympanum, Tím-pa-num; the drum, or cavity of the middle ear.

Typhoid Fever, Tí-fod Fē-ver; a fever differing from the typhus only in the depressed condition of the intestines.

Typhomania, Tī-fō-mā́-ni-a; delirious mutterings during stupor in typhus fever.

Typhus, Tī́-fus; a low continuous fever, with great prostration of the nervous system, and disorder of the secretions.

Typhus Gravior, — Grá-vi-or; malignant typhus, occurring generally in prisons or military camps, and then termed *febris carcerum* (jail fever,) and *febris castrensis*, (camp fever.)

Tyremesis, Tī-rém-ĕ-sis; the curdling and vomiting of an infant's food.

Tysoni Glandulæ, Tī-só-nī Glán-dū-lē; the sebaceous glandules of the *glans penis, labia pudendi;* and *nymphæ.*

U

Ula, Yú-la; *gingivæ*, the gums.

Ulatrophia, Yu-la-tró-fi-a; shrinkage of the gums.

Ulcer, Ul'ser; "a solution of continuity in any soft part;" a purulent sore, resulting from perverted nutrition.

Ulceration, Ul-ser-á-ʃon; the process by which an ulcer is formed.

Ulitis, Yu-lī́-tis; inflammation of the gums.

Ulmus Fulva, Ul'mus Fúl-va; slippery elm; the inner bark is extensively used as a demulcent, and also in the composition of poultices.

Ulna, Ul'na; the under and larger bone of the forearm.

Ulnaris, Ul-ná-ris; applied to two muscles of the forearm, the *flexor* and the *extensor.*

Uloncus, Yu-lón-kus; a swollen condition of the gums.

Ulorrhagia, Yu-lō-rá-ji-a; bleeding of the gums.

Umbilical Cord, Um-bil-i-kal Kerd; the membranous cord that connects the *fœtus in utero* with the placenta, and thereby with the mother.

Umbilical Region, — Rē-jon; that part of the abdomen surrounding the umbilicus.

Umbilicus, Um-bíl-i-kus; the navel; the hilum of a seed.
Unciform, Un′si-fərm; hook-shaped.
Unguentum, Uŋ-gwén-tum; ointment, or salve.
Unguis, Uŋ′gwis; a nail, of a finger or toe.
Unguis Os, — Os; a thin bone, something like a finger-nail, in the orbit of the eye.
Unicorn Root, Yɯ́-ni-kərn Rɯt; *Aletris farinosa.*
Unicorn Root, False, *Chamœlirium luteum*, (*Helonias Dioica*,) a native plant.
Uniparous, Yɯ-níp-a-rus; bringing forth one at a birth.
Univalence, Yɯ-nív-a-lens; having the power to replace an atom of hydrogen.
Urachus, Yɯ́-ra-kus; a tube, or cord, extending from the bladder to the umbilicus.
Uracrasia, Yɯ-ra-krá-si-ɑ; vitiated urine.
Urari, Yɯ-rá-rị; a name for *Curaria.*
Urates, Yɯ́-rets; salts of uric acid, many being found naturally in urine.
Urea, Yɯ-rέ-ɑ; an important constituent of urine, by the formation of which the nitrogen of food is eliminated from the body. [skin.
Uredo, Yɯ-rέ-dω; a heated itching sensation of the
Uresis, Yɯ-rέ-sis; the passage of urine.
Ureter, Yɯ-rέ-ter; the tube that carries the urine from the kidney to the bladder.
Ureteritis, Yɯ-rē-ter-ị-tis; inflammation of the ureter.
Urethra, Yɯ-rέ-ŧrɑ; the tube that carries the urine from the bladder.
Urethralgia, Yɯ-rē-ŧrál-ji-ɑ; pain in the urethra.
Urethritis, Yɯ-rē-ŧrị-tis; inflammation of the urethra, gonorrhœa.
Urethroplasty, Yɯ-rē-ŧrω-plás-ti; the repairing of a lesion in the urethra. flow of urine.
Uretica, Yɯ-rét-i-kɑ; medicines that promote a free
Uric Acid, Yɯ́-rik As′id; an organic acid obtained from urine, known also as *lithic acid.*
Urinary, Yɯ́-ri-nɑ-ri; whatever relates to the urine.
Urine, Yɯ́-rin; a saline fluid secreted by the kidneys.
Urocystitis, Yɯ-rω-sis-tị-tis; inflammation of the bladder. sion of the urine.
Urodialysis, Yɯ-rω-di-ál-i-sis; cessation or suppres-

Urodynia, Yɯ-rɷ-dín-i-ɑ; painful urination.

Urogenital, Yɯ-rɷ-jén-i-tal; appertaining to both the urinary and genital organs.

Urolithus, Yɯ-ról-i-ŧus; calculus from the urinary [bladder.

Urology, Yɯ-ról-ɷ-ji; that branch of medicine which treats of the urine.

Uromancy, Yɯ-rɷ-mán-si; the divination of disease [from inspection of the urine.

Urorrhagia, Yɯ-rɷ-rá-ji-ɑ; diabetes, an immoderate flow of urine.

Urorrhœa, Yɯ-rɷ-rē-ɑ: the involuntary discharge of [urine.

Uroscopia, Yɯ-rɷ-skṓ-pi-ɑ; diagnosing disease by examination of the urine.

Uroses, Yɯ-rṓ-sēz; diseases of the organs of urination.

Urtica Dioica, Ur'ti-kɑ Dį-ɷ-į-kɑ; the common nettle, a stinging weed, the leaves of which are used as a diuretic.

Urticaria, Ur-ti-ká-ri-ɑ; the nettle-rash; a fever attended with small eruptions like those resulting from the stings of the nettle.

Urtication, Ur-ti-ká-ʃon; the stinging of a part with nettles, as a counter-irritation.

Ustilago Maidis, Us-ti-lá-gɷ Má-dis; corn-smut, or corn ergot, a fungus growth on the unripe ears of corn, that is used to contract the uterus.

Ustion, Ust'yon; a burning or combustion.

Uteri, Yɯ́-ter-į; genitive case of *uterus*, "of the womb."

Uterine, Yɯ́-ter-įn; relating to the uterus or womb.

Utero-Gestation, — Jes-tá-ʃon; the period from conception until delivery.

Uterotomy, Yɯ-ter-ót-ɷ-mi; making an incision in the uterus when the lips are closed.

Uterus, Yɯ́-ter-us; the womb, in which the fœtus [grows.

Uterus, (Inversion of,) displacement, and turned inside out by malpractice.

Utricle, Yɯ́-tri-kl; a small cell or vesicle.

Uva Ursi, Yɯ́-vɑ Ur'sį; *Arctostaphylos Uva Ursi*, a small evergreen plant; the leaves are used as a diuretic.

Uvea, Yɯ́-vē-ɑ; the choroid coat of the eye; also applied to the black pigment of the iris.

Uvula, Yɯ́-vɥ-lɑ; the pendulous body above the root [of the tongue.

Uvulitis, Yɯ-vɥ-lį́t-is; inflammation of the uvula.

V

Vaccina, Vak-sį-nɑ; cow-pox, a disease of the cow, attended with eruptions.

Vaccination, Vak-si-ná-ʃon; the introduction of cow-pox virus, under the skin, to prevent the contagion of small-pox.

Vagina, Va-jį-nɑ; "a case;" the passage from the vulva to the uterus.

Vaginal, Váj-i-nal; relating to the vagina.

Vaginate, Váj-i-nat; encased, or sheathed.

Vaginitis, Vaj-i-nį-tis; inflammation of the vagina.

Vagitis, Va-jį-tis: the first cry of a new-born babe.

Vagus, Vá-gus; *Par Vagum*, the pneumogastric nerve.

Valerian, Va-lḗ-ri-an; *Valeriana officinalis*, a European plant, the root of which is extensively used as a nervine.

Valerianates, Va-lḗ-ri-an-ats; salts of valerianic acid.

Valerianic Acid, Va-lē-ri-án-ik As′id; an acid once obtained from valerian root, now made from fusel oil.

Valetudinarian, Val-ē-tų-di-ná-ri-an; an infirm or sickly person.

Valgus, Vál-gus; crooked; bow-legged.

Valley, Vál-i; the fissure in the cerebellum, where the spinal marrow arises.

Vallet's Mass, Vál-et's Mɑs; pill of carbonate of iron.

Valve, Valv; an elongation or fold of the membrane of a canal, which prevents the reflow of its contents; as valves of the heart, valves of the aorta, etc.

Valvula, Vál-vų-lɑ; a small valve.

Valvulæ Conniventes, — Kon-i-vén-tēz; numerous folds of the mucous membrane throughout most of the small intestines.

Vanilla, Va-níl-ɑ; the aromatic fruit of *Vanilla aromatica*, a plant of South America; mostly used for flavoring purposes and as a perfume.

Vapor, Vá-por; the evaporation into fume, or steam, of the essential part of a liquid or solid substance.

Vapor-Bath, Vá-por Baŧ; the application of vapor, medicated or otherwise, to the whole or part of a patient's body.

Vapors, Vá-porz; the colloquial name for hypochondria.

Varicella, Var-i-sél-a; chicken-pox, an eruptive disease.

Varicocele, Vár-i-kω-sēl; a swelling of the spermatic cord, or vessels of the scrotum.

Varicose, Vár-i-kωs; the condition of veins permanently distended with dark-colored blood.

Variola, Var-i-ó-la, or Va-rį-ω-la; the small-pox, a very contagious eruptive disease.

Varioloid, Vár-i-ω-lθd; resembling variola; a mild attack of small-pox, modified by vaccination.

Variolous, Va-rį-ω-lus; having the nature of small-pox.

Varix, Vá-riks; the morbid distension of a vein.

Varus, Vá-rus; acne; a pimple on the face; applied to a crooked or inverted variety of club-foot.

Vas, Vas; (pl; *Vasa;*) a vessel; applied to the membranous tubes and canals of the body.

Vas Deferens, — Déf-er-ens; the canal through which the semen is carried to the ejaculatory duct.

Vas Spirale, — Spį-rá-lē; a vein of the cochlea.

Vasa Brevia, Vá-sa Bré-vi-a: branches of the splenic artery.

Vasa Efferentia, —Ef-er-én-ʃi-a; vessels that convey from a gland; applied especially to a group that ascend back from the testicle.

Vasa Inferentia, — In-fer-én-ʃa; vessels that carry a substance into a gland.

Vasa Vasorum, — Va-só-rum; small nutrient vessels that supply larger veins, etc.

Vasa Vorticosa, — Vθr-ti-kó-sa; ciliary veins of the eye.

Vascular, Vás-kų-lar; relating to or full of vessels.

Vasculum, Vás-kų-lum; a small vessel.

Vastus Externus, Vás-tus Eks-tér-nus; (also *V. Internus;*) two large masses of muscle in the thigh.

Vault, Vθlt: applied to the arch of the cranium, roof of the mouth, etc.

Vauqueline, Vωk-lén; the French for *Strychnia*.

Vegetable Charcoal, Véj-et-a-bl Ꞓár-kωl. See *Carbo Vegetabilis*.

Vegetative, Véj-ē-ta-tiv; relating to growth and nutrition.

Vegeto-Animal, Véj-ē-tō-An'i-mal; vegetable substances that resemble animal matter.

Vegeto-Mineral, — Mín-er-al; applied to substances that resemble both vegetable and mineral structures.

Vehicle, Vé-hi-kl; any liquid or other substance in which a medicine may be conveniently given.

Vein, Van; a long membranous tube that returns the blood to the heart.

Velum, Vé-lum; a veil, or screen.

Velum Pendulum Palati, — Pén-dų-lum Pal-á-tį; the soft pendulous part of the palate.

Velum Pupillæ, — Pų-píl-ē; a membrane that covers the pupil of the eye of the fœtus.

Vena, Vé-na; a vein, which see.

Vena Arteriosa, — Ar-tē-ri-ó-sa; the portal vein; it is like an artery in that it conveys blood for secretion.

Vena Basilica, — Ba-síl-i-ka; the principal vein of the arm.

Vena Cava Inferior, (or *Ascendens;*) Ká-va In-fé-ri-or: one of the great veins which returns the blood to the heart.

Vena Cava Superior, (or *Descendens;*) — Su-pé-ri-or; the great vein which returns the blood from the head, neck, etc., to the heart.

Vena Portæ, — Pór-tē; a vein that unites with most of the organs within the abdomen.

Venæ Cavæ, Vé-nē Ká-vē; the terminations of the *Vena Cava Superior*, and *V. C. Inferior*.

Venenation, Ven-ē-ná-ʃon; poison; poisoning.

Venereal, Ven-é-rē-al; relating to sexual intercourse.

Venereal Disease, — Dis-ēz; syphilis, strictly, but also applied to gonorrhœa.

Venery, Vén-er-i; sexual intercourse.

Venesection, Ven-ē-sék-ʃon; phlebotomy; the opening of a vein in blood-letting.

Venice Turpentine, Vén-is Túr-pen-tįn; the variety of turpentine obtained from the European larch, (*Larix Europœa.*)

Venom, Vén-om; poison, usually that of serpents, etc.

Venous, Vé-nus; pertaining to the veins.

Venter, Vén-ter; the belly; also applied to the womb.

Ventral, Vén-tral; relating to the belly. [heart.
Ventricle, Vén-tri-kl; a cavity of the brain, and of the
Ventricose, Vén-tri-kōs; big-bellied; distended.
Ventriculus, Ven-trík-ụ-lus; a cavity; the stomach.
Venula, Vén-ụ-la; a small vein.
Veratria, or **Veratrin**, Ver-á-tri-a, or Vér-a-trin; an alkaloid obtained from cevadilla seed.
Veratrum Album, Ver-á-trum Al'bum; white hellebore, a poisonous European plant, the root of which is an active emetic and carthartic.
Veratrum Sabadilla, — Sab-a-díl-a; a plant of Mexico that yields cevadilla seed.
Veratrum Viride, — Vir-ị-dī; green hellebore, an indigenous plant, the root of which is used to control the circulation of the blood: poisonous in overdoses.
Verbascum Thapsus, Vɛr-bás-kum Ꞓáp-sus; mullein, a common native weed.
Verbena Hastata, Vɛr-bē-na Has-tá-ta; vervain, a common weed, used in scrofulous affections.
Verdigris, Vɛ́r-di-gris; crude subacetate of copper.
Vermes, Vɛ́r-mīz; worms that infest the intestines.
Vermicular, Vɛr-mík-ụ-lar; having the appearance of worms.
Vermiform Process, Vɛ́r-mi-fōrm Pró-ses; the worm-like connection between the hemispheres of the cerebellum.
Vermifuge, Vɛ́r-mi-fụj; a medicine to expel worms.
Vernonia Fasciculata, Vɛr-nṓ-ni-a Fas-ik-ụ-lá-ta; iron-weed, the root of which is tonic.
Veronica Virginica, Vī-rón-i-ka Vɛr-jín-i-ka; black-root; culver's root; an active cathartic, commonly known as *Leptandra Virginica*. [skin.
Verruca, Ve-rṹ-ka: a wart; any hard projection on the
Verrucose, Vér-ụ-kōs; having many warts.
Vertebra, Vɛ́r-tī-bra; (pl. *Vertebræ;*) one of the twenty-four bones composing the spinal column.
Vertebral Artery, Vɛr-tē-bral Ar'ter-i; one of the arteries of the brain, which takes its name from its passage through the cervical vertebræ.
Vertebral Canal, — Ka-nál; the channel in which the spinal marrow extends through the vertebral column.

Vertebral Column, Vεr-tĕ-bral Kŏl-um; the back-bone.
Vertebral Gutter, — Gút-er; the depression on each side of the back-bone.
Vertebral Nerve, — Nεrv; the trisplanchnic nerve.
Vertex, Vέr-teks; the crown of the head.
Vertigo, Vέr-ti-gω; a swimming sensation of the head.
Vervain, Vέr-van; *Verbena hastata,* which see.
Vesania, Ve-sá-ni-a; mental alienation, or unsoundness.
Vesica, Ve-sį-ka; a bladder; any sac like a bladder.
Vesicants, Vés-i-kants; agents that produce blisters.
Vesication, Ves-i-ká-ʃon; the production of blisters.
Vesicle, Vés-i-kl; a small bladder or blister in the skin; in the plural, small sac-like vessels. [licles.
Vesicles Graaffian,—Grą-fi-an. See Graaffian Fol-
Vesiculæ Seminales, Ve-sik-ų-lĕ Sem-i-ná-lĕz; two seminal canals back of the urinary bladder.
Vessel, Vés-el; a canal, or duct, through which fluids are carried in the body. [ear.
Vestibule, Vés-ti-bųl; a small cavity of the internal
Veterinary, Vét-er-i-na-ri; the treatment of diseases in horses.
Viability, Vį-a-bíl-i-ti: capability of living.
Viable, Vį-a-bl; as applied to a new-born infant, capable of extra-uterine existence.
Viæ Lachrymalis, Vį-ĕ Lak-ri-má-lis; the tear-ducts, both of secretion and excretion.
Vibices, Vi-bį-sĕz; purple spots under the skin, in certain malignant fevers.
Vibriones, Vib-ri-ώ-nĕz; animalcules in putrefying animal fluids.
Vibrissæ, Vį-brís-ĕ; hairs that grow in the nostrils.
Viburnum Opulus, Vį-búr-num Op'ų-lus; cramp-bark; high cranberry, a native shrub, the bark of which is used in spasmodic diseases.
Viburnum Prunifolium, — Prω-ni-fώ-li-um; black-haw, used mostly in uterine diseases.
Vidian Nerve, Víd-i-an Nεrv; third branch of the sphenopalatine nerves. [long soft hairs.
Villose, or **Villous,** Vi-lώs, or Víl-us; shaggy; having
Vinegar, Vín-ĕ-gar; an impure dilute acetic acid, made by fermentation of the juice of fruits.

Vinegar of Squill, Vín-ē-gɑr ov Skwil; a solution made by extracting squill with dilute acetic acid.
Vinum, Vį-num; wine; juice of the grape.
Vinum Antimonii, — An-ti-mɷ́-ni-į; antimonial wine.
Viola Pedata, Vį-ɷ-lɑ Pē-dá-tɑ; a native violet, the root of which is used as an expectorant. [hymen.
Virginale Claustrum, Vɛr-jin-á-lē Klés-trum; the
Virginia Snakeroot, Vɛr-jín-i-ɑ Snák-rɯt; *Aristolochia Serpentaria*, a native plant, the root of which is used as a stimulant.
Virgin's Bower, Vɛ́r-jin'z Bŏ-er; *Clematis Virginica*, a climbing native shrub.
Virile, Vį-ril: relating to man, or manhood.
Virility, Vį-ríl-i-ti; manhood, especially as to his generative power.
Virus, Vį-rus; poison; applied to any product of a disease that will reproduce the disease.
Vis, Vis; force or power.
Vis Formativa, — Fɵr-ma-tį-vɑ; plastic force; the power that is supposed to exist in the body to give nourishment and form to its growth.
Vis Vitæ, — Vį-tē; vital power; irritability.
Viscera, Vís-er-ɑ; the internal organs of the body.
Viscum Flavescens, Vís-kum Fla-vés-ens; synonym for *Phoradendron flavescens*.
Viscus, Vís-kus; any large internal organ, as the liver.
Vita, Vį-tɑ; life; existence. [any organ.
Vita Propria, — Prɷ́-pri-ɑ; vital power peculiar to
Vital Principle, — Prin-si-pl; the undefined power of organized bodies to live.
Vitals, Vį-talz; applied to the heart, lungs and brain.
Vitiligo, Vit-i-lį-gɷ; a disease in which white, glistening patches appear on the skin.
Vitreous Humor, Vít-rē-us Hɥ-mor; the transparent body back of the crystalline lens of the eye.
Vitriol, Blue, Vít-ri-ol, Blɥ; sulphate of copper.
Vitriol, Green, —Grēn; sulphate of iron.
Vitriol, Oil of, — Ŏl ov; sulphuric acid.
Vitriol, White, — Hwįt; sulphate of zinc.
Vivisection, Viv-i-sék-ʃon; the dissection of living animals.

Volatile Alkali, Vól-a-til Al'ka-lį; a name applied to ammonia by the early chemists.
Volatile Oils, — Ơlz. See Oils Volatile.
Volvulus, Vól-vụ-lus. See Iliac Passion. [the face.
Vomer, Vó-mer; part of the *septum narium*, a bone of
Vomica, Vóm-i-ka; an abscess of the lungs.
Vomicus, Vóm-i-kus; relating to vomiting.
Vomit, Vóm-it; an emetic; also the matter discharged.
Vox Abscissa, Voks Ab-sís-a; loss of voice.
Vulnerary, Vúl-ner-a-ri; appertaining to wounds.
Vulpis Morbus, Vúl-pis Mór-bus; death or loss of hair.
Vulva, Vúl-va; the fissure, or *labia pudendi*, opening into the vagina.
Vulva Cerebri, — Sér-ĕ-brį; an aperture of the brain.
Vulvitis, Vul-vį-tis; inflammation of the vulva.
Vulvo-Vaginal Glands, Vúl-vo-Váj-in-al Glandz; a gland at each side of the vulva.

W

Wafer Ash, Wá-fer Aʃ; *Ptelia trifoliata*, the bark of which is used as a stimulant and tonic.
Wahoo, Wą-hú; *Euonymus atropurpureus*, a native shrub, the bark of which is tonic.
Wake-Robin, Wak-Rób-in; a common name for several species of Trillium. [nut, a native tree.
Walnut, (**White**,) Wél-nut; *Juglans cinerea;* butter-
Wart, Wort; *Verruca;* a hard tumor of the skin.
Water Avens, Wé-ter Ȧ'venz; *Geum rivale*, a native plant found in damp places, the root of which is astringent.
Water-Brash, — Braʃ; heartburn, with eructations of insipid water from the stomach.
Water Chalybeate, — Ka-líb-ĕ-at; mineral waters that contain salts of iron.

Water-Cure, Wé-ter Kųr; a method of treating diseases by the use of water; Hydropathy.
Water, Distilled. See Distilled Water.
Water-Lily, — Líl-i; *Nymphæa Odorata*, a water plant, the root of which is used as an astringent.
Watermelon Seed, Wéter-mel-on Sēd; the seed of *Cucurbita citrullus*, a diuretic.
Water of Ammonia, — A-mó-ni-a; a solution of ammonia gas in water.
Water-Pepper, — Pép-er; *Polygonum Hydropiper*, a common weed in the United States and Europe, possessing pungent properties.
Wax, Waks; the comb of the honey bee; when melted it is of a yellow color and known as "yellow wax," *Cera flava.*
Wax Myrtle, — Mér-tl; *Myrica cerifera;* see bayberry.
Weights Atomic, Wats A-tóm-ik; the relative weights of atoms.
Wen, Wen; an encysted tumor, usually sebaceous.
Wharton's Duct, Hwór-ton'z Duct; an excretory duct of the submaxillary gland.
Wheal, Hwēl; an elongated elevation of the skin, like that caused by a stroke from a rod.
Wheezing, Hwéz-iŋ: *Rhoncus;* a rattling in the throat.
Whelk, Hwelk; *Ionthus;* a small tubercle on the face that does not suppurate.
Whisky, Hwís-ki; an alcoholic liquor obtained usually by fermentation of grain.
White Cohosh, Hwįt Kó-hoʃ; *Actæa alba;* an indigenous, herbaceous plant.
White Hellebore, — Hél-ē-bor; *Veratrum album*, a European poisonous plant.
White Indian Hemp, — In'di-an Hemp; *Asclepias. incarnata.*
White Lead, — Led; carbonate of lead.
White Precipitate, — Prē-síp-i-tat; ammoniated mercury.
White Snake-root — Snak-Rut; *Eupatorium ageratoides*, an indigenous plant.
White Swelling, — Swél-iŋ; a scrofulous disease of the bones and joints.
White Vitriol, — Vít-ri-ol; sulphate of zinc.
White Wax, — Waks; *Cera alba*, wax that has been bleached by sunlight.

Whites, Hwįts; the colloquial name for leucorrhœa.
Whitlow, Hwít-lɷ; *Paronychia;* an abscess near the finger nails.
Whooping-Cough, Húp-iŋ-Kef; also spelled Hooping-Cough; *Pertussis;* a contagious disease, attended with fits of violent coughing, terminating with a kind of vomit.
Wild Cherry, Wįld Ҽér-i; *Prunus Serotina*, which see.
Wild Ginger, — Jín-jer; *Asarum Canadense*, Canada snakeroot, a native plant. [*losa.*
Wild Yam; a native herbaceous climber, *Dioscorea vil-*
Willow, Wíl-ɷ: shrubs and trees of the genus *Salix.*
Willow-Herb, Wíl-ɷ-Hɛrb; *Epilobium angustifolium*, a native showy plant. [grape.
Wine, Wįn; a fermented liquor, obtained from the
Wines, Medicated, Wįnz, Méd-i-ke-ted; solutions of medicinal substances in wine.
Wintergreen, Wín-ter-grēn: *Gaultheria procumbens*, a pretty little evergreen shrub.
Wintergreen Oil, — Ơl; an oil obtained from wintergreen herb, used to prepare salicylic acid, as it is mainly methyl-salicylic acid.
Witch-Hazel, Wiç-Hé-zel; *Hamamelis Virginica*, an indigenous shrub with yellow blossoms; the bark and leaves of which are astringent.
Wolffian Bodies, Wúl-fi-an Bód-iz; preliminary or false kidneys, in the third month of the fœtus.
Wolfsbane, Wúlfs-ben; *Aconitum Napellus*, which see.
Womb, Wɯm; the *Uterus*, which see.
Womb, Inflammation of. See *Uteritis.*
Womb, Falling of. See *Prolapsus Uteri.*
Wood Alcohol, (or **Spirit:**) Wud Al'kɷ-hol: methylic alcohol, a liquid produced by destructive distillation of wood.
Wood Charcoal, — Ҽɋr-kɷl; carbon obtained by burning wood with insufficient air for perfect combustion.
Wood Creasote, — Krē-a-sɷt; creasote obtained from pine tar.
Wood Naptha, — Náp-ϑa; wood alcohol.
Wormiana Os, Wur-mi-é-na Os; small bones sometimes found in the sutures of the cranium.

Worms, Wurmz. See *Vermes.*

Wormseed, (**American**,) Wúrm-sed; the seed of *Chenopodium anthelminticum.*

Wormseed, (**Levant**;) the dried flower-heads of a Russian species of *Artemisia*, supposed to be *A. Santonica.*

Wound, Wund, or Wɤnd; a solution of continuity, i. e., a cut or bruise, in a soft part of the body or limbs.

Wourara, or **Wourali**, Wu-rá-ra, or Wu-rá-lį; a name for curaria.

Wrist, Rist; the carpus, composed of eight bones.

Wrist-Drop, — Drop; paralysis of the muscles of the hand, from contact with lead poison.

Wry-Neck, Rį-Nek; *Torticollis*, a permanent inclination of the head to one side.

X

Xanthin, Zán-ŧin; a substance that forms a species of urinary calculus; also applied to the coloring matter of madder.

Xanthodontous, Zan-ŧo-dón-tus; having yellow teeth.

Xanthorrhiza Apiifolia, Zan-ŧo-rį-za Ap-i-fó-li-a; a southern plant, with a yellow root, used as a tonic.

Xanthoxylum Americanum, Zan-ŧóks-i-lum A-mer-i-ká-num; the prickly ash, a native shrub, the berries and bark of which are used as a tonic and stimulant.

Xeroderma, Zer-o-dér-ma; a dry, harsh condition of the skin.

Xerophthalmia, Zer-of-ŧál-mi-a; a dry inflammation of the eyes.

Xiphoid, Zį-fɵd; sword like; applied to the ensiform cartilage of the sternum.

Y

Yarrow, Yár-o; *Achillea Millefolium*, a common weed, used as a tonic.

Yellow Bark, Yél-o Bqrk; the variety of cinchona yielded by *Cinchona Calisaya.*

Yellow Dock, — Dok; *Rumex crispus;* an astringent.

Yellow Jasmine, — Jás-min; *Gelsemium sempervirens*, the fresh root of which is used as an arterial sedative.

Yellow Fever, Yél-ɷ Fḗ-ver; an epidemic, remittent fever, attended with yellow skin, from hepatic disorder; very malignant and fatal in southern localities.

Yellow Parilla, — Pa-ríl-a; *Menispermum Canadense,* the root of which is an alterative.

Yellow Prussiate of Potash, — Prúʃ-i-at ov Pót-aʃ; common name for ferrocyanide of potassium.

Yellow Root, — *Hydrastis Canadensis,* an indigenous plant, the root of which is a valuable remedy.

Yerbe Santa, Yḗr-bē Sán-ta; a Californian plant, *Eriodyction glutinosum,* used in bronchitis.

Z

Zinc, Ziŋk; a metallic element, the salts of which are used in medicine. [sulphuric acid.

Zinc Sulphate, — Súl-fat; a combination of zinc and

Zingiber Officinale, Zín-ji-ber Of-i-si-ná-lē; a plant of India, the source of ginger root.

Zoanthropia, Zɷ-an-ŧrɷ́-pi-a; a monomania, causing the patient to think himself an animal. [life.

Zoismus, Zɷ-ís-mus; animality; the nature of animal

Zona. Zɷ́-na; a zone, or belt; applied to the shingles.

Zoochemical, Zɷ-ɷ-kém-i-kal; relating to animal chemistry.

Zoogeny, Zɷ-ój-en-i; the generation of animal life.

Zoology, Zɷ-ól-ɷ-ji; the science of animal existence.

Zoophyte, Zɷ́-ɷ-fīt; a body once supposed to partake of the nature of both animal and vegetable life.

Zootomy, Zɷ-ót-ɷ-mi; the anatomy of the lower animals.

Zoster, Zós-ter; a species of erysipelas that encircles the body. [on the vertebral bones.

Zygapophysis, Zig-a-póf-i-sis; the yoke-like process

Zygoma, Zi-gɷ́-ma; the cheek bone.

Zygomatic Arch, Zig-ɷ-mát-ik Ȧrç; the arch formed by the junction of the zygomatic process of the malar and temporal bones.

Zygomatic Muscles, — Mús-lz; *major* and *minor,* arising from the cheek bone and connecting with the mouth.

Zymosis, Zi-mɷ́-sis; fermentation; applied to diseases resulting from specific poisons, or bad quality of food.

APPENDIX.

POISONS AND THEIR ANTIDOTES.

For the convenience of the inexperienced student of medicine, the druggist, and others, who may be called upon to render immediate aid in the case of a person who has taken poison, the following list of poisons and their antidotes is here inserted, to enable them to select some remedy without loss of time. The list embraces everything that is known to be fatally poisonous in its effects on the human constitution, including some things for which there is not known to be any positive or reliable antidote.

Most mineral poisons have such qualities as that while they may remain in the stomach for a time, other agents, if promptly administered, will form such chemical union with them, and so change their action that they will be no longer dangerous, and may be removed at leisure by simple means. Such agents are genuine antidotes.

But there are many animal and vegetable products possessing more active properties, whose effect on the system is so sudden and destructive that they must be immediately removed from the stomach, or involved in some albuminous, mucilaginous, or oleaginous substance, that will prevent their absorption into the circulating fluids until means are adopted for their removal. Therefore, when a person has taken poison, there should be administered as soon as possible a small draught of one or the other of the above named remedies, made thick and of the usual temperature of water. Avoid filling the stomach, or relaxing it with warm drinks, which favor the absorption of the poison.

The use of charcoal has been recommended in the treatment of all vegetable poisons whose active principle is alkaloid, as well as in most animal poisons. It has great absorbent powers, and being entirely neutral and harmless may be used freely without any danger. It should be pulverized, and moistened only enough to swallow readily.

The next step is the use of the stomach pump, or, for the want of one, the administration of a promptly acting emetic. Nauseating drugs should be avoided, such as lobelia, ipecac, tobacco, etc., for the reason that they are slow to act, and require a large amount of fluid in the stomach, which promotes the absorption and distribution of the poison; but in preference use common table salt, ground mustard from the caster, sulphate of zinc, sulphate of copper, white vitriol, or tartar emetic. The action of the emetic may be facilitated by tickling the throat with a feather or the finger.

After the stomach has been relieved, another mouthful or two of the demulcent, albuminous, or oleaginous preparation should be given, for the purpose of taking up any remainder of the poison left behind; and shortly afterward a light drink of diluted vinegar or lemonade may be given to advantage.

In the mean time the skillful physician should be called, to give the patient the benefit of his knowledge and experience.

POISONS AND ANTIDOTES.

The Poison precedes the Dash; the Antidote follows.

Poison Unknown—Calcined Magnesia, Pulverized Charcoal, Hydrated Peroxide of Iron, equal parts.

ACIDS.

Acetic Acid—Magnesia; Calcined Magnesia; Chalk; Carbonate of Soda.

Arsenic Acid—Hydrated Peroxide of Iron; dialyzed Iron, followed by a drink of solution of Bicarbonate of Soda.

Arsenious Acid—Same as above.

Carbonic Acid Gas—Open air, Stimulants and douche.

Chlorohydric Acid — Carbonate of Soda; Chlorine inhaled cautiously; Ammonia inhaled cautiously.

Citric Acid—Magnesia; Chalk; Carbonate of Soda; Carbonate of Potassa; Carbonate of Lime.

Muriatic Acid—Carbonate of Soda; Carbonate of Lime; Carbonate of Potassa; Carbonate of Magnesia.

Nitric Acid, (*Agua Fortis*)— Carbonate of Lime; Magnesia.

Oxalic Acid—Carbonate of Lime; Magnesia.

Phosphoric Acid—Ammonia; Chlorinated water; Magnesia; cold water.

Prussic Acid — Ammonia, concentrated; Chlorine, liquid; cold douche to the head; stimulants.

Sulphuric Acid, (*Oil of Vitriol*)—Magnesia; Carbonate of Magnesia: Carb. Lime; Chalk; no water.

Sulphurous Acid Gas—Cold affusions to the head; blood-letting; artificial respiration.

Tartaric Acid— Carbonate of Lime; Carb. Magnesia; Plaster from the ceiling.

Acetate of Copper, (*Verdigris*)—Albumen, (white of egg,) Iron; Milk; no vinegar.

Acetate of Lead, (*Sugar of Lead*)—Sulphate of Magnesia; Phosphate of Soda; Iodide of Potassium.

Acetate of Morphia—Infusion of Galls; Green Tea or Coffee, stimulants, dash of cold water.

Acetate of Zinc—Carbonate of Soda, in solution; Albumen and Milk.

Aconite, (*Monkshood*)—4 or 5 grains Tartar Emetic, or 20 grains Sulphate of Zinc, every fifteen minutes, until vomiting is produced; clysters of strong soapsuds, to clear the bowels; after this, hot coffee, and vinegar diluted should be drank; keep the patient roused.

Actæa Spicata, (*Baneberry*)—Same as for Aconite.

Æsculus Ohioensis, (*Buckeye*)—Ammonia; Alcohol; or same as for Aconite.

Æther, (*Chloric, Nitric, Sulphuric*)—Ammonia by inhalation.

Æthusia Cynapium. (*Common Fool's Parsley*—Same as for Aconite.

Agaricus, (*Mushroom*)—Same as for Aconite.

Alcohol—Solution of Acetate of Ammonia; or emetic of White Vitriol, or Tartar Emetic, with clysters of salt and water; bleeding.

Almonds, Bitter—Same as for Aconite.

Aluminate of Potassium, (*Alum*)—Carbonate of Soda; vegetable acids, such as vinegar, lemon juice, etc.

Amanita, Muscaria, (*Truffles*)—Same as for Aconite.

Ammonia, (*Hartshorn*)—Vinegar; lemon juice, and demulcents.

Ammoniacal Vapor—Vapor of Vinegar; steam.

Amygdalus Communis—See *Almond, Bitter.*

Amygdalus Persica, (*Peach*)—Same as for Aconite.

Anagallis Arvensis, (*Meadow Pimpernel*)—Charcoal; Tannic Acid; Green Tea.

Anda Gomesii—Same as for Aconite.

Anemone Pulsatilla, (*Wind Flower*)—Charcoal; emetic of Sulphate of Zinc; or same as for Aconite.

Antimonial Vapor, (*Vapor of Antimony*)—Vapor of Vinegar, and Antimony.

Antimonii Potassæ Tartras; (*Emetic Tartar*)—Tannic acid; Astringent infusion; Yellow bark; Green Tea.

Antimony—Vomiting by drinking warm water, and tickling the fauces; followed with astringent drinks; Tannic acid; Alkalies.

Antimony, Oxide of—Same as above.

Antimony, Wine of—Same as above.

Apocynum Adrosæmifolium, (*Dog's Bane*)—Charcoal; and same as for Aconite.

Argentum, (*Silver*)—Common Table Salt.

Argenti Nitras, (*Lunar Caustic*)—Common Table Salt.

Argenti Oxidi, (*Oxide of Silver*)—Common Table Salt.

Aristolochia Serpentaria, (*Birthwort*)—Calcined Magnesia; or same as for Aconite.

Arnica Montana, (*Leopard's bane*)—Same as for Aconite.

Arsenicum, (*Arsenic*)—Dialyzed Iron, followed by a draught of solution of Bicarbonate of Sodium; or Tincture of Chloride of Iron one drachm, Bicarbonate of Sodium, (Potash), onedrachm, tepid water a teaspoonful, mix and take; Hydrated Magnesia.

Arseniate of Ammonium—Same as for Arsenic.

Arseniate of Copper—Same as for Arsenic.

Arseniate of Potassium—Same as for Arsenic.

Arseniate of Sodium—Same as for Arsenic.

Arsenite of Ammonium—Same as for Arsenic.

Arsenite of Copper—Same as for Arsenic.

Arsenite of Potassium—Same as for Arsenic.

Arsenic, White Oxide of—Same as for Arsenic.

Arsenic, Black Oxide of—Same as for Arsenic.

Arsenic, Yellow Sulphide of—Same as for Arsenic.

Arum Maculatum, (*Wakerobin*)—Same as for Aconite.

Atropa Belladonna, (*Deadly Nightshade*)—Bromine; Chlorine; Iodine; Stimulants; Lime water: Vinegar.

Atropia—Bromine; Chlorine; Iodine; Stimulants.

Aurum, (*Gold*)—Sulphate of Iron: Mucilage.

Auri Chloridum, *Chloride of Gold*)—Sulphate of Iron; Mucilage.

Barium, Chloride of—Sulphate of Magnesia; Sulphate of Sodium.

Baryta, (*Barytes*)—Sulphuric Acid, diluted; Sulphate of Magnesia; Sulphate of Sodium.

Belladonna Atropa. See *Atropa Belladonna.*

Belladonina—Emetic of Sulphate of Zinc; Iodine.

Bichromate of Potassium—Carbonate of Potassium; Carbonate of Sodium.

Binoxalate of Potassium, (*Salt of Sorrel*) — Lime; Magnesia; Chalk; Plaster from the ceiling.

Bismuth, Subnitrate of — Mucilage; Milk; Eggs; Emetic.

Bromate of Potassium—Albumen; Starch.

Bromine—Albumen; Starch; Magnesia.

Brucea Antidysenterica, (*False Angustura Bark*)—Same as for Aconite.

Bryonia Dioica, (*Bryony*)—If vomiting has resulted, give warm water to facilitate it, and follow with strong Coffee or diluted Vinegar; but in the absence of vomiting treat as for Aconite; or, administer Bromine or Chlorine.

Caladium Seguinum, (*Dumbean*)—Same as for Bryony.

Calla Palustris, (*Water Arum*)—Same as for Bryony.

Calomel—Albumen, from eggs, beaten in milk; or wheat flour mixed with milk or water; Gold dust mixed with Iron filings. [Bryony.

Caltha Palustris, (*Marsh Marygold*)—Same as for

Calx, (*Quicklime*)—Mineral Soda Water; dilute acids.

Camphora, (*Camphor*)—An emetic.

Cantharis Vesicatoria, (*Spanish Fly*)—Whisky; vomiting by Sweet Oil or Linseed Tea; emollient clysters.

Carbonic Acid Gas—Ammonia inhaled cautiously; dashes of cold water.

Carburetted Hydrogen Gas, (*Coal Gas*)—Fresh air; cold effusions to the head; artificial respiration; Chlorine Gas inhaled.

Cerbera, (*Strychnia*)—Same as for Aconite.

Cheese—Charcoal; Emetics.

Chelidonium Majus, (*Celandine*)—Same as for Bryony.

Chenopodium Anthelminticum, (*Woormseed*)—Same as for Aconite.

Chlorine—Ammonia; Ether by inhalation.

Chloroform—Ammonia by inhalation; Galvanic shocks and artificial breathing.

Chromium, (*Chrome*)—Carbonate of Potassium; Carbonate of Lime.

Cicuta Maculata, (*American Hemlock*)—Same as for Aconite.

Cinnabar Vermillion, (*Persulphuret of Mercury*)—Same as for Calomel.

Citrullus Colocynthis—Bromine; Chlorine; Iodine; or same as for Aconite. [Bryony.
Clematis Vitalba, (*Virgin's Bower*)—Same as for
Cocculus Indicus, (*Fish Berries*)—Bromine; Chlorine; Iodine, or same as for Aconite.
Colchicum Autumnale, (*Meadow Saffron*)—Same as for Aconite.
Codeia—Infusion of Galls; and same as for Aconite.
Conium Maculatum, (*Hemlock*)—Same as above.
Conine, (a principle derived from the above)—Galls; Vinegar. [above.
Convolvulus Scammonia, (*Scammony*)—Same as
Copper, Carbonate, or Oxide of—Same as for Calomel.
Copper, Sulphate of—Albumen; Iron filings; Ferrocyanuret of Potassium.
Corrosive Sublimate—Same as for Calomel.
Creasote—Albumen; or Milk and Flour.
Croton Tiglium, (*Purging Croton*)—Same as for Bryony.
Curare, (*Indian War Poison*)—Common Salt; Sugar; or same as for Aconite.
Cyclamen Europæum, (*Sow Bread*)—Charcoal; or same as for Bryony.
Cynanchum Erectum, (*Cynanchum*)—Charcoal; or same as for Aconite.
Cytisus Laburnum, (*Laburnum*)—Bromine; Chlorine; Iodine; or same as for Aconite.

Daphne Gnidium, (*Spurge Flax*)—Charcoal; or same as for Bryony.
Daphne Mezereum, (*Mezereon*)—Same as the last.
Daturia Stramonium, (*Thorn Apple*)—Bromine; Chlorine; Iodine; same as for Aconite.
Daturina, (*Daturia*)—Charcoal.
Delphinium Staphisagria, (*Stavesavre*)—Charcoal, same as for Aconite.
Digitalis Purpurea, (*Foxglove*)—Infusion of Yellow Bark; Stimulants; or same as for Aconite.
Digitaline—Same as last.
Dioica Palustris, (*Swamp Leatherwood*)—Chlorine; Bromine; Iodine, or same as for Aconite.

Elaterium Momordica, (*Squirting Cucumber*)—Bromine: Chlorine; Iodine; or same as for Aconite.
Elatine—Bromine; Chlorine; Iodine. [Bryony.
Equisetum Hyemale, (*Scourgrass*)—Same as for
Ergot, (*Spurred Rye*)—Charcoal; same as for Aconite.
Emetia or **Emetine**—Bromine; Chlorine; Iodine.
Euphorbia Corollata, (*Spurge*)—Same as for Bryony.

Fish, Poisonous or **Decayed**—An Emetic and tickling of the fauces; purgative or a clyster; Charcoal, or Vinegar and water.
Fowler's Solution—Lime water to be freely drank.
Fusel Oil—An active Emetic.

Gaultheria Procumbens, (*Oil of Winter Green*)—Same as for Aconite.
Gelsemium, (*Yellow Jessamine*)—Ammonia; Charcoal; or same as for Aconite.
Glanders, (*Equinia* or *Farcy*)—
Gold, Salts of—Sulphate of Iron; Mucilaginous drinks.

Helleborus Niger, (*Black Hellebore*)—Same as above.
Hydrochloric Acid. (*Muriatic Acid*)—Ammonia.
Hyoscyamus Albus, (*White Henbane*)—Charcoal; Vinegar; Ammonia; or same as for Aconite.
Hyoscyamus Niger, (*Black Henbane*)—Same as last.
Hyoscyamia—Bromine; Chlorine; Iodine; Vinegar.
Hydrargyrum, (*Mercury*)—Albumen; Gluten; Iodine.
Hydrocyanic Acid, (*Prussic Acid*)—Dilute Chlorine Gas; Ammonia; cold douche.

Iodine—Gluten; Wheat Flour; Starch.
Iodides—Gluten; Wheat Flour; Starch.
Ipecacuanha—Bromine; Chlorine; Iodine; same as for Aconite.
Ipomæa Jalapa—Bromine; Chlorine; Iodine; or same as for Bryony.
Iron and its Salts—Carbonate of Sodium.
Iron, Chloride of—Carbonate of Sodium; Magnesia; Mucilage.
Iron, Muriated Tincture of—Carbonate of Sodium.
Iron, Sulphate of—Carbonate of Sodium; Magnesia; Mucilage.

Jatropa Curcas, (*Purging Nut*)—Same as for Bryony.

Juniperus Sabina Oleum, (*Savin, Oil of*)—Same as for Bryony.

Juniperus Virginiana Oleum, (*Red Cedar, Oil of*)—Same as for Bryony.

Kalmia Latifolia, (*Sheep Laurel*)--Same as for Aconite.

Lactuca Virosa, (*Wild Lettuce*)—Ammonia; or same as for Aconite.

Laudanum, (*Opium*)—Four or five grains of Tartar Emetic, or twenty grains Sulphate of Zinc, every fifteen minutes till vomiting results; clysters of strong soapsuds, to be followed with a cup of strong Coffee; the stomach pump is better than the emetic, where it can be used.
[Aconite.

Laurus Camphora, (*Camphor*)—Chlorine; same as for

Laurel Water—Inhalation of Ammonia; Chlorine; Chloroform.

Lead and its Salts—For the solid forms, Dilute Sulphuric Acid; Sulphate of Magnesia and Phosphate of Sodium.
[nite.

Lobelia Inflata, (*Indian Tobacco*)—Same as for Aco-

Lolium Temulentum, (*Darnel*)—Same as for Aconite.

Mercury and its Salts—Albumen from eggs, beaten in milk; or wheat flower mixed in milk or water; Gold finely mixed in dust, with fine iron filings or powder.
nite.

Melia Azederach, (*Pride of China*)—Same as for Aco-

Morphia and its Salts, (*Opium*)—Remove with stomach pump; or give four or five grains Tartar Emetic, or twenty grains Sulphate of Zinc, every fifteen minutes, until vomiting ensues; also clyster of strong soapsuds; avoid giving vegetable acids; after action of the above remedies, give a cup of strong Coffee, and keep the patient roused.

Mushrooms, (*Fungi*)—An emetic followed by Epsom Salts, and stimulating clysters; then give small quantities of brandy and water.

Muriated Acid Gas—Inhalation of Ammonia, cautiously.

Narcotina—Astringents; Coffee: Ammonia.
Nerium Oleander, (*Common Oleander*)—Same as for Aconite.
Nicotiana Tabacum, (*Tobacco*)—Same as for Aconite.
Nux Vomica—See *Strychnos Nux Vomica*.

Oil of Hartshorn, (*Dippel's Animal Oil*)—Fixed Oils; Vinegar; Lemon juice.
Oil of Tobacco—Charcoal; or same as for Aconite.
Oil of Turpentine—Ammonia.
Oleander. See *Nerium Oleander*.
Opium and its Preparations—Same as for Laudanum; or Chlorine; Charcoal; Iodine; Bromine; or same as for Aconite.

Papaver Somniferum, (*Poppy*)—Same as for Aconite.
Paris Green—Same as for Arsenic.
Pastinaca Sativa, (*Common Parsnip*)—Same as for Bryony.
Phosphorous—Tartar Emetic; Copious draughts of Magnesia and Mucilaginous drinks.
Phytolacca Decandra, (*Poke*)—Charcoal; and same as for Bryony.
Picrotoxin—Bromine: Chlorine; Iodine; Charcoal.
Piper Cubeba, (*Cubebs*)—Charcoal; same as for Bryony.
Platinum Chloridum, (*Chloride of Platina*)—Muriate of Ammonia; Soda.
Poppy—Same as for Aconite.
Potassa, (*Potash*)—Fixed Oils; Vinegar; Lemon Juice; Citric Acid in solution.
Potassii Arsenias, (*Arseniate of Potassium*)—Hydrated Peroxide of Iron.
Potassii Bicarbonas, (*Saleratus*)— Lemon Juice; Vinegar.
Potassii Bichromas. (*Bichromate of Potassium*) Carbonate of Potassium; Carbonate of Sodium.
Potassii Bromidum, (*Bromide of Potassium*)—Vegetable acids: Tartaric Acid in solution.
Rotassii Carbonas, (*Pearlash*)—Lemon Juice; Vinegar.
Potassii Nitras, (*Nitrate of Potassium*)—Mucilaginous drinks.

Potassii Cyanidum, (*Cyanide of Potassium*)—Sulphate of Iron in solution.

Potassii Sulphuretum, (*Sulphuret of Potassium*)—Chloride of Sodium; Chlorinated Soda.

Potassii Iodidum, (*Iodide of Potassium*) — Gluten; Wheat Flour; Starch.

Potato Bug, (*Lytta Vittata*)—Emetic of Sweet Oil, Sugar and water, or Linseed Tea with emollient clysters.

Prunus Caroliniana, (*Wild Orange*)—Same as for Aconite.

Prunus Lauro-Cerasus, (*Cherry Laurel*)—Same as for Aconite.

Prunus Nigra, (*Black Cherry*)—Same as for Aconite.

Prunus Virginiana, (*Wild Cherry*)—Same as for Aconite.

Putrid Animal Matter—Ammonia; Tonics, Scutellaria lateriflora.

Rabies Canina, (*Hydrophobia*) — The part bitten should be cut out, even after being healed, then immersed in warm water as long as any blood will flow; then cauterize and poultice; Elecampane root, stewed in a pint of milk, given in small doses, in the mornings, the patient fasting until noon, is said to be a cure.

Ranunculus Acris, (*Crowfoot*)—Charcoal; or same as for Bryony.

Red Precipitate, (*Red Oxide of Mercury*)—Albumen; [Gluten.

Rhododendron, Chrysanthum — Charcoal; or same as for Bryony.

Ricinus Communis, (*Castor Oil plant*) — Charcoal; same as for Bryony.

Robinia Pseudo-Acacia, (*Locust tree*)—Charcoal, or same as for Aconite.

Ruta Graveolens, (*Rue*)—Charcoal; same as last.

Sambucus Canadensis, (*Elder*)—Charcoal; same as for Aconite.

Sausage Poison—Charcoal.

Scilla Maritima, (*Squill*)—Same as for Aconite.

Secale Cornutum, (*Ergot, Spurred Rye*)—Camphor; or same as for Aconite.

Serpent Bites—Apply a cupping glass over the wound, or a tight ligature above it; soak in warm water; then cauterize, and apply lint, saturated with Olive Oil and Hartshorn; frequent draughts of Whisky are efficacious; also, Ammonia, and Scutellaria.

Silver, Nitrate of, (*Lunar Caustic*)—Common table Salt; Albumen. [Lemon Juice.

Sodii Carbonas, (*Carbonate of Sodium*)— Vinegar;

Solanum Dulcamara, (*Bitter Sweet*)—Charcoal; or same as for Aconite.

Spigelia Marilandica, (*Pink Root*)—Charcoal; same as for Aconite.

Stalagmitis Cambogioides, (*Gamboge*) — Charcoal; same as for Bryony. [Flour.

Stanni Chloridum, (*Chloride of Tin*)—Albumen; Milk;

Sting of Insects. See *Insects.*

Strychnia—Same as for Aconite. [Aconite.

Strychnos Ignatii, (*St. Ignatius' Bean*)—Same as for

Strychnos Nux Vomica—Same as for Aconite.

Sulphate of Indigo—Magnesia; Lime; Milk.

Sulphuretted Hydrogen Gas—Chlorine inhalation.

Symplocarpus Fœtida, (*Skunk Cabbage*)—Charcoal; or same as for Aconite.

Tansy, Oil of—Charcoal; or same as for Bryony.

Taxus Baccata, (*Yew*)—Charcoal; same as for Aconite.

Tin, Muriate of—Albumen; Milk, copiously drank.

Turpentine, Oil of—Ammonia.

Turpeth Mineral, (*Sulphate of Peroxide of Mercury*) —Mucilage; Albumen.

Veratrum Alba, V. Niger, V. Viride, (*Hellebore*)— Same as for Aconite.

Virdigris (*Subacetate of Copper*)—Albumen; Milk; Iron filings; Ferrocyanuret of Potassium.

White Precipitate, (*Ammoniated Chloride of Mercury*) —Mucilage; Fixed Oils. [Potassium.

Woorara, (*War Poison of Guiana*)—Iodine; Iodide of

Yew—Charcoal; or same as for Aconite.

Zinc, and **Salts of**—Carbonate of Sodium; Albumen; Tannic Acid; Astringents.

ABBREVIATIONS USED IN PRESCRIPTIONS,

With the Latin Terms in full, and Translated into English.

A.; aa.; or **ana.**;—Of each ingredient.
Abdom., Abdomen;—The belly.
Abs. Febre, Absente febre;—In the absence of fever.
Acm., Acmé;—The hight of the fever.
Ad. or **Add.**, Adde et addatur;—Add; or, to be added.
Ad 2 vic., Ad duas vices;—At twice taking.
Ad Lib., Ad libitum;—At pleasure.
Admov., Admoveatur;—Let there be applied.
Adst. febre, Adstante febre;—When the fever is on.
Agit. vas., Agitato vase;—Shake the phial.
Aliquant., Aliquantillum;—A very little.
Aliquot., Aliquoties;—Some; sometimes.
Altern.; Alternus;—Alternate.
Altern. hor., Alternis horis;—Every second hour.
Altern. dieb., Alternis diebus;—Every alternate day.
Apert., Apertus;—Clear; open.
Aperi., Aperiens;—A gentle purge.
Applic., Applicetur;—Let there be applied.
Aq., Aqua;—Water. Aquæ;—Of water.
Aq. bull., Aqua bulliens;—Boiling water.
Aq. comm., Aqua communis;—Common water.
Aq. dest., Aqua destillata;—Distilled water.
Aq. ferv., Aqua fervens;—Hot water.
Aq. font., Aqua fontana;—Spring water.
Aq. marin., Aqua marina;—Sea water.
Aq. pluv., Aqua pluvialis;—Rain water.
Aq. pur., Aqua pura;—Pure water.

B. A., Balneum arenæ—A sand bath.
Baln. mariæ, Balneum mariæ;—A salt water bath.
Baln. tep., Balneum tepidum;—A warm bath.
Baln. vap., Balneum vaporis;—A vapor bath.
Bals., Balsamum;—Balsam.
B. M., Bene misce;—Mix well.

Bib., Bibe, or bibat;—Drink, or Let him drink.
Bis ind., Bis indies;—Twice a day.
Bol., Bolus;—A pill, or ball.
Bull., Bulliat, or Bulliens;—Let it boil; or, boiling.
Buty., Butyrum;—Butter.

C., Congius;—A gallon.
Calef., Calefactus;—Made warm.
Cap., Capiat;—Let him take.
Cat., Cataplasma;—A poultice.
Cath., Catharticus;—A cathartic.
C. C., Cornu cervi;—Hartshorn.
C. M., Cras mane;—Tomorrow morning.
C. N., Cras nocte;—Tomorrow night.
Cit., Cito; or, Citissime;—Soon; as quickly as possible.
Cochl. Amp., Cochleare amplum;—A large spoonful.
Cochl. Infant., Cochleare infantis;—A child's spoonful.
Coct., Coction;—Boiling.
Col., Colatus;—Strained.
Colat., Colatur;—Let it be strained.
Comp., Compositus:—Compounded.
Conf., Confectio;—A confection.
Cont., Continuo;—To continue.
Cont. Rem., Continuentur remedia;—Let the medicines be continued.
Contu., Contusio;—To bruise, or crush.
Coqu., Coquantur;—Let them be boiled.
Cort., Cortex;—Bark.
Crast.,Crastinus;—For tomorrow.
C. V., Cras Vespere;—Tomorrow evening.
Cuj., Cujus;—Of which.
Cujusl., Cujuslibet;—Of any.
Cyath. theæ., Cyatho theæ;—A teacupful.
Cyath Vina., Cyatho Vinaris;—A wine-glass full.

Deaur. pil.,Deaurentur pilulæ;—Let the pills be gilded.
Deb. spiss., Debita spissitudo;—A proper consistence.
Decub., Decubitus;—Lying down; or retiring to bed.
Decub. Hor, Decubitus Hora;—At bed time.
De d. in d., De die in diem;—From day to day
Dec., Decanta;—Decanted.

Dej. Alv., Dejectionis alvi;—Stools; fæcal evacuations.
Det., Detur;—Let it be given.
Dext. lat., Dextra lateralis;—Right side.
Dieb. alt, Diebnr alternis;—Every other day.
Dieb. tert., Diebus tertiis;—Every third day.
Dig., Digeratur;—Let it be digested.
Dil., Dilutus;—Diluted.
Dim., Dimidus;—One-half.
Div., Divide;—Divide.
Donec alv. sol. fuer., Donec alvus solutas fuerit;—until the bowels are moved.
Drach., Drachma;—A drachm.
Durant. dol., Durante dolore;—While the pain continues.

Ead., Eadem;—The same.
Ed., Edulcora:—Sweeten.
Efferv., Effervesentia;—Effervescence.
Enem., Enema;—A clyster.
Evan., Evanesco;—To disappear.
Extr., Extractum;—Extract.
Exhib., Exhibiatur;—Let it be given.
Ext. sup. alut., Extende super alutam;—Spread on leather.
Ext., Extensus:—Spread.

F., ft., Fiat;—Let a — be made.
F. S. A., Fiat secundum artem;—Let it be made according to the rules of the art.
F. h., Fiat haustus;—Let a draught be made.
F. pil., Fac pillulam;—Make a pill.
Feb. dur., Febre durante;—During the fever.
Fem. intern., Femoribus internis—To the inner part of the thigh.
Flor.; Flores;—Flowers.
Fl., Fluidus;—Liquid; by measure.
Form., Formula;—A prescription.
Fot., Fotula;—A fomentation.
Frust., Frustillatim;—In small pieces.

Garg., Gargarisma;—A gargle.
Gel,, Gelatina;—Jelly.
Gel. quav., Gelatina quavis;—Any kind of jelly.
Glob., Globulus;—A little ball.

Grad., Gradatim;—By slow degrees.
Grat., Grata; Gratum;—Agreeable; pleasant.
G. G. G., Gummi guttæ Gambiæ;—Gamboge.
Gr., Granum;—A grain.
Gtt., Gutta;—A drop. Guttæ;—drops.

Hæc Noct., Hæc Nocte;—This night.
Hor. decub., Hora decubitus;—On going to bed.
Hirud., Hirudo;—A leech.
H. S., Hora somni;—On retiring to rest.
Hor. Un. Spat., Horæ unius spatio;—At the end of an hour.
Hor. interm., Horis intermediis;—At the intermediate [hours.
Hor. ¼, Horæ quadrante;—Quarter of an hour.
Hyd., Hydor;—Water.
Hydr., Hydrargyrum:—Mercury; calomel.

Impon., Imponatur;—Let there be put on.
Impr., Imprimis;—First.
Ind., Indies;—From day to day, or daily.
Indic., Indicaverit;—Indicates.
In pulm.; In pulmentum;—In gruel.
Inf., Infusum;—Infusion.
Infund., Infundatur;—Let there be infused.
Inj. enem., Injiciatur enema;—Let a clyster be given.
Inject., Injectio;—An injection.
Interm., Intermedius;—Intermediate.

Jul,, Julepus;—A mixture.
Jux., Juxta;—Near to.

Lact., Lactis; Lacte;—Of milk; in milk.
Lat. dol., Latere dolente;—To the side affected.
Lb. Libra;—A pound weight, or wine pint.
Lim., Limones;—Lemons.
Lin., Linteum;—Lint.
Liq., Liquor;—Liquor.
Lot., Lotio;—Lotion.
Lumb., Lumborum;—The loins.

M., Misce;—Mix.
Mac., Macera;—Macerate.

Man., Manipulus;—A handful.
Mane pr., Mane primo;—Very early in the morning.
Max., Maximus;—The greatest.
Mat., Matutine;—In the forenoon.
Mediet., Medietas:—Half.
Meli., Melior;—Better.
Mi. pan., Mica panis;—Crumb of bread.
Min., Minimum;—The 60th part of a drachm measure; very small.
Misc., Misceatur;—Let it be well mixed.
Mist., Mistura;—A mixture.
Mitt., Mitte;—Send;—Let there be sent.
Mitig., Mitigatio;—Alleviation.
Mod. præ., Modo præscripto;—In the manner directed.
Mor. sol., More solito;—In the usual way.
Muc,, Mucilago;—Mucilage.

N,, Nocte;—Night.
Nig., Nigrum;—Black.
Ni., Nisi;—Unless.
Nih., Nihil;—Nothing.
No., Numero;—In number.
N. P. S., Nomen proprium signetur;—Write the common name upon the label.
Nup., Nuper;—Lately.

Obst., Obstante;—Preventing.
Oct., Octo;—Eight.
O., Octarius;—A pint.
Ol., Oleum;—Oil.
Ol. lini. s. i., Oleum lini sine igni;—Cold drawn linseed oil.
Omn. alt. hor., Omnibus alternis horis;—Every other hour.
" **hor.**, Omni hora;—Every hour.
" **bid.**, Omni biduo;—Every two days.
" **bih.**, Omni bihorio;—Every two hours.
" **man.**, Omni mane;—Every morning.
" **noct.**, Omni nocte;—Every night.
" **quadr. hor.**, Omni quadrante horæ;—Every quarter of an hour.
O. O. O., Oleum Olivæ Optimum;—Best Olive oil.
Opt., Optimus;—Best.

Ovil. jus., Ovillum jusculum;—Mutton broth.
Ov., Ovum;—An egg.
Ovi. Vit., Ovi vitillum;—The yolk of an egg.
Oxym., Oxymel;—Honey and vinegar.

P., Pondere;—By weight.
P. Æ., Partes æquales;—Equal parts.
Pect., Pectus;—Breast.
Pedil, Pediluvium;—A bath for the feet.
Perg. in us. med., Perga in üsu medicinarum;—Continue to use the medicine.
Perfric., Perfrictus;—Let it be rubbed.
Part. aff., Partem affectam;—The part affected.
Part. dolent., Partem dolentem;—The part in pain.
Part. vic., Partitis vicibus;—To be given a part at a time
Per. op. emet., Peracta operatione emetici;—When the emetic has ceased to operate.
Pil., Pilula; Pilulæ;—A pill; pills.
Pomer., Pomeridianus;—The afternoon.
Post sing. sed. liq., Post singulus sedes liquidus;—After every loose evacuation.
Pro rat. æt., Pro ratione ætatis;—According to the age of the patient.
P. R. N., Pro re nata;—According to the nature of the case.
Pro pot. com., Pro potu communi;—For a common drink.
Pot., Potus;—A beverage.
Postul., Postulent;—May require.
Præp., Præparatus;—Prepared; let them be prepared.
Prim., Primus;—First.
Pug., Pugillus;—A handful.
Pulv., Pulvis;—Powder.
Pulv. Subt., Pulvis Subtillisemus;—The very finest powder.
Pur., Purificatus;—Purified.

Quad., Quadrantis;—Quarter.
Q. P., Quantum placet;—As much as you please.
Q. S. Quantum sufficit;—As much as is sufficent.
Quadrihor, Quadrihorio;—Every four hours.

Quadrupl., Quadruplicato;—Four times as much.
Quamp., Quamprimum;—Immediately.
Quib., Quibus;—To which; with which.
Quiesc., Quiescat;—It may rest.
Q. V., Quantum volueris;—As much as you wish.

R., Recipe;—Take.
Rad., Radix;—Root.
Ras., Rasuræ;—Shavings.
Rat., Ratio;—Proportion.
Rect., Rectificatus;—Rectified.
Red., Reductus;—Reduced.
Red. in pulv., Reductus in pulverem;—Reduced to a powder.
Reg. hep., Regio hepatis;—Region of the liver.
Reg. umb., Regio umbilici;—Region of the umbilicus.
Reli., Reliquus;—The remainder.
Repet., Repetatur;—Repeat; to be repeated.
Retin., Retinendus;—Retained.

S., Signa.—Write; give directions.
S. A., Secundum artem;—According to art.
Sacch., Saccharum;—Sugar.
Sacch. Alb., Saccharum Alba;—White sugar.
Sæp., Sæpe;—Often.
Sæp., Sæpissime;—Very often.
Sang., Sanguis;—Blood.
Sang. miss., Sanguinis missura;—Blood-letting.
Scap., Scapula;—The shoulder blade.
Scrob. cord., Scrobiculus cordis;—The pit of the stomach.
Sec., Secundis;—Second.
Secu., Secundum;—According to.
Sem., Semen;—Seed.
Semih., Semihora;—Half an hour.
Semidr., Semidrachma;—Half a drachm.
Sept., Septimana;—A week.
Seq., Sequens;—Following.
Seq. luce, Sequenti luce;—The following day.
Serv., Serva;—Preserve or keep.
Sesq., Sesqui;—One and a half.
Sesquih., Sesquihora;—One and a half hour.
Sesquinun., Sesquinuncia;—One and a half ounce.

Sesquid., Sesquidrachma;—One and a half drachm.
Si n. val., Si non valeat;—If it does not answer.
Si op. sit, Si opus sit;—If there be occasion.
Si vir. perm., Si vires permittant;—If the strength will bear.
Sig., Signatura;—A label, or direction.
Sign., Signetur;—Let it be marked.
Sig. n. pr., Signetur nomine proprio;—Write upon it the usual name.
Sing., Singulorum;—Of each.
Solu., Solutio,—Solution.
Solv., Solve;—Dissolve.
Som., Somnus;—Sleep.
Som. hor., Somni hora;—Bed time.
Spr., Spiritus;—Spirit.
Ss., Semis;—Half.
St., Stet;—Let it stand.
Stat., Statim;—Directly; immediately.
Sub fin. coct., Sub finem coctionis;—When the boiling is nearly finished.
Subsulp., Subsulphas;—A subsulphate.
Subtep., Subtepidus;—Lukewarm.
Subt,, Subtillis;—To a fine powder.
Sum., Sumo;—To take; to be taken.
Sum. tal., Sumat talem;—Let the patient take one like [this.
Superb., Suberbibo;—To drink after.
S. V., Spiritus vinosus;—Spirit of wine.
S. V. R., Spiritus vinosus rectificatus;—Spirit of wine rectified.
S. V. T., Spiritus vinosus tenuis;—Proof spirit; half alcohol, and half water.
Supr., Supra;—Above.
Syr., Syrupus;—Syrup.

Tenacit., Tenacitus;—Tenacity, or consistency.
Tempef., Tempefactus;—Made warm.
Ter., Tero;—To rub; to be rubbed.
T. O., Tinctura Opii;—Tincture of opium.
T. O. C., Tinctura Opii Camphorata;—Paregoric elixir.
Tr. Tinct., Tinctura;—Tincture.
Trit., Tritura;—Triturate.

Troch., Trochiscus;—A lozenge.
Tuss. mol., Tussis molestante,—When the cough is troublesome.

Ult., Ultimus;—The last.
Ult. præscr., Ultimo præscriptus;—The last ordered.
Umb., Umbilicus;—The navel.
Unc., Uncia;—An ounce.
Unc. c. sem., Unciam cum semisse;—An ounce and a half.
Ung., Unguentum;—Ointment.
Urgen., Urgente;—Urgent.
Urgen. tus., Urgente tussi;—Troublesome cough.
Usq. ut liq. anim., Usque ut liquerit animus;—Until fainting is produced.
U. S. P., United States Pharmacopœia.
Utend., Utendus;—To be used.
Utat., Utatus;—Let him make use of.
Utri. lib., Utrius libet;—Which of the two he prefers.

Vac., Vaccinatio;—The act of inoculating.
Vac. var., Vaccinæ variolæ;—Cowpox.
Vac. lac, Vaccinum lac:—Cow's milk.
Vent., Ventriculus;—The stomach.
V. O. S., Vitello ovi solutus;—Dissolved in the yolk of an egg.
Venes., Venesectio;—Bleeding.
V. S. B., Venesectio brachii;—Bleed in the arm.
Vit., Vitrum;—A glass.
Vom., Vomitio;—A vomiting.

Zz., Zingiber;—Ginger; anciently Myrrh.

♏, Minimum;—a minim.
Gr., Grana;—a grain.
℈, Scrupulum;—a scruple.
ʒ, Drachma;—a drachm.
fʒ, Fluidrachma;—a fluid drachm.
℥, Uncia;—an ounce troy.
f℥, Fluid uncia;—a fluid ounce.
lb, Libra;—a pound.
ss, Semissis;—half.
j, one;—*ij*, two;—*iij*, three;—*v*, five;—*vi*, six, etc.;—*X*, ten; —*xi*, eleven, etc.

THE METRIC SYSTEM OF WEIGHTS,

With a Form of Prescription and Scale of Doses.

The metric, or decimal system, was first suggested by French scientists about the year 1790, with a view of making all measures of length, volume, and weight uniform throughout the world. It comprises the following units of measure:

The *meter*, the unit of length,=the ten millionth part of the terrestrial meridian, or the distance between the pole and the equator=39.370432 inches.

The *liter*, the unit of capacity=a cube of the tenth part of a meter=1.0567454 wine quart.

The *gram*, the unit of weight=the weight of a cubic centimeter of water at its maximum density (4° Cent.)=15.43234874 grains. In medicine, the gram is the unit of weight, and the *cubic centimeter*, or a measure of one gram of water, is the unit of volume; practically the two terms are equivalent, except with very heavy or very light liquids.

The system is the most accurate, consistent, and convenient one known; simpler than others as our money is simpler than pounds, shillings, and pence; multiplying and dividing by a mere shifting of the decimal point to the right or left; giving finer subdivisions than other systems, and saving money in business to such an extent that competent authorities compute that the London and Northwestern Railway alone would annually save £10,000 sterling by the use, in all its computations, of the metric instead of the old system.

There are no tables, scales, or complicated relations, the meter measuring every possible dimension, the liter every capacity, the gram every weight.

Physicians should employ this system because of its great *convenience* in writing and compounding prescriptions, in dividing doses and in computing quantities required during given times; because of its *safety*, due to its *uniformity* and *simplicity*. It may be learned in five minutes. In complexity there is danger, and the resemblance of the signs of the scruple, drachm and ounce has more than once proved fatal to human life. The metric system dispenses with the signs of the quantities, employs Arabic figures instead of Roman numerals, and assures the physician of more competent service because from more educated pharmacists, such being always the first to adopt it. It is decimal, and a perpendicular line instead of the decimal points obviates any possibility of error from this source. It is allied to the change already made by Americans from pounds, shillings and pence to dollars and cents.

The physician should employ the Metric system because of its *delicacy* and *accuracy* for the chemist and the pharmacist; and here the beauty of the system is especially apparent, for it provides denominations of weights applicable to the smallest quantity which the physician can prescribe, the old grain being by far too large and coarse a unit for modern medicine.

Surgeon-General Woodworth, of the U. S. Marine Hospital Service, in 1878 issued a circular, with the approval of Sécretary Sherman, requiring medical officers of the Marine Hospital Service to make use hereafter for all official, medical, and pharmaceutical purposes, of the Metric System of Weights and Measures, which had already, under the act of July 18, 1866, been adopted by this service for the purveying of medical supplies.

To understand the metric system thoroughly, and to

use it intelligently, a person should *forget* the units of length, volume, and weight, to which he has been accustomed, and should, at once and definitely, familarize his senses with the new measures, as they are brought into daily use, irrespective of the old system. It is simply an arbitrary rule which makes a grain of opium a medium dose for an adult; it may be a maximum dose for one and a minimum for another. To supply a practical guide to physicians a list of the minimum and maximum doses of the more common drugs, very nearly equalling the doses usually employed, is given. For those who wish to convert the value of doses in the old system to the new, the following facts and table are given.

Metric Equivalents.

℥i (Troy)=480 grains = 31	103 grams, about 32		
ʒi = 60 grains = 3	888 grams, about 4		
1 grain =	0648 gram, about		06
¼ grain =	016 gram,		016
⅛ grain =	008 gram,		008

The average (household) teaspoon holds 5 and the tablespoon 20 cubic centimeters.

The following prescription illustrates the method of using the system, and the facility of dividing the dose in proportion to the age of the patient, the first column representing the dose for an adult. *The decimal* LINE *instead of* POINTS *makes errors impossible.*

Metrical Prescription.

	(1)	(½)	(¼)	(⅕)	
℞ Potassii Acetatis	8	4	2	1	60
Spiritus Ætheris Nitrosi	16	8	4	3	20
Syrupi Scillæ.	4	2	1		80
Aquæ Menthæ Piperitæ . . .	100	100	100	100	

Misce.

Metric Scale of Doses.

	Minimum		*Maximum*	
Acidum Arseniosum		005		008
Carbolicum		05		20
Gallicum		20	1	90
Hydrocyanicum Dil		10		30
Muriaticum Dil		10	1	00
Nitricum Dil		25	1	00
Phosphoricum Dil		50	4	00
Salicylicum		25	1	00
Sulphuricum Aromaticum		50	2	00
Tannicum		10	1	00
Aconiti Extractum		03		06
Radicus Tinctura		25	1	00
Ætheris, Spiritus Com.	2	00	4	00
Nitrosi	2	00	4	00
Aloe Socotrina		10		50
Aloes et Myrrhæ Tinctura	4	00	8	00
Ammonæ Aqua		50	1	00
Acetatis Liquor	8	00	30	00
Spiritus Aromaticus	1	00	4	00
Ammonii, Bromidum		25	1	00
Carbonas		25	I	00
Chloridum		50	2	00
Valerianus		25		50
Amyl Nitris		10		30
Antimonii Vinum		50	4	00
et Potassii Tartras		002		10
Argenti Nitras		015		15
Assafœtida		25	1	00
Assafœtidæ Tinctura		25	2	00
Belladonnæ Folia		05		15
Extractum		015		06
Tinctura		25	1	25
Bismuthi Subnitras		25	1	00
Buchu Extractum Fluidum	2	00	8	00
Camphora		10		50
Camphoræ Aqua	15	00	30	00
Cannabis Indicæ Extractum		015		06
Tinctura		25	1	00
Cantharidis Tinctura		25	1	00

Metric Scale of Doses.

	Minimum		*Maximum.*	
Capsicum		06		30
Capsici Tinctura		50	1	25
Catechu Tinctura	2	00	8	00
Cerii Oxalas		06		30
Chloral		25	1	25
Chloroformum		25	2	00
Cinchonæ Tinctura Composita	4	00	8	00
Quinia (salts of)		05	1	25
Cinchonia, (salts of)		05	1	25
Cinchonidia (salts of)		05	1	25
Colchici Tinctura		25	1	25
Radicis Vinum		50	2	00
Seminis	2	00	4	00
Colocynthidis Extractum Comp		25	2	00
Conii Extractum		10		25
Tinctura	2	00	4	00
Copaiba	1	00	4	00
Creasotum		05		25
Croton Chloral		05		50
Cupri Sulphas		015		30
Digitalis		05		10
Extractum		03		12
Tinctura		50	2	00
Elaterium		008		10
Ergotæ Extractum Fluidum		50	4	00
Fel Bovinum Purificatum		20		50
Ferri Carbonas Saccharatum		25	2	00
Citras		25		60
Iodidi Syrupus		50	4	00
Pyrophosphas		10		30
Subcarbonas		25	2	00
Sulphas		05		30
Chloridi Tinctura		50	2	00
Ferrum Redactum		06		30
Filicis Oleoresina		50	2	00
Gelsemini Tinctura		05	1	50
Guaiaci Tinctura	2	00	4	00
Ammoniata	2	00	4	00
Guarana		50	2	00

Metric Scale of Doses.

	Minimum		*Maximum*	
Hydrargyri Chloridum Mite		03	1	00
Chloridum Corrosivum		005		015
Iodidum Rubrum		004		015
Pil. Pulvis		05	1	00
Sulphas Flava		015		30
Hydrargyrum cum Creta		10		50
Hyoscyami Extractum		10		25
Tinctura		50	2	00
Iodinii Tinctura		25	1	00
Composita		25	1	00
Ipecacuanha		03	2	00
Ipecacuanhæ Vinum		25	30	00
Jaborandi	2	00	4	00
Jalapa		50	2	00
Jalapæ Tinctura	2	00	8	00
Juglandis Extractum	1	00	2	00
Koosso	10	00	20	00
Kamala	4	00	8	00
Magnesii Carbonas		50	2	00
Sulphas	15	00	30	00
Nucis Vomicæ Extractum		03		10
Tinctura		50	2	00
Strychnia (salts of)		001		005
Oleum Morrhuæ	4	00	15	00
Ricini	4	00	30	00
Terebinthinæ		50	30	00
Oleum Tiglii		03		10
Opium		03		10
Opii Acetum		25		60
Elixir, (Mc. Munn)		25	1	25
Extractum		03		06
Tinctura		50	2	00
Camphorata		50	4	00
Deodorata		50	2	00
Vinum		50	2	00
Morphia (salts of)		008		03
Liquor Morphiæ Sulph. (Mag).		25	1	00
Pulvis Ipecac. Comp.		25	1	00
Pepsina		25	1	00

Metric Scale of Doses.

	Minimum		Maximum.	
Phosphorus		001		002
Plumbi Acetas		10		30
Podophyllum		50	1	25
Potassii Acetas		50	4	00
Arsenitis Liquor		10		50
Bromidum		50	4	00
Chloras		50	2	00
Iodidum		10		50
Nitras		25	1	25
et Sodii Tartras	8	00	30	00
Rheum	1	00	2	00
Rhei Tinctura	2	00	30	00
Salicinum		50	1	00
Santonium		03		12
Scillæ Acetum	1	25	4	00
Tinctura		50	2	00
Sennæ Extractum Fluidum	4	00	15	00
Sodii Carbonas		50	2	00
Hyposulphis		50	1	25
Spigeliæ Extractum Fluidum	4	00	8	00
Stramonii Folia		10		20
Semen		06		12
Tinctura		50	1	25
Uvæ Ursi Extractum Fluidum	2	00	8	00
Valerianæ Extractum Fluidum	2	00	8	00
Veratri Viridis Tinctura		25		50
Zinci Phosphidum		005		01
Sulphas		015	2	00
Valerianas		05		30

Revised and reprinted from The Medical Register for New England, by Francis H. Brown, M.D.

www.ingramcontent.com/pod-product-compliance
Lightning Source LLC
Chambersburg PA
CBHW052107230326
41599CB00054B/4274